Acoustic Immittance Measures in Clinical Audiology

A PRIMER

Acoustic Immittance Measures in Clinical Audiology

A PRIMER

Terry L. Wiley, Ph.D.
Cynthia G. Fowler, Ph.D.

Department of Communicative Disorders
University of Wisconsin–Madison
Madison, Wisconsin

SINGULAR PUBLISHING GROUP, INC.
SAN DIEGO · LONDON

Singular Publishing Group, Inc.
401 West A Street, Suite 325
San Diego, California 92101-7904

Singular Publishing Ltd.
19 Compton Terrace
London N1 2UN, U.K.

e-mail: singpub@mail.cerfnet.com
web site: http://www.singpub.com

Typeset in 10/12 Palatino by SoCal Graphics
Printed in United States of America by McNaughton and Gunn

Library of Congress Cataloging-in-Publication Data

Wiley, Terry L.
    Acoustic immittance measures in clinical audiology : a primer /
Terry L. Wiley & Cynthia G. Fowler.
      p.   cm.
    Includes bibliographical references and index.
    ISBN 1-56593-693-0
    1. Audiometry, Impedance.   I. Fowler, Cynthia G.   II. Title.
    [DNLM: 1. Audiometry—methods. 2. Audiology. 3. Hearing
Disorders—diagnosis.   WV 272 W676a 1997]
RF294.5.I5W55   1997
617.8'0754—dc21
DNLM/DLC
for Library of Congress   97-2454
10 9 8 7 6 5   CIP

Contents

Foreword

As this book evolved the authors sought to create a "teaching primer" for aural acoustic immittance. The final result, however, extends beyond the scope of most primers. The introduction of each new procedure includes a comprehensive discussion of how it is done, why it is done, and how the resultant data can be reported or reduced.

But why should a student learn the basic acoustic principles and mathematical operations that underlie acoustic immittance measurements? A review of historical antecedents and current research data suggests that an audiologist with a superficial grasp of acoustic immittance will neither appreciate nor utilize fully this important tool in the clinic and in the laboratory.

Early contributors to the study of immittance measures were Heaviside, who coined the term impedance in 1886 (Susskind, 1962a) and Steinmetz, who applied complex notation in solving alternating current problems in 1893 (Susskind, 1962b). Webster (1919) usually is credited with extending this work to acoustic circuits and with introducing the concept of acoustic impedance. This innovative analytic technique soon was applied to telephone and acoustic calibration problems.

In human physiological acoustics, static acoustic-immittance measurements initially were used to characterize the normal peripheral auditory system. These baseline data formed a framework for improving the coupling of hearing aids to the ear and for understanding some effects of middle ear disease on the transmission of sound to the cochlea. More recently, laser-Doppler vibrometer measurements and static acoustic-immittance measurements have been compared with models of the pressure transformation required to produce the optimum impedance match between a sound field and a human cochlea. The results of these comparisons highlight at least three important points. First, the mass and the placement of an ossicular-replacement prosthesis can have a major effect on the hearing of a patient postoperatively. Second, a patient with a "pure" sensorineural hearing loss may not have an optimum middle-ear transformer. For this patient, minor middle-ear surgery may provide a greater improvement in high frequency hearing than a typical hearing aid. Third, new clinical applications of this type may never be understood fully by an audiologist who has not mastered the basic concepts that are covered in this book.

Historically, dynamic acoustic-immittance techniques have taken two primary forms. These have involved the measurement of changes in static aural acoustic immittance that accompany changes in the tonus of the middle ear muscles (the acoustic reflex) or changes in air pressure within the closed external ear canal (tympanometry). In their simplest forms, acoustic reflex thresholds and the recording of acoustic reflex adaptation have provided useful clinical information. Multiple-frequency probe signals and multiple-component measurements, however, are required as one begins to study the interaction between the acoustic reflex and the suppression of otoacoustic emissions.

Tympanometry can be evaluated in a similar fashion. In its simplest form, single-component tympanometry with a single low-frequency probe tone also has provided useful clinical data. Again, multiple-frequency probe signals and multiple-component measurements are required to evaluate completely the middle ear function of neonates, the effects of ossicular-chain lesions, and the role of the middle ear in the measurement of otoacoustic emissions.

This foreword has emphasized the need for students to have an understanding of the basic acoustic principles and the mathematical operations that underlie acoustic immittance measurements. A review of the literature suggests that Terry Wiley and Cynthia Fowler are eminently qualified to weave this information into a teaching primer. Their final result reflects not only their grasp of the material but also their ability to teach it.

David J. Lilly
Portland, Oregon

Preface

Over the past 30 years, acoustic immittance measures have evolved from a specialty procedure to a fundamental and routine part of the audiologic evaluation. Since the 1970s, several books have been published dealing with various aspects of acoustic immittance measures. Several book chapters, clinical monographs, conference proceedings, and other published documents also have been devoted to the general topic area. Previous books on acoustic immittance measures, for the most part, have been multiple author publications dealing with the current thinking on the topic at a particular time. Some of the books and other publications have addressed a specific theme, such as middle ear screening, predicting hearing loss from the acoustic reflex, or tympanometry. Many of the available texts are either out of date or devoted to very specific subtopics in the area. Other available materials are written at a more advanced level than is appropriate for students new to the topic area. After several years of experience teaching the bases and clinical applications of acoustic immittance measures, we find that we borrow from a variety of sources for basic reading in the area. The motivation for this book, then, was derived primarily from a perceived void in the availability of a basic teaching primer on acoustic immittance and acoustic immittance measures.

We have aimed our level of topic treatment primarily at students with only a basic background in audiology. Generally, audiology students have been introduced to acoustics, anatomy and physiology of hearing, hearing disorders, and the fundamentals of audiometry before specialty topics such as acoustic immittance and auditory evoked potentials are introduced. This basic level of student background on related audiology topics was our starting point. Experience tells us, however, that student readers may come to the text with more or less than this basic background. Accordingly, we have provided suggestions throughout the text regarding source study material for additional background information on selected topics. We also have included a bibliography on acoustic immittance measures that should be useful for basic and advanced readers seeking greater depth and detail on specific topics.

Our primary goal was the development of a text that introduces the reader to acoustic immittance measures. It is not a comprehensive treatment of all topic areas. Rather, the objective is to provide readers with the fundamentals that are necessary and important for more advanced study on the topic. We have attempted to avoid dense literature citations for the introduction of fundamental concepts. Further, we have avoided lengthy mathematical proofs and descriptions that underlie the basic physics of measurement. At the same time, we have tried to maintain the basic scientific integrity of the explanations. In our attempt to develop a basic teaching text, we have included suggested discussion topics and independent exercises for self-study as well as case examples to embellish basic applications.

Because our goal was a solid introduction to acoustic immittance measures, we have dealt primarily with procedures that are in common clinical use. Procedures that may offer useful diagnostic information in selected cases, but are used only rarely in clinical practice, receive little or no attention. Again, our objective was to get students interested and started, not to fill all of the information needs of practitioners and students at more advanced levels. At the same time, clinicians who use or interpret acoustic immittance measures on a daily basis and students at all levels should find the book useful as a basic reference for more fully understanding the basic characteristics of the measures used in clinical practice.

Acknowledgments

The authors would like to thank the faculty, staff, and student colleagues who reviewed various drafts of our text and offered numerous recommendations for improving the manuscript. In particular, we would like to thank Elizabeth Leigh and Christina Roup for their assistance in preparing selected graphics. Finally, we would like to thank David Lilly for agreeing to write the foreword and for teaching us and many others about the topics covered in the text.

*This book is dedicated to our present
and former audiology student colleagues
who have, directly and indirectly,
provided the foundation and stimulation
for development of the text.*

1

Overview of Clinical Measures

his chapter introduces students to the primary measures and procedures that will be developed in more detail throughout the text. This basic introduction should provide a useful perspective for students as individual topics are developed in greater depth in specific sections of the book which follow.

Acoustic immittance is a general term that indicates either acoustic impedance or acoustic admittance or both. *Impedance* is the opposition to the flow of energy, and *admittance* is the ease with which energy flows through a system. The associated term *acoustic* signifies the character of the energy system under measurement. Acoustic impedance and acoustic admittance are *reciprocal* terms. An acoustic transmission system, such as the human ear, that offers high acoustic admittance to the flow of sound has a low acoustic impedance.

Acoustic immittance measures have become a routine part of an audiologic evaluation. Tympanometry and recording stapedius reflexes for acoustic signals are the two procedures that form the primary set of acoustic immittance measures used in most audiology clinics. These measures will be defined and described in the next section. A primary rationale for the clinical use of acoustic immittance measures is that they are sensitive to middle ear disorders, even in persons who have little or no hearing loss. In many cases of childhood *otitis media* (middle ear infection), for example, the affected children have hearing thresholds within normal limits. In contrast to screening or threshold

1

audiometry, acoustic immittance measures are effective in detecting the presence and character of such middle ear disorders. An additional advantage of acoustic immittance procedures is that they require no behavioral response on the part of the patient. Thus, the measures can be obtained in clinical patients for whom behavioral response techniques are not always feasible (such as very young children).

CLINICAL MEASURES

Tympanometry

Tympanometry is a routine clinical procedure that involves measures of acoustic immittance in the ear canal as air pressure in the canal is varied above (+) and below (−) atmospheric level in the ear canal. Ear canal pressure is expressed in units called *decaPascals* or *daPa*. The graphic representation of acoustic admittance or acoustic impedance as a function of ear canal pressure is called a *tympanogram* (see Figure 1–1). As air pressure in the ear canal is increased or decreased from atmospheric condition (0 daPa) in a person with a normal middle ear, the acoustic admittance is decreased (Figure 1–1, top) or the acoustic impedance is increased (Figure 1–1, bottom). The air pressure changes effectively tense the tympanic membrane and connected ossicular chain, resulting in a stiffening of the middle ear system.

As might be expected, characteristics of the tympanogram are altered in cases of middle ear disorders. In cases of disorders that dampen or stiffen the middle ear system, such as serous otitis media with effusion (liquid), the tympanogram may be reduced in amplitude or flat in configuration (Figure 1–2, tympanogram b). Because the middle ear system is already stiffened by the presence of liquid, there is little or no change in acoustic admittance with alterations in ear canal pressure. In contrast, a discontinuity of the ossicular chain will be associated with a tympanogram having a greater amplitude (higher peak) than normal (Figure 1–2, tympanogram c). The disruption in the ossicular chain results in greater than normal changes in acoustic admittance with variation in ear canal pressure.

Tympanometry also offers an indirect way of evaluating Eustachian tube function. This may be important clinically because Eustachian tube obstruction is often associated with initial stages of otitis media. A rough estimate of the resting pressure within the middle ear is indicated from the pressure location of the tympanogram peak. This is based on the reasonable assumption that sound flow at the tympanic membrane is greatest when the pressure on both sides of the tympanic membrane is equal. In normal subjects with proper Eustachian tube

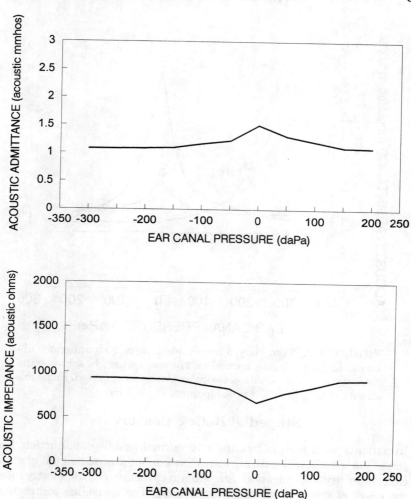

FIGURE 1–1. Acoustic admittance *(top)* and acoustic impedance *(bottom)* tympanograms for a person with a normal middle ear system.

function, the tympanogram peak typically occurs near ambient or atmospheric pressure (0 daPa) (Figure 1–2, tympanogram a). The Eustachian tube maintains pressure equilibrium between the atmosphere and the middle ear. In cases of otitis media, however, the Eustachian tube may be obstructed, resulting in a negative middle ear resting pressure (Figure 1–2, tympanogram d). Tympanometry, then, provides a means of monitoring the ventilatory function of the Eustachian tube.

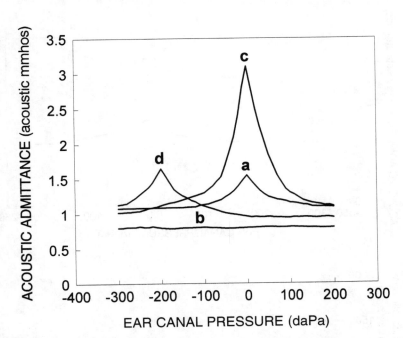

FIGURE 1–2. Exemplary acoustic admittance tympanograms observed in cases of: **a.** a normal middle ear system, **b.** serous otitis media (middle ear liquid), **c.** ossicular chain disruption, **d.** Eustachian tube obstruction. The probe frequency is 226 Hz.

Stapedial Reflex Measures

In patients with normal hearing and normal middle ear function, the stapedius muscle will contract in response to an acoustic signal of sufficient intensity and duration. Stapedial contraction occurs shortly after the onset of the acoustic signal (activator). The stapedius contraction dampens (stiffens) the ossicular chain, resulting in a decrease in acoustic admittance (or increase in acoustic impedance) measured at the tympanic membrane. This chain of events is termed an *acoustic reflex*.

Currently, the following three primary acoustic reflex characteristics are typically evaluated in audiologic practice: (1) presence or absence of an acoustic reflex, (2) acoustic reflex threshold, and (3) acoustic reflex adaptation (or decay). The absence of an acoustic reflex alone may signify potential otic pathology. Absence of the acoustic reflex would mean that no acoustic immittance change was observed with presentation of an acoustic activating signal (such as a tone) at the highest signal level available. Absent acoustic reflexes for various ipsilateral and contralateral signal presentations may be important in the differential diagnosis of both peripheral and central disorders of the auditory system. In cases of *vestibular schwannoma* (tumor of the auditory nerve), for example, acoustic reflexes may be absent in the affected ear even when there is little or no hearing loss.

If an acoustic reflex is present, an *acoustic reflex threshold* can be measured. The reflex threshold is defined as the lowest level of the acoustic activating signal that produces an observable, time-locked (with the activator) change in acoustic immittance. The acoustic reflex threshold for tones in subjects with normal hearing and no pathology of the auditory system occurs at approximately 70–90 dB above the threshold of audibility for the tone. In cases of cochlear and eighth (auditory) nerve disorders, however, acoustic reflex thresholds may be elevated (higher than normal).

If acoustic reflexes are present and the measured acoustic reflex threshold is not extremely elevated, audiologists may measure *acoustic reflex adaptation (or decay)*. Reflex decay is observed as a decline (or relaxation) in reflex contraction during the presentation of a sustained, acoustic activating signal. For reflex decay measures, a sustained acoustic activating signal (usually a low frequency tone of 500 or 1000 Hz) is presented above reflex threshold (usually 10 dB above reflex threshold) for a specified time period (usually 5 or 10 seconds). The acoustic immittance in the ear canal is monitored during presentation of the activator tone. In persons with a normal auditory system, the acoustic immittance in the ear canal remains relatively constant during the presentation of the reflex activating signal. In other words, there is no reflex adaptation or decay for the sustained tone. In contrast, patients with lesions of the cochlea, eighth nerve, or auditory brainstem may evidence abnormal reflex decay. Patients with eighth nerve lesions, for example, usually will demonstrate rapid reflex decay. The acoustic immittance measured in the ear canal steadily changes during presentation of the activating signal and may indicate complete stapedius relaxation (or decay) within a few seconds after the activator is turned on.

2

Principles of Measurement

In order to use acoustic immittance measures effectively in clinical diagnosis, the underlying principles involved in these measures must be understood. Clinicians also must become familiar with the associated terminology, measurement variables, and units of measurement. In this chapter, the concept of acoustic immittance, the underlying mathematical and physical concepts, and the basic measures in clinical use are introduced. Throughout the discussions, we have maintained consistency with the terminology used in the *American National Standards Institute (ANSI) Standard on Aural Acoustic Immittance Measures* (1987). Users of acoustic immittance instruments should familiarize themselves with the material contained in this standard. Selected definitions of terms and measures taken directly from the standard are included as Appendix A. The reader may refer to these definitions as the terms and measures are discussed in sections of the book that follow. Finally, although we will provide background information regarding the relations of acoustic admittance and acoustic impedance measures, the majority of examples, including clinical case studies, are expressed in terms of acoustic admittance. The vast majority of commercially available instruments are based on acoustic admittance measures. Most contemporary clinical studies of acoustic immittance findings in pathologic ears also are based on acoustic admittance measures.

ACOUSTIC IMMITTANCE

As noted in the overview (Chapter 1), acoustic immittance is a general term referring to either acoustic impedance or acoustic admittance. If we are interested in the opposition to the transfer of acoustic energy, we would express such opposition as *acoustic impedance* (Z_a). If we were to express our measures in terms of the resulting energy flow as a result of the transfer of air pressure changes, we would use the term *acoustic admittance* (Y_a). As sound flow increases through a system, such as the human middle ear, the acoustic admittance will increase and the acoustic impedance offered by the system will decrease in a reciprocal manner.

BASICS OF MEASUREMENT

Regardless of the specific instrument or whether the measures are expressed in terms of acoustic admittance or acoustic impedance, the basics of measurement are generally the same. The measurement of acoustic immittance is performed by introducing an acoustic (probe) signal to the ear and measuring the sound pressure level (SPL) of the signal in the ear canal. This is why we refer to our measures in terms of acoustic impedance or acoustic admittance. The measures are based on *acoustic* measurement principles. This accounts for the small *a* subscript for admittance (Y_a) and impedance (Z_a) measures. The *probe signal* introduced into the ear canal is usually a tone, and the SPL of the probe tone serves as an indirect index of acoustic admittance or impedance. The SPL of the probe signal measured at the probe tip is directly proportional to the acoustic impedance offered by the ear at the point of measure. The higher the measured SPL of the probe tone, the higher the acoustic impedance represented by the ear under measurement. Conversely, the higher the SPL of the probe, the lower the acoustic admittance offered by the ear under test. A block diagram of such a system is shown in Figure 2–1.

At least three primary subsystems are fundamental to any instrument used for acoustic immittance measures in human ears. As the measurement technique implies, we must have a sound pressure source and an analysis system for monitoring the SPL of the source or probe signal. We also need a means of varying and monitoring air pressure changes in the ear canal. These three subsystems are depicted in Figure 2–1. An illustration of a child being tested with a screening tympanometer is shown as Figure 2–2. A probe unit surrounded by a soft cuff is *hermetically* sealed (air tight) in the ear canal. The probe tone is introduced into the ear canal from a miniature loudspeaker

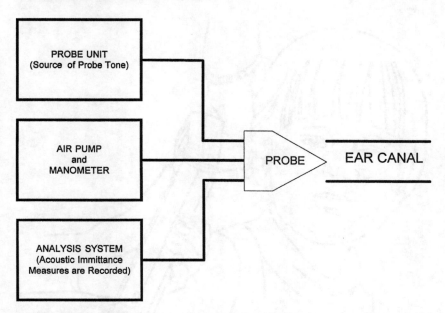

FIGURE 2–1. A block diagram of an electroacoustic immittance instrument. A probe tip is hermetically sealed in the ear canal using a soft rubber cuff that surrounds the probe tip. The probe contains openings connected to the three basic subsystems of the instrument: (1) an air pump used to introduce air pressure in the ear canal and a manometer for monitoring the air pressure, (2) a miniature loudspeaker used for introduction of a probe tone, and (3) a microphone with an analysis system used to monitor the sound pressure level of the probe tone.

housed in the probe unit (see Figure 2–1). The SPL of the tone in the ear canal is monitored via a microphone in the analysis system. As noted earlier, the measured SPL of the tone serves as the referent for acoustic immittance measures. The air pressure subsystem provides a means of increasing or decreasing ear canal pressure via an air pump and provides a means of monitoring the pressure (with a *manometer*).

If acoustic reflex measures are performed, a fourth subsystem providing another signal source would be included in the measurement system (not shown in Figure 2–1). In the case of *ipsilateral* acoustic reflex measures, a second acoustic source would be included in the probe system to allow presentation of acoustic reflex activating signals in the same ear containing the probe unit. We also would need to be able to record acoustic reflexes in the same ear (ipsilateral) by monitoring changes in acoustic immittance. In the case of *contralateral* acoustic reflex measures, the acoustic reflex activating signals are presented in the ear opposite that containing the probe. Contralateral reflex activa-

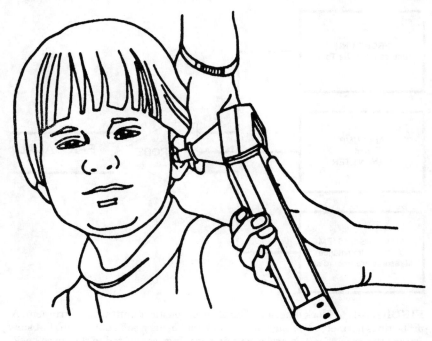

FIGURE 2–2. An illustration of a child undergoing screening tympanometry. (Reprinted with the permission of Welch Allyn, Inc.)

tors may be presented through a conventional earphone encased in a supra-aural cushion or may be presented through an insert receiver (or earphone) that fits in the ear canal. Contralateral acoustic reflex measures involve presentation of an acoustic activator signal to one ear and measuring acoustic immittance changes (indicative of stapedial contractions) in the opposite (probe) ear. According to ANSI (1987) nomenclature for contralateral reflex measures, the ear receiving the reflex activating signal is referred to as the *stimulus* ear and the opposite ear (containing the probe tip) is termed the *probe* ear. In clinical practice, the probe and activator signals must be distinguished in describing acoustic immittance measures. Further, if contralateral acoustic reflex measures are reported, the probe and activator (stimulus) ears must be identified in describing the results of acoustic reflex tests.

Plane of Measurement

As illustrated in Figure 2–1, the tip of the probe unit is the point at which the acoustic immittance analysis system receives input. Thus, the plane (or point) of measurement of the input acoustic immittance of the auditory system is at the probe tip. In terms of ANSI nomenclature, measures referenced to the probe tip are called *measurement plane* measures of acoustic immittance. Although measurement plane measures are useful for specific clinical purposes, such as providing acoustic estimates of the equivalent ear-canal volume, this plane of measurement is remote from the tympanic membrane (eardrum). Because of the manner in which the probe tip is inserted and because of varying conditions within the ear canal, the acoustic immittance at the probe tip is not stable for repeated measures. These measures, for example, will vary with the depth of probe insertion and with differences in ear canal volume across clinical patients. A more optimal point of measurement is at the tympanic membrane because it is an invariable landmark for the individual under test; this plane of measure minimizes differences in depth of probe insertion and differences in the size of the ear canal across clinical patients. Further, it is the middle ear, not the ear canal, that is of primary interest in diagnostic protocols. Disorders of the ear canal often are visible through otoscopic inspection. Disorders of the middle ear, however, often are not apparent based on otoscopic inspection of the tympanic membrane and, thus, require more advanced evaluation techniques.

Although the ideal point of measure is the tympanic membrane, it is not feasible to place a probe tip next to the eardrum using commercially available instruments. Accordingly, definition of the input acoustic immittance of the middle ear system at the tympanic membrane requires extraction of ear canal contributions. Under measurement plane conditions, the observed acoustic immittance includes the contributions of the ear canal, the tympanic membrane, and the entire middle ear system, including the coupling of the ossicular chain to the cochlea. To correct the measurement to the plane of the tympanic membrane, we must subtract the contribution of the ear canal from the total acoustic immittance. The exact subtraction process will vary depending on whether measures are expressed in terms of acoustic impedance or acoustic admittance. In the case of acoustic admittance measures, the contribution of the ear canal is determined by taking acoustic admittance measures with substantial air pressure in the ear canal. The introduction of substantial (positive or negative) ear canal pressure effectively stiffens the tympanic membrane and middle ear transmission system. In the presence of sufficient pressure, the acoustic admittance at the probe tip is approximately equivalent to the acoustic admittance offered solely by the volume of air within the ear canal. This value of acoustic admittance, representing the ear canal, can then be subtracted from the total acoustic admittance at ambient ear-canal pressure to arrive at an estimate of acoustic admittance at the plane of the tympanic membrane. This measure is termed compensated acoustic admittance. The term *compensated* refers to the extraction of ear canal effects.

As a specific example, consider the tympanogram in Figure 2–3. The peak of the tympanogram occurs at ambient (0 daPa) ear canal pressure. The acoustic admittance value at this pressure (point a) represents the contributions of the ear canal, tympanic membrane, and the entire middle ear system. At 200 daPa of ear canal pressure, the observed acoustic admittance value is approximately equal to that offered by the ear canal alone (point b). By simply subtracting the equivalent ear-canal admittance from the admittance at the tympanogram peak (a – b), we obtain an estimate of the acoustic admittance at the lateral surface of the tympanic membrane. This measure is properly termed the *peak, compensated static acoustic admittance of* the ear under test. According to ANSI specifications, compensated measures

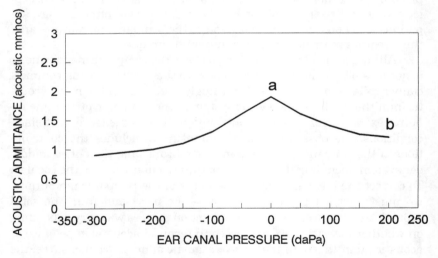

FIGURE 2–3. An exemplary tympanogram illustrating the method for determining peak, compensated static acoustic admittance (Peak Y_{tm}). Peak Y_{tm} is determined by subtracting the acoustic admittance value at 200 daPa (point b) from the acoustic admittance value at the tympanogram peak (point a). The acoustic admittance value at 200 daPa represents the acoustic admittance contribution of the ear canal and the acoustic admittance value at the tympanogram peak represents the acoustic admittance of the ear canal and the entire middle ear system. The subtraction of b from a results in an estimate of the acoustic admittance at the lateral surface of the tympanic membrane.

may be referenced to the pressure corresponding to the tympanogram peak or to ambient ear-canal pressure. So, you can perform either *peak* or *ambient* compensated measures. Peak compensated measures are those most commonly used in clinical practice. In our specific example, the two measures would give the same value because the tympanogram peak occurred at ambient pressure. The term *static* simply indicates that the measure is referenced to a specific ear-canal pressure. If other than peak or ambient pressures are used as a reference for static measures, the specific pressure used should be included in the notation of the static measure. Finally, as will be discussed further under the topic of tympanometry, tympanograms also can be obtained under compensated or measurement plane conditions.

ACOUSTIC IMPEDANCE

Before we continue development of clinical measures, we will examine the physical bases of acoustic impedance and acoustic admittance measures and the relations between the two analysis systems. Our choice of treating acoustic impedance first followed by a discussion of acoustic admittance is based on our experience with the topic. In our view, the impedance approach is intuitively easier to follow at initial stages of study. Our approach makes use of analogies between electrical, mechanical, and acoustical systems. The student is referred to the works of Beranek (1949, 1954) and Firestone (1956) for a more detailed and complete treatment of the topics using dynamic analogies.

As noted earlier, acoustic impedance is a general term referring to the total opposition to sound flow offered by a system. If we were to specify a peak, compensated acoustic impedance value for a human ear, it would represent the total opposition to sound flow offered by the ear under test at the lateral surface of the tympanic membrane. This measure represents the acoustic impedance at the input to the middle ear. The middle ear system, however, is composed of different mechanical structures that react to force (such as an input sound pressure) in a variety of ways (for example, see Dallos, 1973; Lilly, 1973; Zwislocki, 1963, 1976). Energy transfer and changes in state for mechanical structures of the middle ear system do not always occur instantaneously with the applied force. A given acoustic impedance measure is determined by the complex ratio of the applied force (sound pressure) to the velocity (or sound flow). The manner by which different structures oppose sound flow differs in a complex fashion across components of the middle ear. The volume of the external ear canal, the tympanic membrane, the interconnected cavities of the middle ear, the ossicular chain, and the coupling of the stapes footplate to the oval window of the cochlea all contribute in a complex fashion to the overall acoustic impedance measured at the probe tip.

By complex, we mean that different forces are varying together in different directions (phase angles) or at different relative times. When two forces with different phase angles are initiated together, the resultant total force is the vector sum of the two. The vector sum is the total magnitude plus a direction (or phase angle) that results from combining the two divergent forces. Thus, complex forces representing a given acoustic impedance are described by vectors or phasors that have a magnitude and a direction (or phase) of force. The term *phasor* refers to a vector that emanates from the origin of a Cartesian or rectangular coordinate system.

The acoustic impedance of a human ear at the tympanic membrane is determined by the contributions of the mechanical structures of the middle ear system. The acoustic impedance measured at the tympanic membrane is controlled by the mass of the middle ear ossicles, the stiffness of the ossicular ligaments and muscles, the stiffness of the tympanic membrane and round window membrane, the stiffness of the air contained in the tympanum, the mass and friction that result from air movement within the tympanum, and, finally, the impedance (primarily resistance) offered by the coupling of the stapes footplate to the cochlea at the oval window (Lilly, 1973; Zwislocki, 1976). The acoustic impedance at the tympanic membrane, then, is determined by different masses, stiffnesses, and frictions. In terms of the relative contributions of these components to the overall opposition to energy flow, the components may be categorized as *in-phase components* (i.e., those that occur simultaneously with the applied force) and *out-of-phase components* (i.e., those that lead or lag the applied force).

Resistance

The in-phase component of impedance is *resistance* (R). In electrical circuits, electrical energy is converted into heat when a current is passed through a resistance. An example of resistance in a mechanical system is the heat that is produced by rubbing two surfaces together. When the two surfaces are rubbed together, the resulting friction transduces the motion into heat (Figure 2–4). In both electrical and mechanical systems, energy is lost through dissipation of the energy in the form of heat. This resistive dissipation of energy is an in-phase effect that occurs in direct proportion to the force and simultaneous with the applied force. Similar to electrical and mechanical analogs, *acoustic resistance* (R_a) represents the dissipation of acoustic energy. A

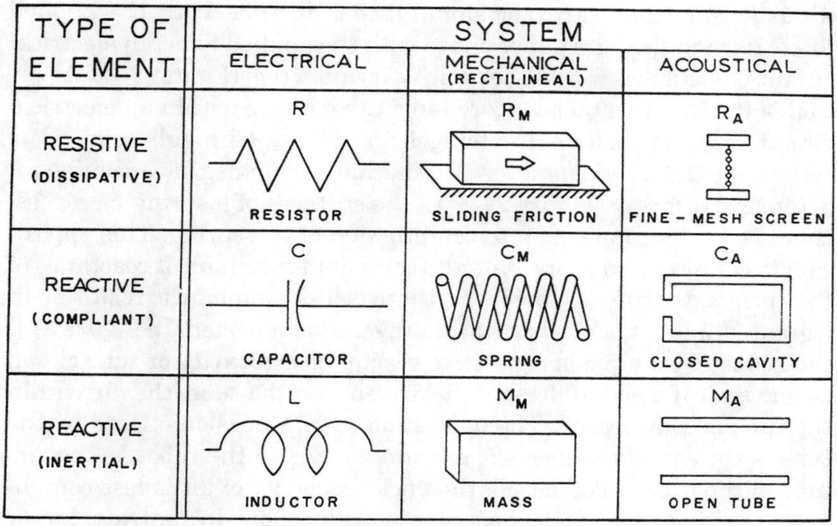

TYPE OF ELEMENT	SYSTEM		
	ELECTRICAL	MECHANICAL (RECTILINEAL)	ACOUSTICAL
RESISTIVE (DISSIPATIVE)	R RESISTOR	R_M SLIDING FRICTION	R_A FINE-MESH SCREEN
REACTIVE (COMPLIANT)	C CAPACITOR	C_M SPRING	C_A CLOSED CAVITY
REACTIVE (INERTIAL)	L INDUCTOR	M_M MASS	M_A OPEN TUBE

FIGURE 2–4. Summary of electrical, mechanical and acoustical analogs of resistive and reactive components comprising an acoustic impedance (From "Acoustic Impedance at the Tympanic Membrane: A Review of Basic Concepts," p. 22, by D. J. Lilly in *Impedance Symposium,* edited by D. Rose and L. W. Keating, 1972. Reprinted with permission of the author.) Further description of the figure components is included in the text.

mesh screen is a physical example of an acoustic resistance (Figure 2–4). The acoustic resistance offered by the screen is inversely proportional to the size of the apertures (openings) in the screen. When a sound pressure from an acoustic source is driven through the screen, the smaller the openings in the screen, the higher the acoustic resistance and the greater the dissipation of acoustic energy. Over the frequency range of probe signals used in clinical acoustic immittance measures, *acoustic resistance remains relatively constant as a function of probe frequency*. The unit of measure for resistance (electrical) is the *ohm*. In referring to mechanical, acoustic, or other systems, the system as well as the unit of measure must be indicated. In acoustic systems, for example, the units for acoustic resistance are *acoustic ohms*.

Reactance

The out-of-phase component of impedance is *reactance* (X). Reactances do not actually dissipate energy. Rather, reactances oppose energy flow by storing the energy for a period of time. Thus, reactive effects on acoustic impedance are not simultaneous in time with the applied force. Rather, they are out of phase with the applied force. In electrical circuits reactances may be capacitive or inductive (Figure 2–4). A portion of the input voltage is stored in a capacitance within an electrical circuit. This opposition to changes in voltage (through storage) is termed *capacitive reactance* (X_c). A mechanical analog of capacitive reactance is a spring (Figure 2–4); as the stiffness of a spring increases, there is greater opposition to compression of the spring. This opposition to compression represents the compliant mechanical reactance of the spring. As stiffness increases, there is less compliance, resulting in a greater amount of mechanical energy that is reflected. In Figure 2–4, the acoustic example of capacitive reactance is a cavity or tube closed at one end. If a sound pressure is driven into the tube, the air within the tube is compressed. The opposition to compression offered by the tube is the *compliant acoustic reactance* ($-jX_a$) of the tube. As the volume of the tube is decreased, the enclosed cavity of air is less compliant, resulting in greater opposition to sound flow. In contrast, larger cavity volumes are more compliant and offer less opposition to sound flow. Compliant acoustic reactance varies with probe frequency; *compliant acoustic reactance is greatest at low probe frequencies and decreases with increases in probe frequency.*

Inductive reactance (X_L) is the opposition to current changes offered by an inductor. Current flow is restricted by an opposite energy flow produced by the inductor. A mass is an example of a mechanical analog for inductive reactance (Figure 2–4). Any physical mass will oppose displacement and the force required for movement of the mass will vary directly with the magnitude of the mass. The opposition to displacement offered by the mechanical mass represents the mass mechanical reactance of the physical mass. The acoustic analog of inductive reactance is *mass acoustic reactance* (jX_a). A physical example of mass acoustic reactance is a column of air in a tube open at both ends (Figure 2–4). In the case of a tube open at both ends, the column of air within the tube may be displaced without compression of the air. As a sound pressure is driven through the tube, the column of air opposes displacement dependent on the characteristics of the air column. This opposition to displacement offered by the air column is termed mass acoustic reactance (jX_a). In reciprocal fashion relative to compliant acoustic reactance, *mass acoustic reactance is greatest at high probe frequencies and decreases with decreases in probe frequency.* So, with changes in probe frequency, one of the acoustic reactance components will increase as the other component decreases. As probe frequency is increased, for example, the compliant acoustic reactance will decrease as the mass acoustic reactance increases. The unit of measure for both compliant and mass acoustic reactance is the *acoustic ohm*.

NUMBERS AND NOTATIONAL SCHEMES

Specific mathematical schemes are used to express how in-phase and out-of-phase components are combined to produce a given acoustic impedance. These schemes require a basic understanding of complex or imaginary numbers and the notational forms used to represent these measures. The following discussion is a brief review of the properties of imaginary numbers and rectangular and polar notational systems. For a more complete explanation of these concepts, the reader may consult a college algebra text for a review of complex numbers and Cartesian or rectangular coordinates. In addition, Lilly (1973) has reviewed the basic concepts and notational schemes important for acoustic impedance measures.

As noted earlier, the total acoustic impedance of a system (such as the human ear) is comprised of resistive and reactive components. These components contribute to the total acoustic impedance at different relative times or phases. Resistance components are in phase with the applied force (sound pressure) and reactive components are out of phase. The total acoustic impedance is determined by the complex summation of these resistive and reactive components. The total of in-phase and out-of-phase components is determined by their relative phase relation (in degrees). These relative phase relations are conventionally represented within a Cartesian coordinate system that employs the use of real and imaginary numbers. When the coordinate system is used to represent acoustic impedance measures, it is termed an acoustic impedance *plane* (Lilly, 1973). An example of such a plot is shown in Figure 2–5. Note that the horizontal axis is used to plot the resistive component and the vertical axis is used to plot the reactive component. Also, note that the resistive axis employs real numbers and the reactive axis employs imaginary numbers. Thus, the real, dissipative (in-phase) effects are represented on the horizontal axis and the storage or imaginary (out-of-phase) effects are represented on the vertical axis. The directed phasor magnitude defined by the resistive and reactive coordinates represents the total acoustic impedance.

As shown in our example, the numbers on both horizontal and vertical axes may have either a positive or negative sign or operator. This sign denotes the direction or phase angle associated with the component that is plotted on the respective axis. Thus, the resistive component, the reactive component, and the total acoustic impedance

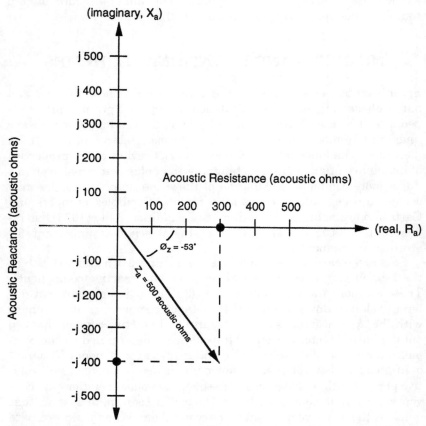

FIGURE 2-5. An example of a rectangular (Cartesian) plot of a complex acoustic impedance plane. The example shown is for an acoustic impedance of 500 acoustic ohms at a phase angle (Φ_Z) of –53 degrees. The total acoustic impedance of 500 acoustic ohms is comprised of an acoustic resistance of 300 acoustic ohms (real axis) and a compliant acoustic reactance of –j400 acoustic ohms (imaginary axis).

values are each represented by a direction (or phase angle) and a magnitude. The actual number on each axis denotes the magnitude of the component and the positive or negative operator denotes the direction or phase of the component with respect to the applied sound pressure. *The + or – sign associated with a reactance refers to the phase angle associated with the reactive component*, not to the value of reactance. Reactances are all equal to or greater than zero;

only the phase angle associated with reactances or impedances may assume a negative operator.

Still another operator, j, is assigned to the positive and negative imaginary axes. This *j operator* used by engineers is the same as the complex number i in mathematics, and is equal to the square root of −1. For purposes of acoustic impedance measures, the j operator refers to the imaginary or storage properties of acoustic reactances and each reactive element is associated with a negative (−90 degrees) or positive (90 degrees) phase angle. Compliant acoustic reactance has a negative phase angle and mass acoustic reactance has a positive phase angle.

In our example (Figure 2–5), we have a single acoustic impedance phasor defined by an acoustic resistance and a total acoustic reactance. The acoustic resistance of 300 acoustic ohms combines complexly with a total acoustic reactance of 400 acoustic ohms to produce a total acoustic impedance of 500 acoustic ohms. The −j operator associated with the acoustic reactance component indicates that the system under measurement is controlled by the compliant reactance component. This does not mean that there was no mass acoustic reactance contributing to the total acoustic reactance. Rather, it indicates that the compliant acoustic reactance was 400 acoustic ohms larger than the mass acoustic reactance. The total acoustic reactance is the simple sum of the two reactive components. Because the two components are directly out of phase, however, the summation process consists of adding a positive and negative number. Thus, the larger component determines the dominant reactive element and determines whether the phase angle is negative 90 degrees or positive 90 degrees. Because the resultant phase angle was negative in our example, the compliant acoustic reactance was the larger of the two components.

Rectangular Notation

One means of representing the total acoustic impedance in Figure 2–5 is as a complex number. In our case, the total acoustic impedance is equal to 300 −j400 acoustic ohms. This complex form is read as 300 negative j400 acoustic ohms. The complex number 300 −j400 includes both a real (300) and an imaginary (−j400) number. This notational method is referred to as *rectangular* notation. *The complex number tells us both the resistive (real) and reactive (imaginary) component that comprise the total acoustic impedance.* Further, because a −j operator is associated with the reactive element, we know that the dominant reactive component was compliant acoustic reactance. Thus, by knowing which reactive component is larger, we can determine whether a system is stiffness (−j) or mass dominant (j). In our example, the total reactance has a –j operator and the system is said to be stiffness-controlled or stiffness-dominant. As discussed earlier, compliant and mass acoustic reactances vary in a predictable manner with changes in probe frequency. In the case of a normal middle ear, compliant acoustic reactance dominates at lower probe frequencies and mass acoustic reactance dominates at higher probe frequencies. As we discuss later (Chapter 4), however, this relation between probe frequency and the frequency at which reactive components dominate is altered in middle ear pathologies.

Polar Notation

The complex number 300 –j400 representing the acoustic impedance in Figure 2–5 also can be expressed as a single number with an associated phase angle. Specifically, 300 –j400 acoustic ohms is equal to the phasor equivalent of 500 acoustic ohms at an angle of –53 degrees. Expression of the acoustic impedance as a single number with the associated phase angle is referred to as *polar notation*. The polar equivalent of a rectangular form can be derived using the mathematical laws governing right triangles. Note that the acoustic resistance and compliant acoustic reactance in Figure 2–5 form the legs of a right triangle. Accordingly, using the Pythagorean theorem, we can derive the magnitude of the vector defined by the rectangular resistive and reactive coordinates. In our example, the magnitude of the acoustic impedance phasor is equal to the square root of the sum of the squared values of acoustic resistance and compliant acoustic reactance. So, the acoustic impedance of 300 –j400 acoustic ohms in rectangular form is equivalent to 500 acoustic ohms in polar form. The phasor magnitude of 500, however, is associated with a unique phase angle. A complete description of acoustic impedance in polar form, then, requires inclusion of the phase angle associated with the phasor magnitude. We can determine the phase angle associated with a phasor using basic trigonometric identities associated with right triangles. The inverse tangent identity is typically used for such derivation. In our case, the acoustic impedance phase angle, or Φ_z, is equal to $\tan^{-1} -jX_a/R_a$. Thus, a complete description of our acoustic impedance in polar form is 500 $\angle-53°$ acoustic ohms. This expression is read as 500 at an angle of negative 53 degrees acoustic ohms.

Just as we used the Pythagorean theorem to convert from rectangular to polar form, we can use another trigonometric law (Euler's theorem) to convert the polar acoustic impedance to its rectangular equivalent. In our example, the acoustic resistance is determined by multiplying the magnitude of acoustic impedance (500) times the cosine of the acoustic impedance phase angle (–53°). In similar fashion, the acoustic reactance is determined by multiplying the magnitude of acoustic impedance (500) times the sine of the acoustic impedance phase angle (–53°).

Thus, we have two notational schemes for presentation of acoustic impedance measures. In rectangular form, the resistive and reactive elements of the total acoustic impedance are expressed and define the total acoustic impedance as a complex number. In polar form, the phasor magnitude of the acoustic impedance is given along with the associated phase angle. In both forms, the dominant reactive component is evident. In rectangular form, for example, the –j operator associated with the reactive element indicates that the compliant reactance is dominant. Similarly, the negative phase angle associated with our polar equivalent indicates a stiffness controlled system.

RESONANCE

As noted earlier, compliant and mass acoustic reactances change in reciprocal fashion as probe frequency is increased or decreased. As probe frequency decreases, for example, the mass acoustic reactance decreases and the compliant acoustic reactance increases. Accordingly, at some specific probe frequency, the two reactances will be equal. Because the two reactances are directly out of phase, they will cancel one another and the resultant total acoustic reactance will be equal to zero. Specifically, the addition of two equal but out-of-phase components will result in a total acoustic reactance of 0 acoustic ohms. At this specific frequency, the system is said to be at *resonance* and the frequency at which this occurs is termed the *resonant frequency*. Because the total acoustic reactance is equal to 0 acoustic ohms at the resonant frequency, the total acoustic impedance is equal to the acoustic resistance offered by the system. Because only acoustic resistance contributes to the total acoustic impedance, the acoustic impedance phase angle is equal to 0 degrees. At the resonant frequency, then, acoustic impedance is at its minimal value and is equal to the acoustic resistance offered by the system under test. Again, *the resonant frequency is that frequency for which the acoustic reactance equals 0 acoustic ohms and the acoustic impedance phase angle equals 0 degrees*. As will be developed in Chapter 4, the resonant frequency of the middle ear transmission system can be estimated through an analysis of acoustic immittance values for probe signals ranging in frequency from low to high. These resonance estimates may be useful diagnostically because the resonant frequency of the middle ear is altered in a predictable way for certain middle ear disorders.

ACOUSTIC ADMITTANCE

As noted in the topic overview, acoustic admittance and acoustic impedance are reciprocal measures: $Z_a = 1/Y_a$ and $Y_a = 1/Z_a$. The vast majority of commercially available clinical instruments provide for acoustic admittance measures. This preference for acoustic admittance measures is primarily due to simpler mathematic and engineering principles associated with acoustic admittance measures as opposed to acoustic impedance measures. The same measurement principles we discussed under acoustic impedance also are fundamental to acoustic admittance measures. The specification of dissipative and storage components and computational methods, however, differ for the two different measurement systems.

Whereas acoustic impedance represents the opposition to the flow of acoustic energy, acoustic admittance represents the ease of sound flow. The measurement unit for acoustic impedance is the acoustic ohm; acoustic admittance measures are expressed in *acoustic mhos (ohm spelled backwards)*. As will be developed more fully later, acoustic admittance measures in human ears are relatively small in magnitude and, accordingly, most clinical acoustic admittance measures are actually expressed in *acoustic millimhos*. Because Y_a and Z_a are reciprocals, the phase angle associated with each term is of the same magnitude but of opposite direction. If the acoustic impedance phase angle is negative, for example, the acoustic admittance phase angle (Φ_y) is positive. This reciprocal relation is illustrated in Figure 2–6. Here, we have replicated the acoustic impedance example from Figure 2–5, but have now included a separate complex acoustic admittance plane illustrating the acoustic admittance equivalent to the acoustic impedance. Note that the phase angles are identical in magnitude but opposite in direction; the acoustic impedance phase angle is negative and the acoustic admittance phase angle is positive. Note also that the value of acoustic admittance is expressed in acoustic mmhos.

Like acoustic impedance, a given acoustic admittance is determined by both in-phase (real) and out-of-phase (imaginary) components contributing to the flow of acoustic energy. There are acoustic admittance equivalents of resistive and reactive components in acoustic impedance measures. The real component of acoustic admittance is *acoustic conductance (abbreviated G_a)* and the imaginary component of acoustic admittance is *acoustic susceptance (abbreviated B_a)*. Like acoustic reactance, acoustic susceptance may be of two types, *compliant acoustic susceptance* and *mass acoustic susceptance*. Acoustic admittance, acoustic conductance, and acoustic susceptance measures are expressed in acoustic mmhos.

The reactive elements of acoustic admittance are plotted on the imaginary (j) axis in the same manner as acoustic reactances associated with an acoustic impedance. Because of the reciprocal relation between admittance and impedance, however, the positive and negative imaginary axes on which the reactive components of admittance are plotted are reversed relative to those for impedance. Specifically, a mass acoustic susceptance is plotted on the negative imaginary axis and a compliant acoustic susceptance is plotted on the positive directed axis (Figure 2–6).

Although acoustic admittance and acoustic impedance are simple reciprocals, acoustic reactance and acoustic susceptance usually are not. Acoustic reactance is the simple reciprocal of acoustic susceptance if, and only if, the value of acoustic resistance is zero. In reality, however, both acoustic resistance and acoustic reactance values are finite (greater than zero) in the case of acoustic impedance measures for human ears. Thus, there is not a simple reciprocal relation between acoustic reactance and acoustic resistance. Rather, a given acoustic conductance or acoustic susceptance is determined by the value of both acoustic resistance and acoustic reactance. This relation is clarified in Table 2–1. The defining equations for acoustic admittance and acoustic impedance terms are shown along with appropriate units of measure and common abbreviations.

Table 2–2 is included as a final step in understanding the relations between acoustic admittance and acoustic impedance measures. Here, tympanometry data are used as a means of calculating compensated, static acoustic admittance. The acoustic admittance values are converted to equivalent acoustic impedance terms for the purpose of illustration. A basic understanding of the calculations and relations between terms is important in understanding the characteristics of clinical acoustic immittance measures. In this regard, the reader is encouraged to confirm each of the calculations and conversions shown in Table 2–2.

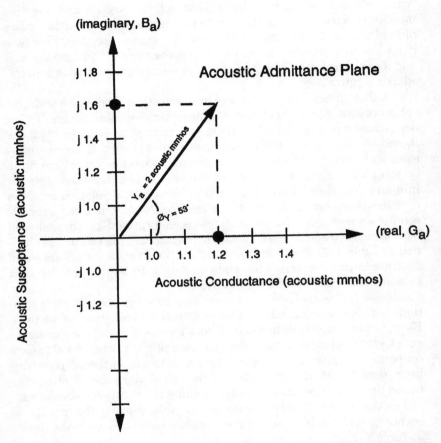

FIGURE 2–6. Cartesian plots of acoustic admittance *(above)* and acoustic impedance *(right)*. Acoustic admittance and acoustic impedance are shown as reciprocal plots; the acoustic admittance phase angle (Φ_y) is 53 degrees and the acoustic impedance phase angle (Φ_z) is –53 degrees. Similarly, the acoustic

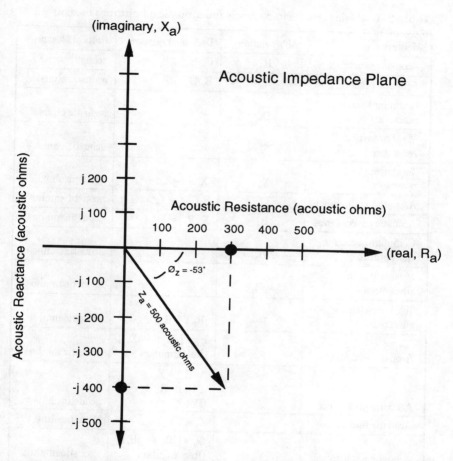

reactance is plotted on the negative axis of ordinates and the acoustic suscep-tance is plotted on the positive axis of ordinates. The units for acoustic admit-tance measures are acoustic mmhos and the units for acoustic impedance measures are acoustic ohms.

Table 2–1. Basic acoustic impedance and acoustic admittance measures.

Measure	Abbreviation	Defining Equation	Units of Measure
Acoustic resistance	R_a	$G_a/G_a^2 + B_a^2$	acoustic ohms
Acoustic reactance	X_a	$B_a/G_a^2 + B_a^2$	acoustic ohms
Compliant acoustic reactance	$-jX_a$		acoustic ohms
Mass acoustic reactance	jX_a		acoustic ohms
Total acoustic reactance	X_a	$jX_a + (-jX_a)$	acoustic ohms
Acoustic conductance	G_a	$R_a/R_a^2 + X_a^2$	acoustic mmhos
Acoustic susceptance	B_a	$X_a/R_a^2 + X_a^2$	acoustic mmhos
Compliant acoustic susceptance	jB_a		acoustic mmhos
Mass acoustic susceptance	$-jB_a$		acoustic mmhos
Total acoustic susceptance	B_a	$jB_a + (-jB_a)$	acoustic mmhos
Acoustic impedance	Z_a	$R_a + [jX_a + (-jX_a)]$ (Rectangular)	acoustic mmhos
Acoustic impedance	Z_a	$\sqrt{R_a^2 + X_a^2} \angle \tan^{-1} X_a/R_a$ (Polar)	acoustic ohms
Acoustic impedance	Z_a	$Z_a = 1/Y_a$	acoustic ohms
Acoustic admittance	Y_a	$G_a + [jB_a + (-jB_a)]$ (Rectangular)	acoustic mmhos
Acoustic admittance	Y_a	$\sqrt{G_a^2 + B_a^2} \angle \tan^{-1} B_a/G_a$ (Polar)	acoustic mmhos
Acoustic admittance	Y_a	$Y_a = 1/Z_a$	acoustic mmhos
Acoustic impedance phase angle	Φ_z	$\tan^{-1} X_a/R_a$	degrees
Acoustic admittance phase angle	Φ_y	$\tan^{-1} B_a/G_a$	degrees

Table 2–2. Estimation of ambient*, compensated acoustic impedance (Z_{tm}) and ambient, compensated acoustic admittance (Y_{tm}) using tympanometric data. In our example, we have used data taken from component (G_a and B_a) measurement plane tympanograms obtained using an acoustic admittance measurement system. For our example, we have chosen the admittance value at 200 daPa as our reference for equivalent ear-canal volume**.

EXAMPLE.　　　　Given: Probe Frequency = 226 Hz

G_{a1} (0 daPa) = 3.7 acoustic millimhos.
G_{a2} (200 daPa) = 0.9 acoustic millimhos.

B_{a1} (0 daPa) = 2.4 acoustic millimhos.
B_{a2} (200 daPa) = 1.2 acoustic millimhos.

Then, acoustic conductance at the plane of the tympanic membrane = G_{tm} = $G_{a1} - G_{a2}$ = 2.8 acoustic millimhos and acoustic susceptance at the plane of the tympanic membrane = $B_{tm} = B_{a1} - B_{a2}$ = 1.2 acoustic millimhos.
And,

　Ambient, compensated static acoustic admittance, in rectangular notation

$$| Y_{tm} | = G_{tm} + jB_{tm} = 2.8 + j1.2 \text{ acoustic millimhos.}$$

And, to find the magnitude in polar notation

$$| Y_{tm} | = \sqrt{[(G_{tm})^2 + (B_{tm})^2]}$$
$$= \sqrt{[(2.8)^2 + (1.2)^2]} = 3.05 \text{ acoustic millimhos.}$$

And, finally, the equivalent acoustic impedance magnitude, or
Ambient, compensated static acoustic impedance***, in polar notation

$$| Z_{tm} | = \frac{1}{| Y_{tm} |} = \frac{1}{.00305}$$
$$= 328 \text{ acoustic ohms.}$$

Up to now, we have only determined the magnitude of the acoustic-impedance and acoustic-admittance phasor in polar notation. We will now compute the acoustic admittance phase angle (Φ_y) and the acoustic-impedance phase angle (Φ_z).

Using the same EXAMPLE:

$$\Phi_y = \tan^{-1} (B_{tm}/G_{tm}) = \tan^{-1} 1.2 / 2.8 = \tan^{-1} (.43) = 23°$$

(continued)

Table 2–2. *(continued)*

And, . $\Phi_z = -23°$,

In polar form, the acoustic admittance is expressed as

$$|Y_{tm}| = 3.05 \angle 23° \text{ acoustic millimhos.}$$

and, the acoustic impedance is expressed as

$$|Z_{tm}| = 328 \angle -23\% \text{ acoustic ohms.}$$

We now have expressed both the magnitude and the phase angle of the acoustic impedance and acoustic admittance phasors. The phase angle of the acoustic impedance phasor will be negative and the reciprocal acoustic admittance phase angle will be positive.

Because we can transform acoustic susceptance and acoustic conductance to reciprocal quantities of acoustic reactance and acoustic resistance, we can also solve for Z_{tm} in rectangular notation using our acoustic resistance and acoustic reactance equivalents.

Using the same EXAMPLE again,

$$R_{tm} = G_{tm} / [G_{tm}^2 + B_{tm}^2] = .0028 / [.0028^2 + .0012^2]$$
$$\approx 302 \text{ acoustic ohms.}$$

$$X_{tm} = B_{tm} / [G_{tm}^2 + B_{tm}^2] = .0012 / [.0028^2 + .0012^2]$$
$$\approx 129 \text{ acoustic ohms.}$$

Ambient, compensated static acoustic impedance, in rectangular form is

$$|Z_{tm}| = R_a + jX_a = 302 - j129 \text{ acoustic ohms.}$$

We have now determined both ambient Y_{tm} and Z_{tm} in both rectangular and polar notation. As a final check on our mathematical relations, we can use our rectangular components to redetermine our ambient, compensated acoustic Impedance in polar form.

$$|Z_{tm}| = \sqrt{[(Rtm)^2 + (X_{tm})^2]}$$
$$|Z_{tm}| = \sqrt{[(302)^2 + (129)^2]} = 328 \text{ acoustic ohms}$$
$$\Phi_z = \tan^{-1} X_{tm} / R_{tm} = \tan^{-1} 129 / 302 = \tan^{-1} (0.43) \approx -23°$$

Again,

$$|Z_{tm}| = 328 \angle -23° \text{ acoustic ohms}$$

Notes

* The examples shown are for ambient, compensated static measures; the process is the same for peak, compensated static computations except acoustic immittances at the tympanometric peak are used in place of values at ambient pressure.

** In determining $|Z_{tm}|$ and $|Y_{tm}|$, we must compensate for the contributions of the volume of the external auditory meatus. This is mathematically an easier process with acoustic admittance terms. Effectively, the acoustic susceptance at the plane of the tympanic membrane is approximately equal to the acoustic susceptance at ambient pressure (B_1 at 0 daPa) minus the acoustic susceptance at a pressure that stiffens the middle-ear system (B_2 at 200 daPa):

i.e., $B_{tm} = B_1 - B_2$.

The same is true with acoustic conductance at the plane of the tympanic membrane

$G_{tm} = G_1 - G_2$,

where

$G_1 = G_a$ at 0 daPa, and

$G_2 = G_a$ at 200 daPa.

*** Acoustic admittance measures in millimhos must be converted to equivalent values in mhos before equivalent Z_a values are computed.

DISCUSSION ITEMS FOR SELF-STUDY

1. Briefly define the following terms. Provide a physical example for each term and list the appropriate units for each.
   acoustic resistance
   compliant acoustic reactance
   mass acoustic reactance
   acoustic admittance
   compliant acoustic susceptance
2. Briefly describe the relation between the volume and the acoustic admittance for an enclosed volume of air.
3. Define what is meant by the term Peak Y_{tm}. How is this measure determined from an acoustic admittance tympanogram?

SUGGESTED EXERCISE FOR SELF-STUDY

Obtain measurement-plane acoustic conductance and acoustic susceptance tympanograms for one ear of one participant (you may serve as your own participant) using a 226 Hz probe. Using the tympanograms, compute peak, compensated static acoustic admittance, and peak, compensated static acoustic impedance for the ear under test. Present your compensated data in both rectangular and polar form. Check your work using the equations and examples given in Table 2–1. How does your Peak Y_{tm} value agree with ASHA norms (see Chapter 4)?

3

Calibration of Acoustic Immittance Instruments

Basic calibrations are critical to valid and reliable clinical acoustic immittance measures in human ears. Our purpose here is to summarize briefly the basic calibrations necessary for acoustic immittance instruments. The discussions are based primarily on calibration procedures and tolerances detailed in the 1987 American National Standards Institute (ANSI) standard for aural acoustic-immittance measures. In addition to this standard, the user should be familiar with the ANSI (1996) standard on audiometer specifications and with the instrument specifications and recommended calibrations supplied by the manufacturer of the specific acoustic immittance device. Additional references on the calibration of acoustic immittance instruments and related issues are available in the bibliography on acoustic immittance measures published by the American Speech-Language-Hearing Association (ASHA, 1991). (See Appendix B.)

The calibration of acoustic immittance instruments involves an evaluation of the basic subsystems discussed earlier in describing the function of these measuring instruments (Chapter 2). The four subsystems that were reviewed must be evaluated to assure the user that each is functioning properly. These four systems include (1) the probe unit, (2) the acoustic immittance analysis system, (3) the air pressure system, and (4) the acoustic reflex signal (activator) system. In each case, *the purpose of calibration is to determine that the specifications for each subsystem meet or exceed ANSI specifications.* It should be noted that ANSI specifications differ depending on the specific acoustic immittance instrument under test. ANSI S3.39 defines four types (1–4) of acoustic immittance instruments that range in application from basic screening to more advanced measurement applications. The specific calibration requirements and measurement tolerances differ across the four instrument types. The user must verify that the calibration routine and tolerances are appropriate for the type of instrument under evaluation. In the discussion of basic calibrations that follows, the fundamental purpose and approach to instrument calibration are discussed. The reader is referred to ANSI (1987) for full details on specific calibrations and tolerances.

PROBE UNIT

As noted earlier, the probe unit provides an acoustic signal (probe signal) that serves as the reference for acoustic immittance measures. For the vast majority of instruments, the probe signal is a tone of a specified frequency and SPL. Although there are instruments that provide for multiple probe frequencies, almost all commercially available instruments include a 226 Hz tone as a probe signal. *The purpose of calibrating the probe unit is to confirm that the probe signal is accurate in frequency, at the specified level, and free of unwanted distortion and noise.* Measures of these probe signal characteristics are performed by coupling the probe tip with a standard 2 cubic centimeter (cm^3) coupler (HA-1). The coupler, in turn, is connected to a microphone and sound measuring instrument, such as a sound level meter. The acoustic signal developed in the coupler may then be monitored with the sound level meter. The instrumentation complement required for these measures is illustrated in Figure 3–1. The user can determine the specific output level for the probe signal and check the measured output against that specified by the instrument manufacturer and the tolerances required by ANSI.

The frequency of the probe tone also should be evaluated for accuracy. This evaluation is usually done by monitoring the probe tone with a digital frequency counter. For example, with the SPL of the probe being monitored with a sound level meter, the output of the sound level meter can be directed to a frequency counter (Figure 3–1). The frequency counter provides a direct digital display of the measured probe signal frequency. This measure allows determination of the accuracy of the probe signal frequency.

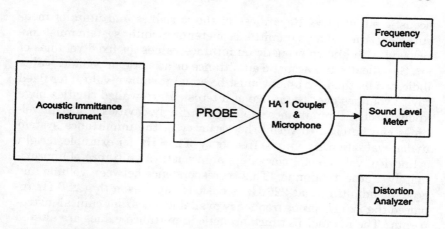

FIGURE 3–1. An illustration of the general instrumentation complement used for calibration of an electroacoustic immittance instrument. Details regarding specific calibrations are provided in the text.

Finally, the probe tone should be evaluated to make sure that it is free of unwanted harmonic distortion and noise. That is, the purity of the probe tone must be evaluated. In reality, there is almost always some harmonic distortion and noise present in the probe signal, but the level of any distortion or noise should be much lower in level than the probe signal itself. Again, ANSI (S3.39-1987) specifies allowable levels of distortion and noise for acoustic immittance probe units. The measurement of harmonic distortion and noise can be done with a distortion analyzer. The SPL developed in the HA-1 coupler (e.g., out of the sound level meter) is directed to the input of a distortion analyzer (Figure 3–1). The distortion analyzer has the capability of monitoring signal levels for different discrete frequency regions. For example, the energy present at each successive harmonic of the probe signal can be monitored individually with the distortion analyzer.

ACOUSTIC IMMITTANCE ANALYSIS SYSTEM

The purpose of calibration for the analysis system is to confirm that the acoustic immittance value indicated by the instrument is accurate. This is done by measuring the acoustic immittance for calibration cavities (right cylinders) of known and specified volumes. As noted earlier (Chapter 2), the volume of a cavity is directly related to the acoustic admittance offered by the cavity; larger cavities offer higher values of acoustic admittance. Regardless of the variables and units of measurement, the acoustic immittance meter or monitor system must correspond with known acoustic immittance values for fixed volumes of air. Specifically, the acoustic admittance or acoustic impedance value indicated by the instrument must be equal to known values for fixed cavity volumes over the range of interest. Hard-walled cavities have known acoustic immittance values; accordingly, cavities of specific volumes can be used to verify the accuracy of the immittance system under evaluation. At a probe frequency of 226 Hz, for example, a right cylindrical volume of 1 cm^3 offers an acoustic admittance of approximately 1 acoustic mmho. (This correspondence between volume and acoustic admittance at 226 Hz is basic to the reason that 226 Hz replaced the 220 Hz probe frequency available on earlier clinical instruments.) The manner in which acoustic immittance values are altered to bring them within ANSI tolerances varies with the instrument design. Some instruments, for example, provide trim pots that may be adjusted with a small screwdriver. Computer-based instruments provide for correction of calibration errors through software commands.

The exact test cavities and tolerances should conform to those supplied by the manufacturer. ANSI S3.39-1987 specifies the number and volumes of calibration cavities that must be supplied with instruments meeting ANSI standards and the tolerances for corresponding acoustic immittance values. It is particularly important that the atmospheric conditions (i.e., altitude and barometric pressure) common to the specific location be accounted for in the calibration procedure. The acoustic immittance offered by a given volume of air differs with different geographic locations dependent on the altitude and barometric pressure. Lilly and Shanks (1981) have provided a detailed discussion of the way users may correct for the specific atmospheric condition at their respective facilities. Selected manufacturers provide preset calibrations for each purchaser that account for the local conditions.

AIR PRESSURE SYSTEM

The primary purposes of calibration for the pneumatic system are to (1) determine that the readings on the air pressure indicator (manometer) are correct, and (2) to confirm that the rate of air pressure changes are accurate. As with other calibrations, the user should confirm that the accuracy of the manometer is within tolerances specified by the manufacturer and meets ANSI (1987) specifications. Calibration of the air pressure system is usually performed with an external manometer (e.g., U-tube) graduated in known steps. The probe unit of the instrument is connected via a small tube to the U-tube manometer. As the pressure setting on the acoustic immittance instrument is changed up and down, the exact pressure corresponding to the pressure setting on the instrument is read on the U-tube manometer. The accuracy of the air pressure system is determined by comparing the pressure indicated on the instrument with the actual pressure measured with the U-tube manometer. It is important that the U-tube manometer used for calibration have available pressure steps that are smaller than the unit accuracy of interest. If the user wants to calibrate in 10 daPa steps of pressure, for example, the U-tube manometer should have calibrated steps less than 10 daPa.

Because tympanogram characteristics for human ears vary with the rate of air pressure change, the specific rate or pump speed must be determined. The pump speed is usually specified in decaPascals per second (daPa/s). The rate of air pressure changes can be determined by timing the completion of a tympanogram over a specified pressure range. If it takes 2.5 seconds for the instrument to trace a tympanogram from 200 to −300 daPa, for example, the pump speed would be 200 daPa/s. Some commercially available acoustic immittance instruments provide an auxiliary output voltage that corresponds in magnitude to the pressure output of the air pump. This auxiliary output voltage can be connected to an oscillographic recorder or other time-calibrated plotter for purposes of recording the pump speed characteristics.

In most contemporary clinics, tympanometry is performed automatically with the tympanogram recorded on some form of chart recorder (e.g., a printer or X-Y plotter). The user must account for the characteristics of the recording device during calibration. Specifically, as ear canal pressure is changed during tympanometry, the manometer readings and the corresponding pressure readings indicated on the recorder chart should be the same. Finally, the user should determine that the changes in air pressure at the output of the air pump are linear in direct proportion to the steps indicated on the manometer.

ACOUSTIC REFLEX SYSTEM

The specification and calibration of acoustic reflex-activating signals should be evaluated in a manner similar to that used in the specification of acoustic test signals for audiometers (see ANSI S3.6-1996).

Melnick (1991) and Robinette et al. (1982) provide basic tutorial information on audiometer calibration. In the case of contralateral activators delivered through earphones, the applicable sections of ANSI S3.39-1987 regarding frequency accuracy, output levels, attenuator linearity, harmonic distortion, and other required specifications should be evaluated. These measures should be performed in a standard NBS 9-A (6 cm³) coupler and presented in a form consistent with that used in the specification of tones used in audiometry. If available and used as reflex activating signals, the specifications for broadband and band-limited noise should be consistent with ANSI and manufacturer specifications. Wherever possible, the frequency response characteristic (including bandwidth and slope measures) of the noise should be provided. If insert receivers are used for the presentation of activator signals, the appropriate ANSI methods (e.g., see ANSI S3.6-1996) specific to insert receivers should be conducted for calibration of output measures.

The characteristics of ipsilateral acoustic activators typically are evaluated by measuring the acoustic output of the activating signal with the probe unit housed in a standard HA-1 (2 cm³) coupler. This procedure is generally the same as that used for the specification of signals presented via insert receivers for audiometry or for signals used in contralateral acoustic reflex measures. The level of ipsilateral reflex-activating signals may be expressed in terms of dB SPL (coupler) or in dB hearing level (HL) based on manufacturer or local norms. It is important that ipsilateral and noise activators be clearly referenced in terms of sound pressure level (SPL) or hearing level (HL). In addition, the reference for HL designations should be clearly stated.

If the instrument under evaluation is used to measure the latency and recovery times of acoustic reflexes, the response time of the unit must be measured and specified. The various on and off latencies of the unit can be determined by measuring the output of the unit in response to an instantaneous signal presented at the probe unit. The probe unit can be coupled to a calibration cavity that also contains an input from a miniature transducer (e.g., a hearing aid receiver). The miniature loudspeaker is used to produce a signal (having a frequency equal to the probe signal) with an instantaneous rise-fall characteristic. The output of the acoustic immittance unit in response to this pulsed signal can be used to evaluate the on and off times inherent to the unit. As with tympanometry, if a recording device is used for recording acoustic reflex responses, the time constants must account for the response times of the recorder. The work of Lilly (1984) provides a more detailed review of the temporal characteristics of acoustic reflexes and the issues involved in instrumental time constants.

DISCUSSION ITEMS FOR SELF-STUDY

1. Why is calibration of acoustic immittance instruments necessary? Can you think of a case in which improper calibration of a clinical instrument could result in inappropriate diagnosis and treatment for a patient?
2. List the primary calibrations necessary for any acoustic immittance instrument.

4

Tympanometry and Compensated Static Measures

Tympanometry is the dynamic measurement of acoustic immittance in the external ear canal as a function of changes in air pressure in the ear canal (ANSI, S3.39-1987). The primary reason for performing tympanometry on a patient is to determine the existence and potential cause of a middle ear disorder. There are several tympanometric methods ranging from vector (single-frequency, single-component) tympanometry to multi-frequency, multi-component tympanometry. *Vector* tympanometry is the most common method of evaluating the middle ear, but it is also the most limited. This method involves the use of one low-frequency probe tone (typically 226 Hz) and the measurement of one component, generally the acoustic admittance vector. As noted in Chapter 2, two numbers are required to specify an acoustic admittance measure; you must specify either the admittance vector (magnitude) and the phase angle (direction, or degree of mass or stiffness control) or alternatively you must specify the acoustic susceptance (magnitude and sign) and the acoustic conductance (magnitude). Because vector tympanometry provides only one value, the magnitude of the acoustic admittance, the diagnostic information from the relative contributions of mass and stiffness components that would be provided with the phase angle is not available.

Further, by using only one probe-tone frequency, the view of the middle ear is quite limited, almost as if you were to try to estimate hearing sensitivity by testing thresholds at only one frequency. Disorders that exert an influence on middle ear mechanics only at the high frequencies, such as those adding mass to the system, will not be evident using only the low-frequency probe tone. Despite these limitations, vector tympanometry is the most common method of tympanometry and will be discussed first. Following this discussion, we will discuss more complex tympanometric measures in light of the additional information they add to the diagnostic process. Screening applications are treated separately in Chapter 7.

VECTOR TYMPANOMETRY

For the present purposes, *vector tympanograms* are single-component (acoustic admittance) tympanograms measured at a single probe-tone frequency (226 Hz). A typical, normal vector tympanogram is shown in Figure 4–1. Ear canal pressure is varied from a positive pressure (200 daPa) to a negative pressure (–300 daPa), and the resulting changes in acoustic admittance are measured and plotted as a tympanogram. At the extremes of pressure, the tympanic membrane and middle ear system stiffen and the ear canal effectively becomes a hard-walled cavity. Little acoustic energy passes through the tympanic membrane; instead, the majority of the acoustic energy is reflected into the ear canal. At the pressure extremes, therefore, the acoustic admittance of the middle ear is minimal, and the acoustic admittance measured is essentially that contributed by the trapped volume of air in the ear canal. As the ear canal pressure approaches atmospheric pressure (0 daPa), less energy is reflected and more passes into the middle ear. Near atmospheric pressure, the normal tympanic membrane passes most of the acoustic energy into the middle ear; therefore, the acoustic admittance is at its highest value. The normal vector tympanogram, therefore, has a single, positive peak near atmospheric pressure. Because the normal middle ear system is dominated by compliant acoustic susceptance, manufacturers commonly call the single component *compliance*, although in actuality the single component is the vector component, *acoustic admittance*. These terms are discussed in Chapter 2.

To determine if the tympanogram is normal, several characteristics may be measured, including tympanometric amplitude or compensated static acoustic admittance (Y_{tm}), tympanometric width (TW) or gradient, equivalent ear canal volume (V_{ea}), and tympanometric

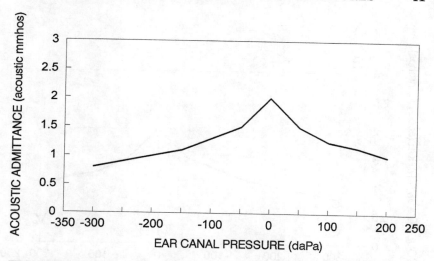

FIGURE 4–1. Typical vector tympanogram recorded with a 226 Hz probe tone from an adult with a healthy middle ear system. Ear canal pressure is shown on the abscissa and acoustic admittance is shown on the ordinate. The tympanogram shows the acoustic admittance increasing as the ear canal pressure is decreased from 200 daPa to 0 daPa and then decreasing as the ear canal pressure is further decreased to –300 daPa.

peak pressure (TPP). These characteristics are shown in Figure 4–2a and 4–2b. Each of these measures is discussed below.

Tympanometric Amplitude or Compensated Acoustic Admittance

The tympanometric amplitude or *peak compensated static acoustic admittance* (Y_{tm}) is of interest because disease processes can increase or decrease the height of the tympanometric peak. Tympanometric measures are taken in the plane of the probe (measurement plane) and include measures of Y_{tm} as well as the acoustic admittance of the volume of air in the ear canal (Y_{ec}). Because we are interested only in Y_{tm}, we need to eliminate the Y_{ec}. As discussed in Chapter 2, we can eliminate Y_{ec} from the admittance measure by subtracting the acoustic admittance at the tail of the tympanogram from the acoustic admittance at the tympanometric peak.

Subtracting the effect of the ear canal volume results in the tympanometric amplitude or compensated static acoustic admittance (see Chapter 2). The term *compensated* means that the effect of the ear

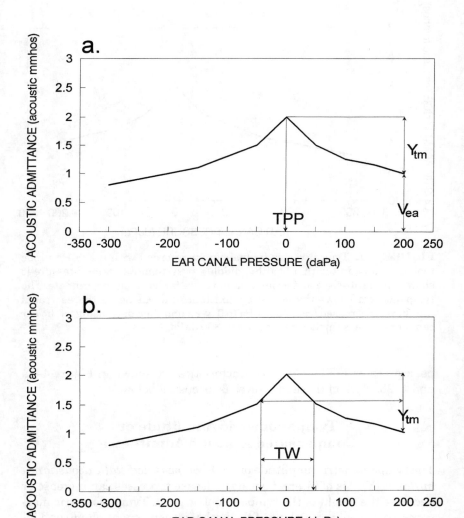

FIGURE 4–2. Typical vector tympanograms showing the characteristics that are commonly measured. Figure 4–2a shows the way that peak compensated static acoustic admittance (Y_{tm}), equivalent ear canal volume (V_{ea}), and tympanometric peak pressure (TPP) are determined. Y_{tm} is the height of the tympanogram from the peak to the tail. V_{ea} is determined by the height of the tail. TPP is the pressure location of the peak. Figure 4–2b shows tympanometric width (TW), which is the width of the tympanogram at half the height between the peak and the tail.

canal is removed from the measurement plane values; consequently, the compensated measure estimates the acoustic admittance at the plane of the tympanic membrane and reflects the acoustic admittance of the tympanic membrane and the middle ear system combined. The term *static* means that the measure is taken at only one pressure, not as a function of varying pressures as in tympanometry. The tympanometric amplitude or compensated static acoustic admittance (Y_{tm}), therefore, is the amplitude of the tympanogram measured at the plane of the tympanic membrane.

The Y_{tm} can be measured at the peak of the tympanogram (peak compensated) or at ambient or atmospheric pressure (0 daPa) (ambient compensated). The rationale for the peak measure is that the peak of the tympanogram occurs at the pressure at which the middle ear functions most efficiently. A peak measure, therefore, provides an estimate of the best possible function of the middle ear system. Further, it is a reliable measure that is not affected by small, normal fluctuations in the peak pressure caused by swallowing and respiration.

The rationale for measuring Y_{tm} at ambient pressure is that the middle ear system actually functions under ambient pressure, and thus this measure represents the function of the system under everyday conditions. The actual pressure at the tympanometric peak, however, is variable, even in people with normal middle ear systems, and changes with swallowing and respiration. Because the tympanogram slopes steeply near the peak, slight fluctuations in middle ear pressure can produce shifts in pressure location of the peak that can result in substantial reductions in the acoustic admittance measured at ambient pressure. The magnitude of the peak, regardless of the pressure location, therefore, is the more stable value and is the preferred measure for clinical use.

Although there are no universally accepted norms for Y_{tm}, interim values for adults and children have been reported. For preschool children, the mean is 0.5 acoustic mmho, with a 90% range from 0.2–0.9 acoustic mmho. For adults, the mean is 0.8 acoustic mmho, with a 90% range from 0.3–1.4 acoustic mmho (ASHA, 1990; Margolis & Heller, 1987). These values were derived from tympanometric data taken from children and adults who showed no evidence of middle ear disease. Data were obtained using a screening tympanometer at two pump speeds, with ear canal estimates taken at 200 daPa.

ASHA (1997) screening guidelines, using both normal and pathologic cases, suggest that normal Y_{tm} values should be >0.2 acoustic mmho for infants and >0.3 acoustic mmho for older children. The addition of findings from pathologic cases in the ASHA (1997) guidelines is an important advance over the previous screening guidelines. The comparison of normal and pathologic cases allows us to determine the sensitivity and specificity of the measures based on the amount of overlap between the normal and pathologic populations. These data are still preliminary, so exact sensitivity and specificity values are not yet available.

There is variability in the norms, and some sources of the variability can be attributed to measurement and recording parameters. First, the interim norms show data taken at different pump speeds, with the faster pump speeds exhibiting higher peak values. Second, the choice to use either the positive or negative pressure tail for determining the contributions of the ear canal clearly changes the measurement of the peak height. Tympanograms typically are asymmetrical on the positive and negative sides, and the lower tail of the tympanogram generally occurs with the negative pressure. The discrepancy between the estimates of ear canal volume taken from the negative and positive tails increases with increasing asymmetry in the shape of the tympanogram. Consequently, Y_{tm} will be smaller when referenced to the positive tail, and correspondingly the variability associated with the smaller Y_{tm} mean will be less than when Y_{tm} is referenced to the negative tail. It is important to note that, if the normative values from the ASHA (1997) guidelines are used, the procedures should be identical to those used for collecting the norms, including the use of the positive tail for determining ear canal volume and Y_{tm}. Most screening instruments provide an estimate of equivalent ear canal volume at 200 daPa, which is at the positive tail of the tympanogram.

Some of the variability in Y_{tm} values can be attributed to variability across different clinical populations. There are significant differences in Y_{tm} by gender; women have lower Y_{tm} values than men (Jerger, Jerger, & Mauldin, 1972; Wiley et al., 1996; Zwislocki & Feldman, 1970). There are also significant changes in Y_{tm} with age; children have lower Y_{tm} values than adults (Margolis & Heller, 1987), as reflected in the ASHA (1990; 1997) guidelines. After adulthood, however, the Y_{tm} values do not change significantly with age through the age of 90 years, although the gender difference remains (Wiley et al., 1996).

Pathologic conditions alter the shape of the tympanograms; the goal of the diagnostic use of tympanometry is to separate the changes that are caused by pathologic conditions from the changes that are associated with normal variability. Pathologic changes seen with vector tympanograms generally are manifested by reduced Y_{tm}, although increased Y_{tm} and notching of the tympanogram also occur. Reduced Y_{tm} can result from stiffening conditions, resulting in an overall decrease in the acoustic admittance (see Chapter 2). Some causes of reduced acoustic admittance include otosclerosis and the presence of middle ear liquid. *Otosclerosis* involves a growth of spongy bone around the stapes which anchors it in place and effectively stiffens the ossicular chain. This may be reflected as reduced Y_{tm}. Middle ear liquid reduces the volume of air in the middle ear cavity, and dampens the ossicular chain, thus increasing the stiffness of the middle ear system. When the middle ear is completely filled with liquid, the middle ear system is unable to function normally and acts as a hard-walled cavity. The extreme case of reduced Y_{tm}, such as that seen when the middle ear is completely filled with liquid, is a flat tympanogram with a peak Y_{tm} value approaching 0 acoustic mmhos.

Although the most common condition producing a flat tympanogram is the presence of liquid in the middle ear, flat tympanograms also can result from impacted cerumen or tympanic membrane perforations. Cerumen may be hard enough to yield acoustic admittance results similar to those for a hard-walled cavity when it occludes the ear canal; therefore, peak Y_{tm} values approximate 0 acoustic mmhos with cerumen impaction. With a tympanic membrane perforation, the compensated acoustic admittance measured is no longer from the tympanic membrane and the term Y_{tm}, is not strictly accurate. Instead, the acoustic admittance measured includes the ear canal and the middle ear cavity, which approximates a hard-walled cavity. This condition produces a flat tympanogram with a peak value of 0 acoustic mmhos. Ear canal volume measurement may help distinguish among the possible causes of flat tympanograms, as described later in the section on equivalent ear canal volume.

Single peaked high amplitude tympanograms that are characterized by increased Y_{tm} can result from pathologic conditions that add mass to the middle ear system (see Chapter 2). As mass increases, high amplitude vector tympanograms may notch, although notching is more commonly seen in component tympanometry (see Component Tympanometry later in this chapter). Some causes of increased acoustic admittance include ossicular discontinuity, ear drum pathology such as external otitis, or even cerumen or water adhering to the surface of the tympanic membrane. With ossicular discontinuity, the ossicles that remain attached to the tympanic membrane may add mass. With external otitis, pus and debris deposited on the tympanic membrane may add mass. Similarly if cerumen adheres to the surface of the tympanic membrane, it adds mass. Finally, droplets of water remaining on the tympanic membrane following irrigation of the ear canal also may add mass. Mass effects are better evaluated with component tympanometry and probe frequencies higher than 226 Hz.

Unfortunately, the diagnostic use of Y_{tm} has been limited because there is substantial overlap in the range of values recorded from normal and diseased ears (Shanks & Shelton, 1991). Because ethical constraints prevent studies that require surgical exploration of normal ears, no studies have compared Y_{tm} in normal and diseased middle ears that have been confirmed by surgical procedures such as myringotomy. Nozza, Bluestone, Kardatzke, and Bachman (1992) studied a group of children who had a history of chronic otitis media and were scheduled for tympanotomy tubes. In the ears that were found to have liquid (effusion) at surgery, the 90% range for peak Y_{tm} was 0.10 to 0.60 acoustic mmho; whereas in the ears that were found to be dry at surgery, the 90% range was 0.01 to 1.95 acoustic mmho. The ranges for the two groups significantly overlapped with each other, making it difficult to distinguish children with effusion from children without effusion. Both groups of patients, however, had histories of middle ear pathology, and therefore neither group could be considered to have normal middle ear function. The Y_{tm} values could have been altered by the presence of chronic middle ear disease in all the children. The data of Nozza et al. (1992), however, also overlapped with the data of Margolis and Heller (1987) for children with normal middle ear function. The explanation for this overlap may lie, in part, in the different reference values chosen for eliminating ear canal effects. The Nozza et al. study used compensated measures at 300 daPa rather than the 200 daPa used in the Margolis and Heller data. The different reference values used can alter the Y_{tm} measures so that the data reported in the two studies are not directly comparable.

Nozza, Bluestone, Kardatzke, and Bachman (1994) used several different cutoff values to estimate sensitivity and specificity of the Y_{tm} measure. They reported that Y_{tm} had a sensitivity of 46% and a specificity of 92% using a cutoff value of 0.2 acoustic mmho, as suggested in the ASHA (1990) guidelines, in separating a group of children with and without middle ear effusion. Sensitivity improved to 70%, but specificity dropped to 85% with a cutoff value of 0.3 acoustic mmho. The children in this study also had histories of chronic middle ear disease and were evaluated with myringotomy, but may have had abnormal middle ear systems even when no liquid was detected at surgery. Nozza et al. (1994) suggested that the addition of other measures, such as the tympanometric width or gradient and the acoustic reflex, could improve the diagnostic value of tympanometry. Clearly, more research is needed on children with normal and pathological middle ears to define the best cutoff values to use for Y_{tm} as well as the best combination of tympanometric measures to separate the normal and pathological groups.

Tympanometric Width (TW)

Tympanometric width (TW) is the width of the tympanogram (in daPa) measured at half of the height from the peak to the tail. ASHA (1990, 1997) guidelines specify that the tail value is to be estimated from the tympanogram at 200 daPa. TW has been reported to be reliable and to have a low correlation with Y_{tm} (Koebsell & Margolis, 1986). A low correlation between Y_{tm} and TW suggests that the TW measure adds further information to the admittance examination beyond that provided by the Y_{tm} measure alone. The TW measure is not used widely, due to the lack of normative values and its variability within the normal population. No gender differences have been noted (Margolis & Heller, 1987; Wiley et al., 1996), although TW does increase with advancing age in the adult population (Wiley et al., 1996).

Pathologic conditions of the middle ear system can change the TW. Stiffening pathologies, such as otosclerosis, can narrow the tympanometric width (Ivey, 1975). The general application of TW, however, is in identifying pathologies that increase the width, especially otitis media. The presence of liquid in the middle ear tends to increase tympanometric width, although there is still significant overlap between values measured for TW in ears with and without middle ear liquid. There is still uncertainty about the cutoff value for determining normal and pathologic conditions. The ASHA (1990) guidelines suggested that TW exceeding 150 daPa in children or 110 daPa in adults should be considered abnormal. The ASHA (1997) guidelines, however, increased the cutoff for normal, and suggested that widths exceeding 235 daPa in infants, 200 daPa in older children, and 300 daPa in children with a high prevalence of middle ear disorders should be considered abnormal. These data were based on results from children with normal middle ear function (Roush, Bryant, Mundy, Zeisel, & Roberts, 1995) and children with chronic middle ear disease who underwent surgery and were found to have either dry ears or middle ear effusion at surgery (Nozza et al., 1994). The ASHA (1997) guidelines do not provide TW limits for adults, because the payoff for immittance screening in adults is expected to be extremely low due to the low prevalence of middle ear disease in the adult population.

Sensitivity and specificity data have been calculated for the TW measures. In a group of children undergoing myringotomy, Nozza et al. (1994) reported a sensitivity of 81% and a specificity of 82% using a criterion of >275 daPa in separating children with and without middle ear effusion. They identified this variable as the single best tympanometric variable for separating these two groups of children. All of these children had chronic middle ear disease and, on the average, wider

TW than a group of children with no history of middle ear disease. More studies using data from populations with a wide variety of middle ear disorders are needed to substantiate the value of this measure in separating normal from abnormal populations.

Tympanometric Gradient

Tympanometric gradient is a measure that refers to the slopes of the sides of the tympanogram near the region of the peak pressure. Although there are several methods for calculating gradient, a common method is to calculate the difference in the acoustic admittance between the tympanometric peak and the average of the acoustic admittance at 50 daPa on the positive and negative sides of the peak pressure (deJonge, 1986). Several investigations have suggested that the presence of middle ear liquid decreases the gradient of the tympanogram (Brooks, 1969; Nozza et al., 1992; Paradise, Smith, & Bluestone, 1976), suggesting the possible use of this measure to distinguish between normal and liquid-filled middle ears. Subsequent studies (deJonge, 1986; Koebsell & Margolis, 1986), however, have reported that the gradient measure is highly correlated with peak Y_{tm} and thus provides no additional information. Peak Y_{tm} is an easier, straightforward calculation, and therefore is preferred over gradient measures. The ASHA (1990, 1997) guidelines do not advocate gradient measures in screening for middle ear diseases.

Tympanometric Peak Pressure (TPP)

Tympanometric peak pressure (TPP) is the pressure at which the peak of the tympanogram occurs, and provides an estimate of the middle ear pressure. Y_{tm} is at its highest value when the pressures on both sides of the tympanic membrane are equal. The value of measuring TPP is that it can detect the presence of negative pressure in the middle ear. If the Eustachian tube becomes blocked by disease, negative pressure develops in the middle ear prior to the development of effusion as the liquids from the tissues surrounding the middle ear are drawn into the middle ear. The presence of negative middle ear pressure, therefore, can indicate a problem with Eustachian tube function that requires medical intervention. As middle ear effusion resolves, the tympanogram progresses from flat, to negative peaked, to normal. Monitoring the TPP following a bout with middle ear effusion, therefore, allows an objective measure of the restoration of normal middle ear function. Eustachian tube function can be measured with tympanometric procedures whether the tympanic membrane is intact or perforated. These procedures are discussed in Chapter 5.

Although tympanometric peak pressure has received much attention in the past, currently it is considered to have little clinical value for screening purposes. For normal adult ears, the tympanometric estimate of middle ear pressure is generally within 30 daPa of the actual value in normal ears (Eliachar & Northern, 1974). The pressure peak can vary, however, with recording parameters such as recording speed, direction of pressure change, and number of tympanograms measured sequentially (Wilson, Shanks, & Kaplan, 1984). In patients with tympanic membrane abnormalities, such as monomeric membranes (thin patches on the tympanic membrane from healed perforations), the discrepancy between the tympanometric estimate and the actual middle ear pressure may be large. The discrepancy, therefore, is the greatest in those patients for whom the measure is most needed (Shanks, Lilly, Margolis, Wiley, & Wilson, 1988).

A further difficulty, especially in screening applications, is that the tympanometric peak pressure does not adequately separate normal ears from ears with middle ear effusion. The tympanometric pressure varies widely in children with normal middle ear systems, with as many as 25% of children having values of –250 daPa during some seasons (Lildholdt, 1980). Because of the amount of normal pressure variation, therefore, reliance on middle ear pressure measures may lead to overreferral rates in screening programs (Roush & Tait, 1985). Current screening guidelines suggest that TPP not be used as a referral criterion (ASHA, 1990, 1997).

Tympanometric pressure measures may have uses other than screening and determining the normality of the tympanogram. Some clinicians monitor the progression of or recovery from middle ear effusion by monitoring serial TPP measures over time and between ears in an individual child, with the expectation that the pressure peak will move toward atmospheric pressure as the problem resolves. Tympanometric pressure measures also are used in testing Eustachian tube function and, in this capacity, may be used for predicting which children are likely to develop middle ear effusions and for predicting the outcome of middle ear surgical procedures. These uses are discussed in Chapter 5.

Equivalent Ear Canal Volume (V_{ea})

The *equivalent ear canal volume* (V_{ea} or V_{ec}) is an estimate of the volume between the probe tip and the tympanic membrane. The appropriate abbreviation for equivalent ear canal volume is V_{ea} (ANSI, 1987), although the abbreviation V_{ec} is also used (ASHA, 1990, 1997). V_{ea} is derived from the admittance of the volume of air trapped between the probe and the tympanic membrane. This measure is called equivalent ear canal volume because, under reference conditions, a given volume of air has a known admittance. If we measure the admittance, we can calculate that equivalent volume of air. The calculation is rather straightforward with a 226 Hz probe tone because a 1 cm^3 volume of air has an admittance of 1 acoustic mmho under reference conditions (Lilly & Shanks, 1981). If the admittance of the volume of air trapped between the probe and the tympanic membrane is 2 acoustic mmho, then the equivalent volume is 2 cm^3, and the ear canal volume estimate is 2 cm^3.

Tympanometric estimates of V_{ea} are best measured from the height of the lower tail (either negative or positive) of the tympanogram (Shanks & Lilly, 1981). This method assumes that the introduction of negative or positive pressure stiffens the tympanic membrane and middle ear system and removes the effect of their combined admittance from the measure. To determine the best method to estimate ear canal volume, Shanks and Lilly (1981) compared several tympanometric estimates with the actual canal volume measured directly by filling the ear canal with alcohol. The tympanometric estimates included susceptance measures at −400, −200, +200, and +400 daPa for 220 and 660 Hz probe tones. All tympanometric estimates exceeded the direct measure, but the greatest error occurred at 200 daPa. As the pressure was decreased from 200 to −400 daPa, the amount of the error also decreased. The lower tail of the tympanogram, which was generally at −400 daPa, provided the more accurate estimate of the true ear canal volume. Further, with the −400 daPa pressure, the susceptance value at the 660 Hz probe tone (divided by 3) provided a more accurate V_{ea} estimate than did the 220 Hz probe. The V_{ea} measure at 200 daPa, therefore, was contaminated by ear canal and middle ear effects. The recommended procedure, then, was to use the lower tympanometric tail, generally at −400 daPa with the 660 Hz probe tone (if available) or, secondarily, with the 220 Hz probe tone.

Clinically, the most common measure of V_{ea} is from the tympanometric tail at 200 daPa measured with the 226 Hz probe tone. The 226 probe tone is the most commonly used for tympanometry and is present on all admittance screening instruments. The screening instruments automatically measure V_{ea} from the tail value at 200 daPa, and the ASHA (1990, 1997) screening guidelines are based on this measure. The resulting V_{ea} estimate is larger than it would be if the negative tail were used.

Some immitance instruments provide a *baseline correct* function that will automatically remove the effect of the ear canal volume.

When the tympanogram is plotted as it is recorded in the measurement plane, the plotted tympanogram includes the admittance from the compensated tympanogram as well as the admittance from the ear canal volume. The baseline correct function subtracts the effect of the ear canal volume and plots only the compensated tympanogram, with tympanometric tail values that equal or approximate 0 acoustic mmhos. Most instruments will allow the user to choose the pressure at which the correction will occur. Tympanogram tails that descend below 0 acoustic mmhos are indications that the ear canal volume was better approximated at another pressure. For example, if the pressure at 200 daPa is selected for compensation and the negative tail appears below 0 acoustic mmhos, the tympanogram is asymmetrical and the negative tail is lower than the positive tail. If the tympanogram is run again with the pressure at −300 daPa selected for compensation, the negative tail will be at 0 acoustic mmhos and the positive tail will have a slightly positive value.

The normal range for V_{ea} is dependent on age, with 90% ranges including volumes from 0.3–0.9 cm^3 in young children (Shanks, Stelmachowicz, Beauchaine, & Schulte, 1992). These ranges were determined from a sample of 334 children, aged 6 weeks to 6.7 years, who underwent insertion of tympanostomy tubes. Equivalent ear canal volumes were measured pre- and postoperatively. With intact tympanic membranes, the 90% range for V_{ea} was 0.4–0.9 cm^3, in close agreement with range of 0.4–1.0 cm^3 reported by Margolis and Heller (1987). Shanks et al. (1992) further showed that, in the presence of patent tympanostomy tubes, the 90% range for V_{ea} was from 1.0 and 5.5 cm^3, or an increase in volume of 0.4 cm^3 as compared to the V_{ea} with intact tympanic membranes. The V_{ea} was stable through the age of 4.9 years with intact tympanic membranes, whereas the V_{ea} increased with age with patent tympanostomy tubes, reflecting the growth of the middle ear cavity.

V_{ea} is larger in adults than in children, ranging from 0.63–1.46 cm^3 in adults (Margolis & Heller, 1987). Older adults have larger ear canals than younger adults, but as aging progresses into the 9th decade, ear canal volumes tend to decrease (Wiley et al., 1996). Women have smaller ear canal volumes than men do at all ages (Wiley et al., 1996). Separate norms for young children as well as for men and women, therefore, are advisable. When there is a question regarding the normalcy of the ear canal volume, the volume between the two ears of an individual can be compared; barring obvious unilateral pathology or surgery, the ear canal volumes should be similar.

The measurement of the ear canal volume, sometimes called the *physical volume test* (PVT), is important in the interpretation of flat tympanograms. Three flat tympanograms with different ear canal volume measures are shown in Figure 4–3. If the volume is normal, then the probe is adequately situated and the flat tympanogram may be due to liquid behind the tympanic membrane or to lateral ossicular fixation. If the volume is small, the flat tympanogram may be due to the cerumen filling the ear canal or to the probe resting against the canal wall. If the volume is large, the flat tympanogram may be due to a perforation of the tympanic membrane or to the presence of a patent PE *(pressure equalization) tube*. In this case, the measure may include the volume of all or some of the middle ear. An exception to this final case occurs when there is a tympanic membrane perforation with an accumulation of liquid or cholesteatoma filling the middle ear. In these cases, the volume measure may be within the normal range and will fail to identify the perforation (Margolis & Shanks, 1985).

Tympanometric Types

Liden (1969) and Jerger (1970) used the basic shape of the 226 Hz tympanogram to devise a method of assigning tympanograms into one

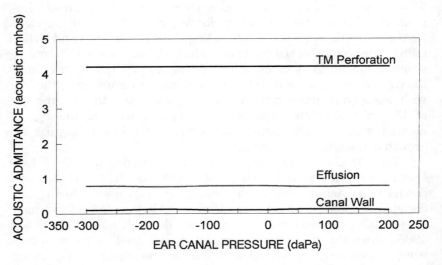

FIGURE 4–3. Three flat tympanograms with three different equivalent ear canal volume measures resulting from three different causes. For middle ear effusion (effusion), the V_{ea} is within normal limits for the probe against the ear canal wall (canal wall), the V_{ea} is below normal limits and for a tympanic membrane perforation (TM perforation), the V_{ea} is above normal limits.

of several descriptive categories, as shown in Figure 4–4. Type A is the tympanogram for a normal middle ear and is characterized by a single peak of normal height at or near atmospheric pressure. Two abnormal subcategories of type A exist; type A_S refers to a "shallow" tympanogram with a reduced peak height present at normal pressure, and type A_D refers to a "deep" tympanogram with an increased peak height present at normal pressure. Type A_S may occur with low-lying middle ear liquid, otosclerosis, or ossicular fixation. Type A_D may occur with disorders as disparate as ossicular disarticulation or tympanic membrane pathology. Type B is a flat tympanogram, characteristically seen with cases of middle ear liquid, tympanic membrane perforation, or cerumen occlusion. Type C refers to a tympanogram with a peak of normal height that occurs at significant negative pressure and is suggestive of negative middle ear pressure.

There are several difficulties with the use of these types. First, they were devised over 25 years ago and were based on the qualitative measures that were in use at the time. Qualitative measures are difficult to duplicate and compare across clinics. Second, the types only apply to vector tympanograms recorded at 226 Hz, and not to the more complex multi-frequency, multi-component tympanograms that can

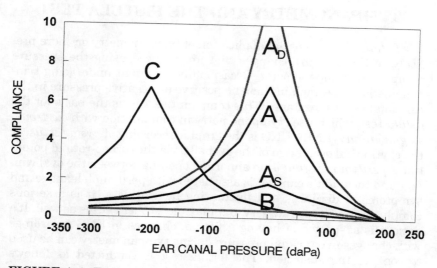

FIGURE 4–4. Five tympanograms that illustrate typing based on descriptive categories from Liden (1969) and Jerger (1970). Ear canal pressure is on the abscissa and compliance in arbitrary units is on the ordinate. Type A is normal, type A_S is shallow with a decreased height, type A_D is deep with an increased height, type B is flat, and type C has a peak at a negative pressure.

be recorded today. Third, the original types were based on tympanograms recorded in impedance using arbitrary units, which varied in magnitude with the size of the ear canal volume and the sensitivity of the recording instrument. For example, increasing the sensitivity of the instrument would increase the amplitude of the tympanogram, possibly changing it from a type A to an A_D. Fourth, because these types are purely descriptive, the distinction among the types in particular is ambiguous. There are, for example, no clear boundaries between A and A_S, A and A_D, or A and C. Increased objectivity may be achieved if the types are used in conjunction with the other admittance measures, such as Y_{tm} and tympanometric width (Margolis & Heller, 1987). Fifth, despite their long history of use, no sensitivity and specificity data are available for the tympanogram types. Finally, given the shift away from the importance of negative middle ear pressure as measured tympanometrically, especially in screening, the significance of labeling a tympanogram a type C is not clear. For these reasons, use of this classification system is not recommended. Quantification of the tympanometric measures and the use of standard measurement units will facilitate the development of appropriate norms and comparisons of tympanometric data across clinics.

TYMPANOMETRY AND THE FISTULA TEST

The *fistula test* is a special application of tympanometry or, more precisely, of the pressure changes that are induced using the pressure pump of the tympanometer. Occasionally, a patient undergoing tympanometry will complain that the positive or negative pressure in the ear canal causes dizziness. This complaint serves as the basis for the *fistula* test, which uses tympanometry in combination with *electronystagmography* (ENG). ENG is the graphic recording of *nystagamus*, or the rhythmical oscillation of the eyeballs, via the corneo-retinal potential. A *perilymph fistula* is an abnormal opening between the oval window and the middle ear that is associated with perilymph leakage and symptoms of dizziness and fluctuating hearing loss. It is a serious complication of stapes surgery, but may have other causes as well. If a patient is suspected of having a fistula, changes in ENG recordings with changes in ear canal pressure during tympanometry can be used to confirm the suspicion. The fistula test is conducted as follows (Causse, Causse, & Bel, 1983):

1. The patient is prepared as for an electronystagmography test. The patient is seated in a comfortable chair and electrodes are attached next to the eyes in horizontal and vertical arrange-

ments to record any nystagmus. The patient is instructed to keep his or her eyes closed during the test and to indicate any sense of imbalance or dizziness. The recorder is started and any spontaneous nystagmus that is present before the test begins is noted.

2. The acoustic admittance probe is placed in the patient's ear and the ear canal pressure is increased to 400 daPa and held for 20 seconds. Then the ear canal pressure is decreased to −400 daPa and held for 20 seconds. Finally, the pressure is released quickly.

3. A positive test is indicated by the presence of nystagmus to negative or positive pressure. A negative test is indicated by the lack of nystagmus for either condition.

The results of the fistula test have proven to be quite variable. Causse et al. (1983) had no positive results from people with normal ears. Of the patients in their group who were found to have a fistula at surgery, 18 had a positive result and 12 had a negative result. Of the group found not to have a fistula at surgery, 16 had a positive result and 14 had a negative result. Further, 7 of 10 poststapedectomy ears of people who were asymptomatic produced a positive result. The authors concluded that the larger the perilymphatic leak was from the fistula, the smaller the response was on the fistula test. In contrast to these findings, Daspit et al. (1980) reported that, in 91% of their cases, fistula test results (positive or negative) were consistent with surgical findings (fistula present or not present). Clearly, more data are needed on this procedure before it can be used routinely and with confidence in diagnosis of a perilymph fistula.

COMPONENT TYMPANOMETRY

Component tympanometry refers to measurement of the two components (susceptance and conductance, or admittance and phase angle) that provide an adequate view of the magnitude and direction of the admittance. Manufacturers typically do not provide a direct measure of *phase angle*, but do provide the remaining three components, any two of which may be used to calculate phase angle if necessary. These components include acoustic *admittance* (Y_a), *susceptance* (B_a), and *conductance* (G_a). Conversions from rectangular (susceptance and conductance) to polar (admittance and phase angle) forms were discussed in Chapter 2. Evaluation of the two components is more important for the interpretation of tympanograms measured with high frequency probe tones than for tympanograms measured with the 226 Hz probe tone because of the variety of tympanometric shapes that occur in normal as well as abnormal ears at higher probe frequencies. The various shapes indicate the relative contribution of mass and stiffness to the admittance tympanogram and, as discussed in the next section, and are used to (a) separate normal from pathological tympanograms and (b) determine the cause of the abnormalities reflected in the tympanogram. Knowing whether a tympanogram has increased mass or stiffness allows the clinician to identify the probable cause of the middle ear disorder that has resulted in the changes in the tympanograms.

Multi-frequency Component Tympanometry

Multi-frequency tympanometry refers to the procedure in which the tympanogram is measured at two or more probe frequencies, and it is done in order to measure the admittance characteristics of the ear across a broad spectral range. The broad range, determined by more than one probe tone frequency, enables the measurement of potential changes in mass and stiffness components of the acoustic admittance as compared to the normal middle ear system, and it may enable a determination of *resonant frequency*, or the frequency above which the middle ear is mass controlled and below which the middle ear is stiffness controlled. As discussed below, quantifying these changes across frequency provides more detail on the admittance characteristics of the middle ear system than is possible using only one probe frequency. Increases in mass or stiffness provide clues to the cause of abnormal acoustic admittance measured on the tympanograms and, therefore, to the cause of a conductive component.

The tympanometric shapes considered normal for multi-frequency component tympanometry are more varied than those for single-component tympanometry. Consequently, the descriptors (peak amplitude, width, and pressure) used for vector tympanometry are not useful in classifying these tympanograms. Vanhuyse, Creten, and Van Camp (1975) and Van Camp, Creten, Vanpeperstraete, and Van de Heyning (1980) proposed a classification system to be used with tympanograms recorded with high frequency probe tones. In their system, shown in Figure 4–5, the numbers of extrema or peaks (positive or negative) in the tympanograms are specified. Thus, a single peaked tympanogram is a type 1B1G (Figure 4–5a), because there is only one extremum each for the B and G components. More complex shapes also occur, such as 3B1G (Figure 4–5b), in which the B component has two positive extrema and one negative extremum, and the G component has one positive extremum. The remaining two types are 3B3G

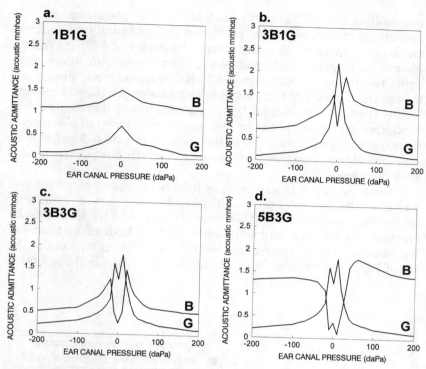

FIGURE 4–5. Tympanometric types for normal middle ears based on the Vanhuyse et al. (1975) model. **a.** Type 1B1G, with a single extremum for the acoustic susceptance (B) and acoustic conductance (G) tympanograms. **b.** Type 3B1G, with three extrema for the acoustic susceptance tympanogram (B) and one extremum for the acoustic conductance tympanogram (G). **c.** Type 3B3G, with three extrema for the acoustic susceptance (B) and acoustic conductance (G) tympanograms. **d.** Type 5B3G, with five extrema for the acoustic susceptance tympanogram (B) and three extrema for the acoustic conductance (G) tympanogram.

(Figure 4–5c) and 5B3G (Figure 4–5d). These four types are a result of a simple and orderly interaction of reactance and resistance (Vanhuyse et al., 1975).

The tympanogram of a normal adult ear will progress though the four types as the probe frequency increases. The simplest type, 1B1G, occurs in almost all normal adult middle ears tested with a probe frequency of 226 Hz. Consequently, a notched tympanogram at 226 Hz is abnormal in an adult ear. As the probe frequency increases, the tympanometric pattern becomes more complex in adults, including sequentially types 3B1G, 3B3G, and 5B3G. The percentage of tympanograms of each type recorded from a group of adults with normal middle ear function and using a probe frequency of 678 Hz (Wilson, Shanks, & Kaplan, 1984) is shown in Figure 4–6. This figure highlights two important facts about 678 Hz tympanograms. First, even though the majority of 678 Hz tympanograms are 1B1G, all types are found in normal ears. Second, tympanograms recorded in the direction of positive to negative pressure sweeps generally have simpler shapes than tympanograms recorded in the opposite direction. For this reason, clinical tympanograms usually are recorded in the positive to negative direction.

Tympanometric shapes seen in infants are different from those seen in adults. In adults with healthy middle ear systems, virtually all tympanograms recorded at 226 Hz are of the type 1B1G. In infants, by contrast, the 1B1G pattern is the least common. Instead, up to 83% of the susceptance (B_a) tympanograms recorded from infants under the age of 130 hours show notching (Sprague et al., 1985). In these infants

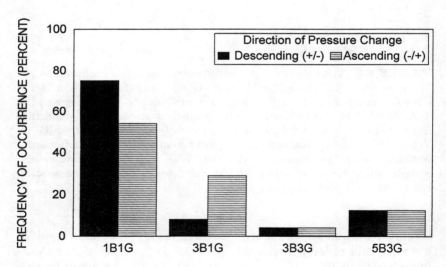

FIGURE 4–6. Frequency of occurrence for the four tympanometric types (1B1G, 3B1G, 3B3G, 5B3G) in normal middle ears depending on direction of pressure change used during the recording (Data from "Tympanometric Changes at 226 Hz and 678 Hz across 10 Trials and for Two Directions of Ear Canal Pressure Change," by R. H. Wilson, J. E. Shanks, and S. K. Kaplan, 1984. *Journal of Speech and Hearing Research, 27*, p. 258. Copyright 1984 American Speech-Language-Hearing Association.)

with theoretically normal middle ear systems, 26% had no discernible peak for the 660 Hz acoustic susceptance (B_a) tympanogram, which again is a rare finding in normal adult ears (Sprague et al., 1985). The tympanometric patterns seen in infants also included irregular shapes, B and G peaks occurring at different pressure locations, and monotonically rising acoustic susceptance tympanograms (Holte, Margolis, & Cavanaugh, 1991; Sprague et al., 1985). As infants age, they show fewer complex tympanometric shapes for the 226 Hz tympanograms. Holte et al. (1991) reported that, by the age of 2 months, healthy infants yielded tympanograms that were 3B3G or simpler, and by the age of 4 months, all of the infants yielded tympanograms that were 1B1G. Because the infant ear canal is cartilaginous, it cannot be modeled as a hard-walled cavity as it is in adults. Consequently, the models that have been developed for adult ears may not apply. More data are needed on the ears of infants with confirmed middle ear disease before we know the best way to distinguish normal from pathological ears in this important group of patients.

The most commonly used version of multi-frequency tympanometry involves two frequencies, typically 226 and 678 Hz. For tympanograms elicited at 678 Hz, Vanhuyse et al. (1975) listed the following criteria for the tympanograms to be considered normal: (a) there should be no more than five B and three G peaks, (b) the G peaks must fall within the B peaks, and (c) the distance between the B peaks must not be more than 75 daPa if there are three B peaks or more than 100 daPa if there are five B peaks. Tympanograms that fall outside of these criteria are considered abnormal (Van de Heyning, Van Camp, Creten, & Vanpeperstraete, 1982). For example, disarticulation of the ossicular chain increases the mass loading on the tympanic membrane; the result might be an abnormally notched tympanogram with more than five B peaks with outer peaks that are spaced more than 100 daPa apart.

Because acoustic susceptance (B_a) is the algebraic sum of positive (stiffness) and negative (mass) components, it can be used to determine whether the middle ear system is dominated by mass components, stiffness components, or is at resonance, as shown in Figure 4–7. Recall that the acoustic admittance at the tympanic membrane is determined by subtracting the effects of the ear canal from the measurement plane tympanogram. Doing this effectively makes the tail of the acoustic susceptance (B_a) tympanogram a new zero line, as indicated by the light horizontal lines drawn on the acoustic susceptance tympanograms in Figure 4–7. The sign of the peak of the acoustic susceptance tympanogram, then, provides information on the condition of the middle ear system. If the peak is positive (above the tail of the

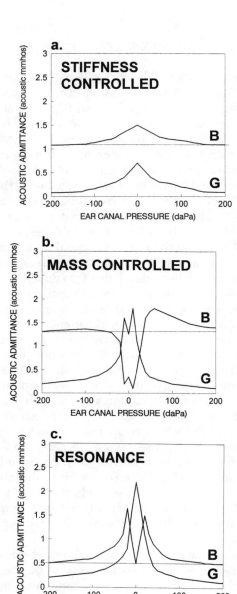

FIGURE 4–7. Tympanograms for middle ears that are: **a.** stiffness controlled, **b.** mass controlled, and **c.** at resonance. The acoustic susceptance tympanogram (B) and the acoustic conductance tympanogram (G) are shown. The thin line drawn at the tail of the acoustic susceptance tympanogram represents the correction for ear canal volume. If the peak of the acoustic susceptance (B) tympanogram is above the line, the middle ear is stiffness controlled; if the peak is below the line, the middle ear is mass controlled; and if the peak is on the line, the middle ear is at resonance.

acoustic susceptance tympanogram), the ear is stiffness controlled as shown in Figure 4–7a. This fact is true even for notched tympanograms. If the peak is negative (below the tail of the acoustic susceptance tympanogram), then the ear is mass controlled, as shown in Figure 4–7b.

Finally, if the peak of the acoustic susceptance (B_a) tympanogram is at 0 acoustic mmhos in the compensated tympanogram (i.e., at the level of the tail of the acoustic susceptance [B_a] tympanogram), then the system is at *resonance* and the probe frequency producing that situation is the resonant frequency of the middle ear transmission system, as shown in Figure 4–7c. At the *resonance frequency*, the stiffness components (positive) are equal to the mass components (negative), and they effectively cancel each other. The result of this cancellation is an acoustic susceptance (B_a) value of 0 acoustic mmhos in the rectangular coordinate system or a phase angle of 0° in the polar system (see Chapter 2). The acoustic admittance at resonance is equal to the value of the acoustic conductance. Any probe frequency chosen above the resonant frequency will produce tympanograms that show mass effects, and any probe frequency chosen below the resonant frequency will produce tympanograms that show stiffness effects for that ear. Note that the acoustic conductance (G_a) tympanogram is not used in determining if the ear is stiffness or mass controlled.

Pathological conditions produce two effects on the tympanograms; both the shape and the resonance frequency may be affected. First, the patterns produced by the tympanograms can be evaluated with reference to the normal criteria identified by Vanhuyse et al. (1975); any tympanograms that do not meet these criteria are considered abnormal and are suggestive of middle ear pathology. Second, the resonance frequency is compared to the resonance frequency of normal ears. Using these criteria, pathologies that increase the mass component, such as external otitis and ossicular discontinuities, may produce tympanograms with more extrema, more widely spaced extrema, and irregular ordering of B_a and G_a extrema as compared to normal tympanograms. An example of the tympanogram produced by an ossicular discontinuity is shown in Figure 4–8a. Pathologies that increase the stiffness component, such as middle ear effusions and ossicular fixations, may produce tympanograms with components that are widely spaced with a low amplitude. An example of a tympanogram from an ear with effusion is shown in Figure 4–8b. If the middle ear system is completely stiffened by effusion or ossicular fixation, a flat tympanogram may result for the multi-frequency tympanograms, as shown in Figure 4–8c. Note that the interpretation of the flat tympanogram for higher frequency probe tones is not substantially differ-

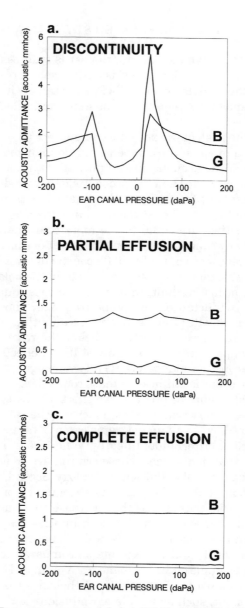

FIGURE 4–8. Tympanograms recorded at 678 Hz that fall outside of the normal categories of the Vanhuyse et al. (1975) model. **a.** The effect of ossicular discontinuity for which the peaks of the acoustic susceptance (B) tympanogram are broadly spaced and deeply notched due to an increase in the mass component. **b.** The effect of middle ear effusion that has not completely filled the middle ear, with low amplitude and broadly spaced peaks in the acoustic susceptance (B) tympanogram. **c.** The effect of middle ear effusion that has completely filled the middle ear, with flat acoustic susceptance (B) and acoustic conductance (G) tympanograms.

ent from the interpretation of flat tympanograms recorded with low frequency probe tones.

Additional information, however, can be gleaned from ears with tympanic membrane perforations using high frequency probes (678 Hz) in component tympanometry. The expected finding with a tympanic membrane perforation is a flat tympanogram with a large equivalent volume. The large volume results from the combined volume of the ear canal and middle ear spaces. If, however, the middle ear spaces are filled with a cholesteatoma, glue, or debris, the volume will not be larger than normal, and the distinction between an intact and perforated tympanic membrane will not be obvious with tympanometric measures. In ears with tympanic membrane perforations and otherwise normal middle ear systems, there may be a reversal of the acoustic susceptance (B_a) and acoustic conductance (G_a) tympanograms, with the acoustic susceptance tympanogram near or below 0 acoustic mmho. These findings are seen more frequently with 678 Hz probe frequencies, but may be seen with 226 Hz probe frequencies as well. The low value of the acoustic susceptance suggests that these ears have an increase in resistance and mass as compared to the usual findings in ears with perforated tympanic membranes (Shanks, 1984).

In addition to increasing the stiffness or mass components, middle ear pathologies also may shift the resonance frequency of the middle ear. Normally the resonance occurs between 800–1200 Hz (Shanks, Wilson, & Cambron, 1993). A stiffening pathology (such as otosclerosis) may increase the resonance frequency of the middle ear, whereas a mass loading pathology (such as ossicular disarticulation) may decrease the resonance frequency of the middle ear. With multi-frequency tympanometry that employs a sufficient number of probe frequencies, the resonance frequency can be identified as the frequency at which the mass and stiffness components are equal, resulting in an acoustic susceptance (B_a) value of 0 acoustic mmhos in the compensated tympanogram. This method, unfortunately has not yet proven to be clinically effective due to the large normal range of resonant frequencies and the significant overlap between normal and pathologic groups. Further, recording methods, such as pressure for ear canal estimation, speed of recording, recording direction, and sensitivity of the instrument, can significantly alter the estimate of resonant frequency. Standard procedures are not in use. Finally, current equipment cannot measure acoustic admittance with probe frequencies above 2000 Hz, which limits the number of cases in which the resonant frequency can be identified, given that resonant frequencies can occur at frequencies above 2000 Hz (Shanks et al., 1993).

TYMPANOGRAMS AND AUDIOGRAMS

One challenge in determining the causes of middle ear pathology is that there is not always a direct relation between the effect of the pathology on the tympanogram and auditory thresholds shown on the audiogram. These two measures of middle ear function, however, can be used together to provide more information than can be gathered from either measure alone. The audiogram reflects any reduction in the air conducted signal as compared to the bone conducted signal in the presence of a conductive pathology. The tympanogram, on the other hand, reflects only the admittance of the lateral-most pathological change in the flow of energy through the middle ear system (Chesnutt, Stream, Love, & McLarey, 1975). The tympanogram, therefore, is not a measure of the admittance of pathology affecting the entire middle ear system or even of the most significant pathology. Because of this, the exact structure producing the conductive pathology cannot always be identified with tympanometry. For example, if a patient has a significant conductive hearing loss and dual pathologies, such as external otitis and otosclerosis, the cause of the conductive loss may be difficult to determine. If the otosclerosis alone produces a stiffness controlled tympanogram (1B1G) and the external otitis alone produces an abnormally mass-controlled tympanogram (e.g., 7B5G), the patient will present with an abnormally mass-controlled tympanogram (7B5G). The otosclerosis, however, is the pathology that actually causes the air-bone gap. Despite the fact that the otosclerosis is actually producing the conductive hearing loss, the tympanogram reflects the outermost disorder, the external otitis. Whereas the otitis externa can be confirmed with otoscopy, the otosclerosis may remain hidden. The effect of the otosclerosis on the admittance of the middle ear system is completely obscured by the more lateral tympanic membrane pathology.

Because the tympanogram and audiogram provide different measures of the conductive mechanism, the tympanogram sometimes will identify a medically significant disorder that is not evident on the audiogram. Some disorders will produce minimal air-bone gaps, or none at all, and yet the patient will have an active pathology that requires medical referral. For example, if a patient has external otitis, the auditory thresholds are likely to be normal. Only an abnormal tympanogram (such as 7B5G) will indicate that the middle ear system is pathological. The tympanogram will confirm otoscopic findings, but not the audiometry.

In some cases, the audiograms and tympanograms can be used together to determine the cause of a middle ear pathology, particularly when either measure alone does not provide adequate discriminative information. Similar conductive losses indicated on audiograms may be accompanied by a variety of different tympanograms. Conversely, similar tympanograms may be accompanied by a variety of audiometric findings. In the first instance, audiograms showing similar degrees of air-bone gaps can result from middle ear disorders that produce significantly different tympanograms. A substantial air-bone gap can be caused by otosclerosis and yield a relatively normal tympanogram, by ossicular discontinuity, and yield an abnormal mass component or by a traumatic tympanic membrane perforation and yield a flat tympanogram with a large ear canal volume. In the second case, similar tympanograms may be accompanied by a wide variety of audiometric configurations. For example, external otitis and ossicular discontinuity both may produce abnormally notched tympanograms (e.g., 7B5G), but the ossicular discontinuity will have a substantial audiometric conductive component, whereas the eardrum pathology will not. The audiogram and tympanogram together, therefore, can be used to rule out the ossicular discontinuity if there is not a significant air-bone gap or to rule it in if there is a significant air-bone gap.

Finally, because there is a large range for normal tympanograms, and it is not always easy to determine whether the tympanogram recorded from a particular patient is normal for that patient, even if it falls within the range that would generally be considered normal. In these cases, the audiogram can sometimes be used to provide audiometric confirmation of any potential tympanometric abnormality. If the stiffening effects seen on the tympanogram are accompanied by a low frequency conductive component, there is additional support to predict that the patient has a stiffness-producing middle ear pathology. If, on the other hand, an increase in the mass component on the tympanogram is accompanied by a high frequency conductive component, there is additional support for the presence of a mass-producing middle ear pathology. The conductive component indicated on the audiogram, therefore, may provide confirmation of the presence of a clinically significant pathology. In all of these cases, it is the combination of the tympanogram and the audiogram that will allow the audiologist to arrive at the appropriate cause for any middle ear disorder.

DISCUSSION ITEMS FOR SELF-STUDY

1. Equivalent ear canal volume (V_{ea}) is derived from tympanograms for use in the determination of causes of flat tympanograms. What procedures are recommended for determining V_{ea} and how are they used clinically?
2. What are the advantages and disadvantages of using tympanometry in determining the cause of a conductive hearing loss?

SUGGESTED EXERCISES FOR SELF-STUDY

1. Run an acoustic admittance (Y_a) tympanogram on your ear. Use a 226 Hz probe and a positive-to-negative direction of pressure change. Using the tympanogram, compute the tympanometric indices of middle ear function that can be derived from your tympanogram. Compare the values from your tympanogram to the norms of ASHA (1997). Is your tympanogram within normal limits?
2. Run acoustic susceptance (B_a), acoustic conductance (G_a), and acoustic admittance (Y_a) tympanograms on yourself using a 226 Hz probe. Using the tympanograms, calculate the Y_a and phase angle from B_a and G_a. How close was your calculated Y_a to your measured Y_a? Check your work using the equations and examples in Table 2–1. What are some reasons that might cause the measured and calculated values to differ?

5

Eustachian Tube Function

*O*ne primary function of the Eustachian tube is to ventilate the mid-*dle ear*, which is critical to normal middle ear function. Using tympanometric measures, we can measure the ventilatory function of the Eustachian tube with either intact or perforated tympanic membranes. The major rationale for performing clinical measures of *Eustachian tube function* with intact tympanic membranes is based on the association of dysfunction of the Eustachian tube with the development of otitis media (Bluestone, 1975; Bluestone & Cantekin, 1981). The major rationale for measuring Eustachian tube function with a perforated tympanic membrane is to predict outcomes for middle ear surgeries (Holmquist & Bergstrom, 1978).

A normally functioning Eustachian tube provides equalization of air pressure between the middle ear space and the surrounding atmosphere. A nonfunctioning Eustachian tube may lead to negative middle ear pressures that are associated with middle ear disorders. Children who have a premyringotomy resting pressure that is substantially negative show a high incidence of recurrent acute otitis media with effusions. As resting pressures become increasingly negative, the percentage of cases with effusion increases. About 75% of children with resting pressures from −100 to −400 daPa have been reported to show middle ear effusions (Bluestone, 1975). Although these data should be viewed with caution given the amount of variability in the pressure fluctuations in children, they suggest that Eustachian tube function should be monitored in children who are prone to middle ear infections.

The cause of the high negative pressures in the middle ear that are associated with middle ear effusion is not entirely known. It has been assumed that obstruction of the Eustachian tube followed by absorption of gases by the middle ear mucosa is responsible for the negative pressure, but this theory has not been proven clinically. An alternate theory is that negative middle ear pressure results from sniffing in people who also have Eustachian tube dysfunction (Magnuson, 1981). Children who dislike blowing their noses sniff frequently. Many adults who suffer from chronic middle ear disease or patulous Eustachian tubes may become habitual sniffers. The Eustachian tube dysfunction that leads to middle ear disease in these people consists of (a) failure of tubal closure that causes evacuation of gases from the middle ear and (b) failure of tubal opening with swallowing that prevents subsequent pressure equalization. This dual failure results in the development and persistence of negative middle ear pressure, which is the ideal set of conditions for the development of middle ear effusion and its sequelae (Falk & Magnuson, 1984).

Eustachian tube function can be used in monitoring aspects of middle ear disease including prediction of onset, recovery, and prevention. Eustachian tube function tests eventually may help identify children who are at risk for the development of middle ear disease. One encouraging report showed that children who were able to resolve negative middle ear pressure by inflating their middle ears were less likely to develop middle ear problems than those who were not. They inflated their middle ears with either Valsalva (by holding their noses, closing their mouths, and gently blowing) or a special balloon and tube designed for this purpose. These results were short term, however, indicating that continued inflation is necessary to maintain health of the middle ear (Strangerup, Sederberg-Olsen, & Balle, 1992). Monitoring of Eustachian tube function in children who are at risk for developing otitis media may allow nonsurgical intervention early enough to prevent the effusion in a significant number of cases.

As a preoperative measure for patients who have tympanic membrane perforations, Eustachian tube function may be tested to predict the outcome of surgery of the tympanic membrane and the middle ear. Holmquist and Bergstrom (1977) indicated that fewer than half of the patients with poor Eustachian tube function had successful surgical repair of their tympanic membranes, whereas up to 80% of patients with good Eustachian tube function had successful outcomes. Although good Eustachian tube function prior to surgery is predictive that the surgical repair of the tympanic membrane will not fail, the prediction is not perfect. The relation between Eustachian tube function before and after tympanoplasty is an area that requires more study to present a definitive answer.

TEST PROCEDURES

The most common measures of Eustachian tube function are derived from tympanometric measures. These techniques are based on the assumption that the pressure location of the tympanometric peak approximates the resting pressure in the middle ear space. Initially, a pretest baseline tympanogram is obtained. Next the subject is instructed to perform a maneuver, such as swallowing, that normally results in opening the Eustachian tube. A postmaneuver tympanogram is then obtained to assess tubal opening. Shifts of the peak pressures of the tympanogram typically are used as an index of tubal function. The lack of a pressure shift indicates tubal dysfunction.

Three techniques commonly used as tests of Eustachian tube function in intact tympanic membranes are the Inflation-Deflation procedure, the Toynbee procedure, and the Valsalva procedure (Bluestone, 1975). A fourth test, the sniff test (Falk, 1982), is used less commonly but may also be useful clinically. Descriptions of these techniques follow.

1. Inflation-Deflation Procedure
The *Inflation-Deflation* procedure is a pressure-swallow technique for assessment of Eustachian tube function. The test sequence is as follows:
a. A pretest, baseline tympanogram is obtained.
b. A high positive (Inflation) or negative (Deflation) air pressure is introduced into the external ear canal and the patient is instructed to swallow several times.
c. A posttest tympanogram is obtained after swallowing.

Tubal opening is indicated by a shift in pressure location for the posttest tympanometric peak relative to the pretest peak. The shift in pressure typically is in the opposite direction from the applied ear canal pressure. For example, in the Inflation technique, a positive pressure is applied and the normal peak shift is in the negative direction. Pre- and posttest tympanograms for the Inflation procedure are shown in Figure 5–1 and for the Deflation procedure in Figure 5–2. These changes may be small and difficult to interpret in a clinical population.

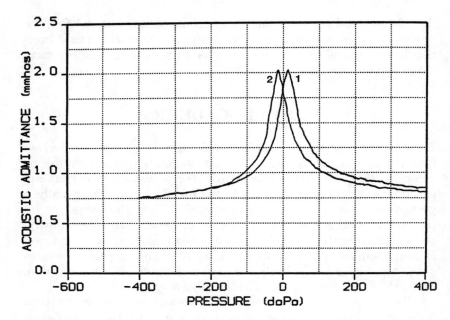

FIGURE 5–1. Tympanograms before and after a successful Inflation test. The initial tympanogram has a slightly positive peak (1). After positive pressure is introduced into the external ear canal and the patient swallows, the pressure peak of the tympanogram shifts in a negative direction (2). (From "Tympanometric Measures of Eustachian Tube Function," by C. L. Riedel, T. L. Wiley, and M. G. Block, 1987. *Journal of Speech and Hearing Research, 30,* p. 210. Copyright 1987 American Speech-Language-Hearing Association. Reprinted with permission.)

2. Toynbee

The *Toynbee* procedure is designed to introduce a negative middle ear pressure via the Eustachian tube. The test sequence is as follows:

a. A pretest baseline tympanogram is obtained.

b. The patient is instructed to pinch the nose and swallow.

c. A posttest tympanogram is obtained.

A successful Toynbee maneuver will cause the tube to open and will evacuate air from the middle ear, resulting in a tympanometric peak that is shifted in the negative direction. A successful Toynbee maneuver is shown in Figure 5–3. An unsuccessful Toynbee maneuver will not shift the tympanometric peak.

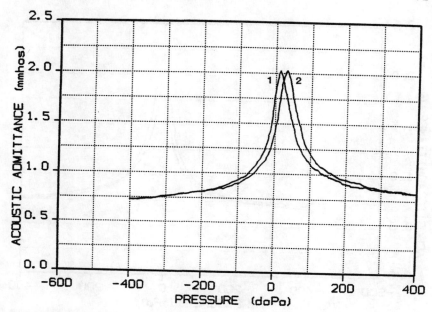

FIGURE 5–2. Tympanograms before and after a successful Deflation test. The initial tympanogram has a slightly positive peak (1). After negative pressure is introduced into the external ear canal and the patient swallows, the pressure peak of the tympanogram shifts in a positive direction (2). (From "Tympanometric Measures of Eustachian Tube Function," by C. L. Riedel, T. L. Wiley, and M. G. Block, 1987. *Journal of Speech and Hearing Research, 30,* p. 210. Copyright 1987 American Speech-Language-Hearing Association. Reprinted with permission.)

3. Valsalva

The *Valsalva* procedure is designed to introduce a positive middle ear pressure via the Eustachian tube. Steps a and c are identical to those of the Toynbee procedure. In step b, however, the patient is instructed to close off the nose and mouth and blow gently. A successful Valsalva maneuver will cause the tube to open and allow air to be forced into the middle ear, resulting in a posttest tympanometric peak that is shifted in the positive direction. This result is shown in Figure 5–4. An unsuccessful Valsalva maneuver will not cause the tympanometric peak to be shifted. Caution must be exercised because the maneuver may cause the probe to become dislodged in the ear canal and a pressure leak in the ear canal may be confused with a change in the pressure in the middle ear.

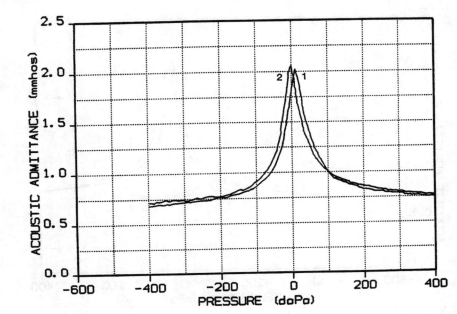

FIGURE 5–3. Tympanograms before and after a successful Toynbee test. The initial tympanogram shows a slightly positive pressure peak (1). After the patient pinches the nose and swallows, the pressure peak of the tympanogram shifts in a negative direction (2). (From "Tympanometric Measures of Eustachian Tube Function," by C. L. Riedel, T. L. Wiley, and M. G. Block, 1987. *Journal of Speech and Hearing Research, 30,* p. 210. Copyright 1987 American Speech-Language-Hearing Association. Reprinted with permission.)

4. Sniff Test

The *sniff test* is designed to determine if sniffing induces significant negative pressure in the middle ear. The procedure is as follows:

a. The patient performs a Valsalva maneuver.

b. A baseline tympanogram is recorded.

c. The patient is asked to close off one nostril with a finger and to take several sharp sniffs.

d. A second tympanogram is recorded.

If the test is positive, the second tympanogram will have a peak that is shifted in the negative direction (Falk & Magnuson, 1984).

Eustachian tube function can also be measured with an Inflation-Deflation procedure on ears in which the tympanic membrane is not intact (Bluestone, 1975). First, the positive pressure is increased to 200–400 daPa and the patient is asked to swallow. Then, the negative

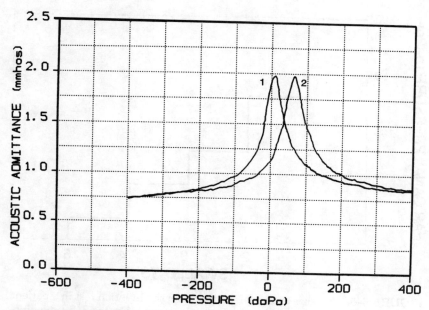

FIGURE 5–4. Tympanograms before and after a successful Valsalva test. The initial tympanogram shows a slightly positive pressure peak (1). After the patient closes off the nose and mouth and gently blows, the pressure peak of the tympanogram shifts in a positive direction (2). (From "Tympanometric Measures of Eustachian Tube Function," by C. L. Riedel, T. L. Wiley, and M. G. Block, 1987. *Journal of Speech and Hearing Research, 30,* p. 210. Copyright 1987 American Speech-Language-Hearing Association. Reprinted with permission.)

pressure is decreased to –200 daPa and the person again is asked to swallow. If the Eustachian tube function is normal, the pressure will return to 0 daPa after several swallows, as shown in Figure 5–5. If the Eustachian tube function is not normal, one of two patterns will occur. For the first pattern, with positive ear canal pressure, a pressure, called the opening pressure, will cause the Eustachian tube to open and the ear canal pressure to return to a level closer to 0 daPa. Subsequent swallows may allow the pressure to approach, but not reach, 0 daPa. For the negative pressure, swallows will not cause the Eustachian tube to open to equalize the pressure. The recorded ear canal pressure, therefore, will not change and the recording will remain at a negative pressure. For the second abnormal pattern, swallowing will not cause the Eustachian tube to open whether there is negative or

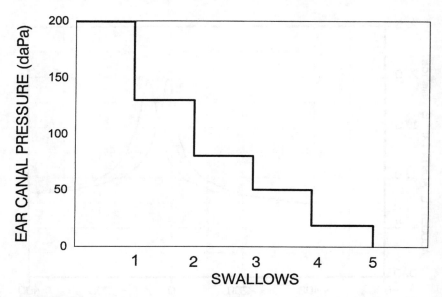

FIGURE 5–5. Pressure changes resulting from the Inflation test in a patient with a tympanic membrane perforation and adequate Eustachian tube function. Positive pressure (200 daPa) was introduced into the ear canal and the patient was asked to swallow five times. Each swallow produced a decrement in the pressure in the ear canal. The fifth swallow brought the ear canal pressure to 0 daPa.

positive pressure in the ear canal. The result is that the recorded ear canal pressure will not change with either positive or negative ear canal pressures. Similar procedures can be used with the Toynbee and Valsalva maneuvers.

CLINICAL APPLICATION

Tests of Eustachian tube function are not performed on every patient. If the tympanometric peak is near atmospheric pressure, there is no reason to suspect dysfunction of the tube. If the peak is significantly negative, the simplest test is to have the patient swallow or Valsalva and then to repeat the tympanogram. If the peak moves to or near atmospheric pressure, tubal function can be assumed to be normal. The above tests then are reserved for patients for whom swallowing is not sufficient to open the Eustachian tube. If the above tests then are successful, you have learned that the tube can open with sufficient pressure, but unfortunately you have learned nothing about the functional capability of the tube in everyday living situations.

Some patients will exhibit oscillatory changes in the admittance during tympanometry. If these changes are synchronous with breathing, then the Eustachian tube is considered to be *patulous*, or constantly open. This condition may occur in people with chronic middle ear disease. People with this problem often complain that their voices sound hollow.

Although these tests are simple and fast to perform and despite the strong link between Eustachian tube dysfunction and middle ear disease, tests of Eustachian tube patency and function have not received widespread clinical acceptance (Bluestone & Cantekin, 1981; Givens & Seidemann, 1984). The primary reasons they are not used are the lack of normative data and standardized protocols and procedures for each test. Normal confidence limits, for example, which are critical to the definition of normal and abnormal Eustachian function, are not available. Values obtained with 220 Hz probe tones in both ears of 24 young adults are shown in Table 5–1 (Riedel, Wiley, & Block, 1987) for the Inflation-Deflation, Toynbee, and Valsalva procedures. Norms are needed from people across the age span, including children who are a high-risk group for Eustachian tube dysfunction. Clinical validation on people with abnormal middle ear function and abnormal Eustachian tube function also is needed.

DISCUSSION ITEMS FOR SELF-STUDY

1. What is the function of the Eustachian tube?
2. Who is a good candidate for Eustachian tube function tests?
3. How well do positive Eustachian tube function tests predict successful tympanoplasties? Why is this prediction not 100% accurate?

SUGGESTED EXERCISE FOR SELF-STUDY

Perform the Valsalva and Toynbee procedures on the ear of a young adult with a normal tympanogram. Compare the peak pressures of the baseline and post-test tympanogram and the amount of shift with the values given in Table 5–1. Did your values agree with the values in the table? If your values did not agree, what could account for the differences?

Table 5–1. Means, standard error of the mean, and confidence intervals for the peak pressure (in daPa) of the baseline tympanogram and the posttest tympanogram, and the amount of shift produced for the Valsalva, Toynbee, Inflation, and Deflation procedures for adults with normal tympanograms.

Test	Mean	Standard Error of the Mean	95% Confidence Interval
Valsalva			
Baseline	9	1	7 to 11
Experimental	72	8	55 to 87
Shift	63	8	47 to 79
Toynbee			
Baseline	9	1	7 to 11
Experimental	−6	5	−17 to 5
Shift	−15	5	−26 to −4
Inflation			
Baseline	8	1	6 to 10
Experimental	−3	1	−6 to 0
Shift	−11	1	−13 to −8
Deflation			
Baseline	8	1	6 to 10
Experimental	23	2	20 to 26
Shift	15	2	12 to 18

Source: From "Tympanometric Measures of Eustachian Tube Function," by C. L. Riedel, T. L. Wiley, and M. G. Block, 1987. *Journal of Speech and Hearing Research, 30*, p. 209. Copyright 1987 American Speech-Language-Hearing Association. Reprinted with permission.

6

Stapedial Reflex Measures

ANATOMY AND PHYSIOLOGY OF THE MIDDLE EAR MUSCLES

There are two small muscles contained in the middle ear that are functionally related to the middle-ear transmission system, particularly the ossicular chain. For a more detailed treatment of middle ear anatomy and physiology, the reader is referred to the texts of Dallos (1973), Schuknecht (1993), and Zemlin (1988). The *tensor tympani* muscle arises (originates) from the wall of the Eustachian tube and inserts (connects) on the upper margin of the manubrium of the malleus. The tensor tympani is innervated by Cranial Nerve V (Trigeminal). The tensor tympani contracts as a part of a general startle response and the muscle also can be activated by tactile stimulation of the orbital area. Pulling upward on the eyebrow or directing an air puff to the orbital area, for example, will result in a contraction of the tensor tympani. Contraction of the tensor tympani muscle draws the malleus inward which, in turn, tenses the tympanic membrane. This tensing of the tympanic membrane may result in an increased acoustic impedance (decreased acoustic admittance) at the lateral surface of the tympanic membrane due to a resultant stiffening of the ossicular chain. Or, contraction of the tensor tympani may cause a decrease in acoustic impedance at the tympanic membrane due to a resultant enlargement of the external auditory meatus. Specifically, the tensor tympani contraction may pull the malleus and attached tympanic membrane medially (inward), enlarging the external ear canal. Most clinical diagnostic protocols do not include an evaluation of tensor tympani responses; thus, the major discussions that follow will deal only with stapedius muscle reflexes.

The second middle ear muscle, the *stapedius,* originates in a small bony canal adjoining the facial canal and inserts on the head of the stapes. *The stapedius muscle is innervated by the motor or stapedial branch of Cranial Nerve VII (Facial).* There are two primary means of eliciting a contraction of the stapedius muscle, acoustic and non-acoustic. Uniquely, the stapedius muscle will contract in response to an acoustic signal of sufficient intensity level and duration. As noted earlier, this stapedial contraction is called an *acoustic reflex.* Other than in association with general startle responses, the tensor tympani does not contract in response to acoustic signals. Thus, clinical acoustic reflex measures are a result of stapedius contractions alone. The stapedius also will contract in response to tactile or electrocutaneous stimulation of the facial area surrounding the pinna. This area of the face is referred to as the *reflexogenic skin zone* and includes the orbital area. So, stimulation of the orbital area typically elicits a contraction of both the stapedius and the tensor tympani.

Functionally, a contraction of the stapedius (for both acoustic and nonacoustic activators) pulls the stapes down and out of the oval window. As the head of the stapes is drawn back, the anterior base of the stapes is tilted toward the tympanic cavity. This angular movement of the stapes results in stiffening of the ossicular chain with a corresponding decrease in acoustic admittance at the lateral surface of the tympanic membrane. There is little or no change in ear canal volume with stapedius contraction; the major change in acoustic admittance is a result of the stiffened middle-ear transmission system. Clinically, *this time-locked (with the activating signal) change in acoustic admittance comprises our measure of stapedius muscle response.*

In normal ears, contraction of the stapedius muscle is bilateral for both acoustic and nonacoustic activators. That is, if the stapedius muscle on one side contracts, the opposite stapedius muscle contracts as well. Thus, a stapedius muscle reflex can be obtained for either ipsilateral or contralateral activating signals. In the case of *ipsilateral* stapedius reflex measures, an activating signal is presented to the same ear in which acoustic immittance changes are being measured. With *contralateral* stapedius reflex measures, an activator is presented to one ear (referred to as the *stimulus or activator ear*) and acoustic immittance changes are measured in the opposite ear (referred to as the *probe ear*). The arrangement for ipsilateral and contralateral acoustic reflex measures is illustrated in Figure 6–1.

The acoustic stapedius reflex is slightly stronger for ipsilateral (or homolateral) activators than it is for contralateral activators. Specifically, a slightly lower activator level (3–5 dB) is required for elicitation of an ipsilateral acoustic reflex relative to the signal level required for a comparable contralaterly elicited acoustic reflex. The nonacoustic stapedius reflex is *substantially* stronger for ipsilateral activators. Accordingly, clinical applications of tactile or electrocutaneous reflexes

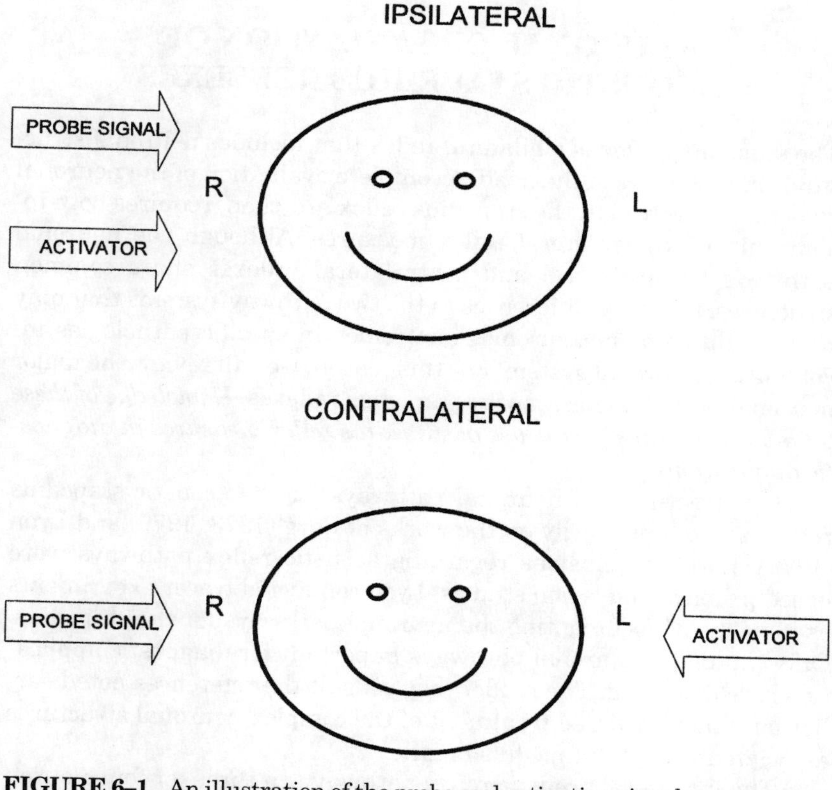

FIGURE 6–1. An illustration of the probe and activating signal arrangement for measures of ipsilateral *(top)* and contralateral *(bottom)* acoustic reflexes. In the case of ipsilateral acoustic reflex measures, the probe and activating signals are both presented to the same ear. For contralateral acoustic reflex measures, the probe signal is presented to one ear (probe ear) and the activating signal is presented to the other (stimulus) ear.

typically involve only ipsilateral measurements. A major problem with clinical application of tactile reflexes is the movement artifact associated with stimulation. Care must be taken to avoid physical contact with the pinna and the area of the head surrounding the acoustic-immittance probe unit and the patient must remain still during the stimulation procedures. In addition, it is difficult to time lock the tactile stimulus and response recording system. These problems, in large part, account for why nonacoustic reflex measures have not received widespread clinical application. Accordingly, we have restricted our remaining treatment of stapedius reflex measures in diagnostic audiology to acoustic reflex measures.

NEURONAL ORGANIZATION OF ACOUSTIC STAPEDIUS REFLEXES

The stapedius reflex is a bilateral reflex that includes neuronal structures on both sides of the head. A complete evaluation of the neuronal structures involved in the stapedius reflex arc, then, requires both ipsilateral and contralateral reflex measures. Although the neuronal pathways for ipsilateral and contralateral reflexes share common structures, there are differences in the two pathway systems that may produce different measurement outcomes in specific pathologies involving the neuronal system. For this reason, we will review the major neuronal pathways for acoustic stapedius reflexes. *Knowledge of these pathways is critical to the use of stapedius reflex measures in diagnostic applications.*

Our treatment of neuronal pathways for the acoustic stapedius reflex is based primarily on the works of Borg (1973, 1976) and Lyon (1978). Borg's conclusions regarding acoustic reflex pathways were based primarily on lesion studies; Lyon conducted tracer experiments as a means of documenting the neuronal pathways for the stapedius. Only the major neuronal pathways important for diagnostic applications are discussed. The reader may consult the references noted earlier for a more detailed treatment of the complex neuronal structures associated with the stapedius muscle.

The ipsilateral acoustic reflex pathway is a three- or four-neuron system as illustrated in Figure 6–2. As noted earlier, ipsilateral acoustic reflex measures require presentation of an acoustic activating signal to the same ear in which acoustic immittance changes indicative of stapedius contractions are measured. That is, the activator (stimulus) ear and the probe ear are the same. Neuronally, the prima-

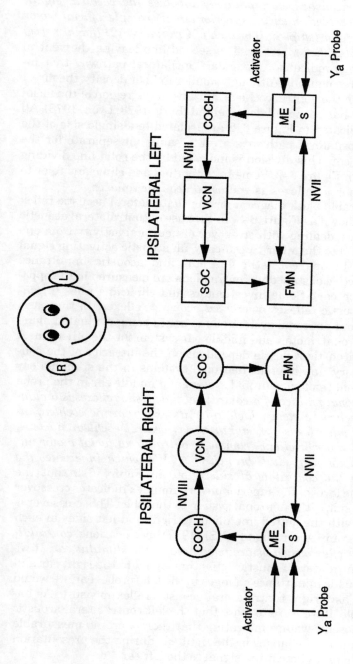

FIGURE 6-2. A block diagram showing the primary neuronal pathways for ipsilateral (uncrossed) acoustic reflexes. Separate diagrams are included for the right and left ears. Circles are used to indicate structures for the right ear and squares represent companion structures for the left ear82. The key for abbreviations is as follows: COCH: cochlea, ME: middle ear, VCN: ventral cochlear nucleus, SOC: superior olivary complex, FMN: facial motor nucleus, NVIII: cranial nerve eight (auditory), NVII: cranial nerve seven (fa-

81

ry *ipsilateral acoustic reflex pathway involves the cochlea, eighth nerve, ventral cochlear nucleus, superior olivary complex, facial motor nucleus, and motor (stapedial) branch of Cranial N. VII (facial nerve) which innervates the stapedius.* The second line leaving the ventral cochlear nucleus indicates a secondary ipsilateral pathway that involves only three neurons. Although smaller in fiber density, the direct fiber tract from the ventral cochlear nucleus to the region of the facial motor nucleus has been well-documented (Borg, 1973; Lyon, 1978). All structures indicated in Figure 6–2 are isolated to a single side of the head; these ipsilateral pathways are the same but separate for the right and left ear. This division is indicated by the solid line dividing the two ears in Figure 6–2. Some investigators and clinicians refer to *ipsilateral* acoustic reflexes as *uncrossed* acoustic reflexes.

A comparable block diagram for the contralateral acoustic-reflex pathways is shown as Figure 6–3. In the case of contralateral acoustic reflexes, we are dealing with crossover of neuronal activity from one side of the head to the other. Specifically, an acoustic activating signal is presented to one ear (stimulus ear) and acoustic immittance changes reflective of stapedius contractions are measured in the opposite ear (probe ear). Some investigators and clinicians refer to *contralateral* acoustic reflexes as *crossed* acoustic reflexes. In this case, the sensory and neuronal system of one ear is being evaluated along with the neuronal, motor, and middle ear system for the other ear. A measurable acoustic reflex is dependent on the integrity of the conductive, sensory, and afferent neuronal systems in the stimulus ear and the efferent (motor) neuronal system and middle ear in the probe ear. *The neuronal pathway for contralateral acoustic reflexes is a mandatory four-neuron system which, after its exit from the cochlea, includes the cochlea (sensory), eighth nerve, ventral cochlear nucleus, contralateral superior olivary complex, contralateral facial motor nucleus, and motor (stapedial) branch of N. VII which innervates the stapedius on the contralateral side.* Note in Figure 6–3 that the synapse at the level of the superior olivary complex indicates crossover from the one side of the neuronal system to the other. This crossover is highlighted with the dotted line dividing right and left sides in each pathway diagram. According to ANSI (1987) specifications, *contralateral acoustic reflex measures are referenced to the stimulus ear.* If we present a contralateral acoustic activating signal to the right ear and measure acoustic immittance changes in the left (probe) ear, we would refer to this as a right contralateral acoustic reflex measure. As another example, if we were to state that the left contralateral acoustic reflex was absent, we are indicating that there were no measurable acoustic immittance changes in the right ear during the presentation of an acoustic reflex activating signal to the left ear.

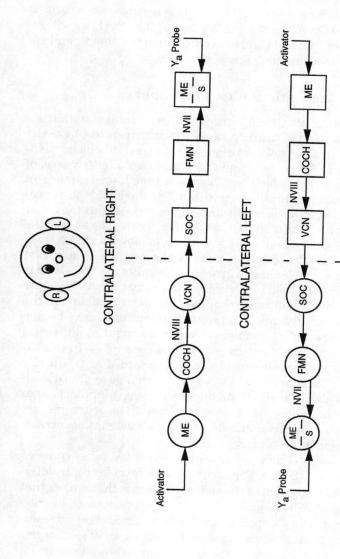

FIGURE 6–3. A block diagram showing the primary neuronal pathways for contralateral (or crossed) acoustic reflexes. Separate diagrams are included for the right and left ears. Circles are used to indicate structures for the right ear and squares represent companion structures for the left ear. The key for abbreviations is as follows: COCH: cochlea, ME: middle ear, VCN: ventral cochlear nucleus, SOC: superior olivary complex, FMN: facial motor nucleus, NVIII: cranial nerve eight (auditory), NVII: cranial nerve seven (facial), S: stapedius muscle. The dotted vertical line indicates the division (crossover) point for structures on the right and left sides of the head.

83

CLINICAL ACOUSTIC REFLEX MEASURES

The following three primary acoustic-reflex measures are used in typical clinical protocols: (1) presence or absence of the reflex, (2) acoustic-reflex thresholds, and (3) acoustic-reflex adaptation (decay). The presence or absence of the acoustic reflex usually is restricted to screening applications and will be discussed in a later section. Next, we will review acoustic reflex threshold and decay measures and the general applications of each measure in diagnostic audiology.

Acoustic Reflex Threshold

The concept of threshold for an acoustic reflex is similar to that for hearing thresholds. In the case of acoustic reflex thresholds, however, we are dealing with a physiologic response, not an overt behavioral indication of hearing. We are searching for the lowest intensity level of an activating signal for which we observe a time-locked change in acoustic immittance. Clinically, acoustic reflex thresholds are measured by monitoring acoustic immittance in the probe ear as the tester presents acoustic activating signals at specified levels. The level of the activating signal is systematically varied up or down in prescribed steps (e.g., 5 dB), and the tester searches for the lowest activator level that produces a noticeable change in acoustic immittance. This level is the acoustic reflex threshold for the activating signal used. The tester may monitor acoustic immittance changes on a meter available on the acoustic immittance instrument or acoustic immittance may be displayed on a chart recorder. A sample recorder tracing that illustrates an acoustic reflex threshold search is shown as Figure 6–4. In this example, the acoustic reflex threshold would be recorded as 90 dB HL. Levels below 90 dB HL do not result in a visible change in acoustic admittance. Levels above 90 dB HL produce increasingly larger changes in acoustic admittance in proportion to the level of the activating signal. The stapedius is a *graded* muscle; contraction magnitude increases with increases in activator signal level.

In most audiology clinics, acoustic reflex thresholds are expressed in hearing level (i.e., dB HL). The zero reference level for contralateral acoustic activators presented through earphones is the same as that (ANSI, 1996) used in audiometry for the measurement of hearing thresholds. As noted in Chapter 3, the basis for ipsilateral HL measures differs with the transducer used and is often a set of local norms furnished by the manufacturer of the acoustic immittance instrument or transducer (e.g., insert receivers). These norms generally are acoustic reflex thresholds for tonal activating signals in a group of lis-

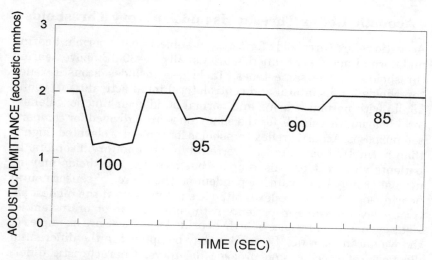

FIGURE 6-4. An exemplary plot of acoustic admittance measures used for determination of an acoustic reflex threshold. Changes in acoustic admittance (in acoustic mmhos) are shown as a function of time (in seconds). The level of the acoustic activating signal is in dB HL and is indicated at the bottom of each acoustic reflex event. In this example, the acoustic reflex threshold is 90 dB HL. Further explanation is included in the text.

teners with normal hearing and normal middle ear function. Most of the available data sets on acoustic reflex thresholds are based on acoustic immittance measures for a probe frequency of 220 or 226 Hz. In keeping with the objectives of this book, we will deal primarily with acoustic reflex threshold data that are consistent with these conditions. It should be understood, however, that probe frequency, activator spectra, transducers, measurement procedures, and other factors may influence acoustic reflex thresholds. Further, the population being tested may require alterations in the typical measurement protocol. If acoustic reflex measures are performed in newborns, for example, examiners will want to select a probe frequency higher than 226 Hz. Research has shown that acoustic reflexes in newborns are present more frequently for a 660 Hz probe than for a 220 Hz probe (McMillan, Bennett, Marchant, & Shurin, 1985; Sprague et al., 1985). (This and other issues concerned with middle ear screening in newborns are discussed in Chapter 7.) For more information on these issues, the reader is referred to more advanced treatments of the topic (see Silman, 1984, and Appendix B for other references).

Acoustic Reflex Thresholds and Auditory Thresholds

Acoustic reflex thresholds for tones in subjects with normal hearing and normal middle ear function are usually 70–80 dB above hearing thresholds for the same tones. Table 6–1 includes acoustic reflex thresholds for ipsilateral and contralateral tonal activators in young adults with normal hearing and normal middle ear function. Behavioral hearing thresholds for the same tones are provided for comparison purposes. Acoustic reflex thresholds for tones are elevated (higher than normal) in patients with certain types of auditory disorders. In patients with cochlear disorders, acoustic reflex thresholds may be normal or may be elevated dependent on the degree of sensorineural hearing loss. Acoustic reflexes often are not present at the highest activator level possible in patients with eighth nerve or brainstem lesions even in the presence of little hearing loss. These are examples of the way acoustic reflex thresholds may be applied in the differential diagnosis of specific otoneurologic disorders. Characteristic differences in acoustic reflex thresholds with various auditory disorders are covered later in this chapter.

Because they do not require a behavioral response, acoustic reflex measures are used as an indirect means of estimating hearing sensitivity (thresholds) in selected patients for whom behavioral measures are either not feasible or reliable. Specifically, physiologic acoustic reflex measures may be used in estimating hearing sensitivity for (a) hard-to-test patients such as very young children and others who are unable to perform tasks necessary for behavioral assessment of hearing abilities and (b) patients who are not willing to respond appropriately in behavioral audiometry, such as patients who may be feigning a hearing loss. In these clinical patients, predictions of hearing sensi-

Table 6–1. Mean auditory (hearing) thresholds and acoustic reflex thresholds for young adults with normal hearing and normal middle ear function.

Frequency	Auditory Threshold	Ipsilateral Acoustic Reflex Threshold	Contralateral Acoustic Reflex Threshold
500 Hz	1.2	79.9	84.6
1000 Hz	−0.5	82.0	85.9
2000 Hz	−0.7	86.2	84.4
4000 Hz	2.4	87.5	89.8

Source: The data are taken from Wiley, Oviatt, and Block (1987) and were based on a subject pool of 77 women and 50 men.

Note: All thresholds are in dB HL.

tivity can be made from acoustic reflex thresholds obtained from the patients. The predictions of hearing sensitivity are based on reported acoustic reflex thresholds for tones and noise activating signals in patients with normal hearing and in patients with verified degrees of sensorineural hearing loss. The prediction of auditory thresholds from acoustic reflex measures is limited primarily to patients with cochlear disorders because (a) the neuronal pathways of the acoustic stapedial reflex are restricted to structures at and below the auditory brainstem and (b) acoustic reflexes typically are absent for patients with lesions of the eighth nerve and auditory brainstem.

Normal acoustic reflex thresholds for a broadband noise, which has a wider bandwidth than a tone, are approximately 20–25 dB lower than acoustic reflex thresholds for tones. This difference between acoustic reflex thresholds for narrow bandwidth (e.g., tones) and wide bandwidth (e.g., broadband noise) activating signals is decreased in patients with sensorineural hearing loss, and the amount of decrease is roughly related (inversely) to the amount of hearing loss. *As the degree of sensorineural hearing loss in dB increases, the difference in acoustic reflex thresholds for tones and noise decreases.* In addition, acoustic reflex thresholds for tones occur at predictable levels that are related to behavioral auditory thresholds for the same signals. Patients with substantial sensorineural hearing losses have elevated acoustic reflex thresholds for tones.

As an example of the way clinicians apply these normative relations for acoustic reflex thresholds, consider the issue of diagnosis in cases of *pseudohypoacusis* or *functional hearing loss.* If a clinical patient is suspected of feigning a hearing loss, acoustic reflex thresholds may provide support for the suspected diagnosis. Specifically, if a patient volunteers behavioral thresholds that are worse than corresponding acoustic reflex thresholds for the same acoustic signals, the diagnosis of pseudohypoacusis is supported. It is not physiologically possible for the patient to truly have behavioral thresholds worse (higher) than acoustic reflex thresholds for tonal activating signals.

Various prediction algorithms have been developed for predicting the degree of hearing loss from acoustic reflex measures. Most of the algorithms are based on normative reflex-threshold values and on the difference in acoustic reflex thresholds for tones and for a broadband or band-limited noise. (The reader is referred to the works of Popelka [1981] and Silman, Gelfand, Piper, Silverman, & van Frank [1984] for details on the topic.) Although the degree of precision varies with the algorithm used, predictions of hearing sensitivity based on acoustic reflex thresholds generally are quite gross and there is a good deal of variability inherent to the procedure in clinical patients. In cases of sensorineural hearing loss for which audiometric thresholds are 50 dB HL or less, for example, patients may present normal or near normal acoustic reflex thresholds. (This relation between auditory thresholds and acoustic reflex thresholds in cochlear disorders is discussed in more detail later in this chapter under Cochlear Disorders.) Presently, most audiologists use acoustic reflex measures only to make gross predictions regarding the presence or absence of hearing loss. The approach is much less efficacious in making specific predictions of hearing loss in dB or in predicting the configuration of hearing loss across audiometric frequencies.

Acoustic Reflex Adaptation (Decay)

Acoustic reflex adaptation or decay is defined as a perstimulatory decline in acoustic reflex contraction for a sustained acoustic activating signal. Under specific conditions, the acoustic reflex may decline in magnitude over time during the presentation of a sustained activating signal. This relaxation of the stapedius muscle over the time course of the activating signal presentation is termed *acoustic reflex adaptation* or *acoustic reflex decay*. Acoustic reflex decay is the more popular term in clinical practice and will be used in the discussions that follow.

As with acoustic reflex threshold measures, acoustic reflex decay is observed by monitoring changes in acoustic immittance measures over time. A sample recorder tracing that demonstrates acoustic reflex decay is shown as Figure 6–5. Note that, shortly after the onset of the acoustic reflex activating signal, the acoustic admittance at the probe decreases, consistent with a contraction of the stapedius muscle and stiffening of the middle ear transmission system. As time proceeds during presentation of the activating signal, however, the acoustic admittance begins to increase, indicating that the stapedius muscle is relaxing over time. The extent of reflex decay increases over the time course of the sustained activating signal. A primary index of acoustic reflex decay that is used clinically is the *reflex half life*. Reflex half life is the time required for the acoustic reflex response to decline in magnitude by one half. In terms of our measurement variable, it is the time required for the acoustic admittance to decline to a value 50% between peak and baseline (no reflex) values. The method used for determining reflex half life is illustrated in Figure 6–5. The computation of reflex half life provides a single number index of acoustic reflex decay that can be used in differential otoneurologic diagnosis.

Clinically, acoustic reflex decay is usually measured for 500 Hz and/or 1000 Hz tonal activating signals at 10 dB above the acoustic reflex threshold for the tone. The duration of the activator stimulus is

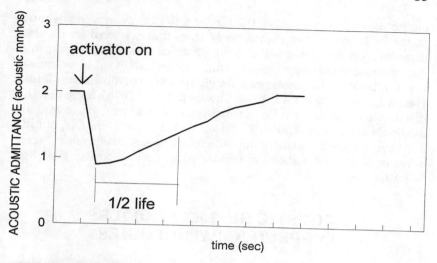

FIGURE 6–5. A sample recording of acoustic reflex decay illustrating the method for determining reflex half-life. The reflex half life in seconds is shown at the bottom of the tracing. In this example, reflex half life is 3 seconds.

typically 10 or 5 seconds, although some testers have reported the use of a 30-second activator duration. Low-frequency (500 or 1000 Hz) tonal activators are used because persons with a normal auditory system do not demonstrate significant acoustic reflex decay at those frequencies. At higher activator frequencies (e.g., 2000 and 4000 Hz), persons with a normal auditory system as well as persons with auditory pathologies may demonstrate acoustic reflex decay. Accordingly, clinical measures of acoustic reflex decay are limited to low-frequency activators. As with acoustic reflex threshold measures, the stimulus ear is the ear for which acoustic reflex decay measures are being made. If we present the sustained activator to the left ear and record acoustic immittance measures in the right ear, for example, we are recording acoustic reflex decay for the left ear. Specifically, our example would be a contralateral acoustic reflex decay measure for the left ear.

As noted in the overview of clinical measures (see Chapter 1), acoustic reflex decay is a characteristic sign of specific auditory disorders (e.g., tumors of the VIII cranial nerve). *Rapid and dramatic acoustic reflex decay is typically observed with sustained tonal activators presented to an ear with an eighth nerve tumor* (Anderson, Barr, & Wedenberg, 1969; Olsen, Noffsinger, & Kurdziel, 1975). Acoustic reflex decay also may be observed in cases of cochlear lesions, but the magnitude of reflex decay is usually less than that observed for cases of eighth nerve disorders. Also, the rate of reflex decay is typically much faster for lesions of the eighth nerve than that observed for cochlear disorders (Cartwright & Lilly, 1976). Based on this characteristic finding, investigators have suggested that a reflex half life of 10 seconds or less is a positive diagnostic sign for eighth nerve involvement (Jerger, Harford, Clemis, & Alford, 1974; Sheehy & Inzer, 1976). More detailed discussions of acoustic reflex decay in normal and pathologic ears are available elsewhere (Fowler & Wilson, 1984; Wilson, Shanks, & Lilly, 1984). In the sections that follow, the use of acoustic reflex decay measures in diagnostic audiology is reviewed for specific classes of auditory pathologies.

ACOUSTIC REFLEX PROFILES
IN SPECIFIC PATHOLOGIES

The purpose of this section is to present basic acoustic reflex findings typically observed for selected disorders of the auditory system. As noted earlier, knowledge of the neuronal pathways of the stapedius is important for diagnosticians and is fundamental to the discussions that follow. For additional information on the reflex pathways and reflex findings in various disorders, the reader is referred to the works of Jerger (1980), Jerger and Hayes (1980), and Wiley and Block (1984). In the examples that follow, we have exemplified clinical findings in single and specific disorders of the auditory system. The reader should understand that, in clinical practice, a patient may present with disorders to more than one primary neuronal site. In the case of combined neuronal disorders, the specific circumstances of each case will have to be considered in making diagnostic predictions of the presenting problem based on acoustic reflex findings.

The basic neuronal pathways for ipsilateral and contralateral acoustic stapedius reflexes have been reconfigured as Figure 6–6. We will use this basic block diagram as a means of illustrating the basis for acoustic reflex findings in various disorders. The primary structures involved in both ipsilateral and contralateral neuronal pathways for right and left ears are included in Figure 6–6. As detailed earlier, the ipsilateral acoustic reflex pathway for each ear ascends through the cochlea, Cranial Nerve (N.) VIII, and the ventral cochlear nucleus. The primary pathway includes an ascending tract to the superior olivary complex on the same side; a smaller, less dense fiber tract bypasses the superior olivary complex and descends directly from the ventral cochlear nucleus to the facial motor nucleus. The descending portion of the ipsilateral acoustic reflex arc, beginning at the output of either the superior olivary complex or the ventral cochlear nucleus, involves the facial motor nucleus, the motor branch of Cranial N. VII and the stapedius muscle on the same side. The contralateral acoustic reflex pathway crosses from one side to the other at the level of the superior olivary complex and involves the ascending system (cochlea, Cranial N. VIII and ventral cochlear nucleus) for the stimulus or activator ear and the superior olivary complex and descending (efferent) system (facial motor nucleus, Cranial N. VII and stapedius) for the probe ear.

It is important to note that the middle ear transmission system is integral to both ascending and descending pathways. Any significant conductive hearing loss, for example, will potentially attenuate the level of an activating signal to a level insufficient for producing an acoustic reflex. Also, any disorder that compromises the function of the middle ear transmission system may also compromise measures of acoustic immittance changes indicative of stapedial reflexes in the probe ear. Finally, it should be understood that the possible clinical outcomes for reflex measures are numerous, depending on the number, size, extent, and location of pathologies (see Wiley & Block, 1984). As noted earlier, our basic discussions here are limited to discrete, single-entity lesions for purposes of illustration. In each disorder section, we present expected acoustic reflex findings under specific conditions followed by selected case examples for discrete abnormalities. Throughout the discussions, we have used terminology consistent with the current ANSI standard on acoustic immittance measures (ANSI, 1987). Specific to contralateral acoustic reflex measures, ANSI terminology references contralateral reflex measures to the ear receiving the activating signal (stimulus ear), not to the ear containing the acoustic immittance probe.

Middle Ear Disorders

Typically, acoustic reflexes are absent in cases of middle ear pathology. This general rule, however, needs to be applied individually for each ear. *In cases of bilateral middle ear pathology, acoustic reflexes are typically absent for ipsilateral and contralateral activating signals in both ears.* The middle ear disorder in each ear prohibits the examiner from observing acoustic immittance changes reflective of stapedial contractions. This situation is illustrated in Figure 6–7. Recall that, in the case of ipsilateral acoustic reflex measures, the activator (stimulus) and probe signals are presented to the same ear. Consider the case of bilateral otitis media with effusion. Here, the liquid in the middle ear cavity stiffens the middle ear transmission system. Even if the pre-

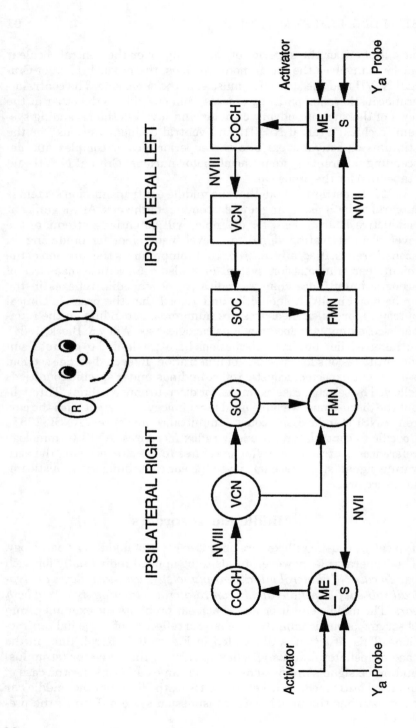

IPSILATERAL LEFT

IPSILATERAL RIGHT

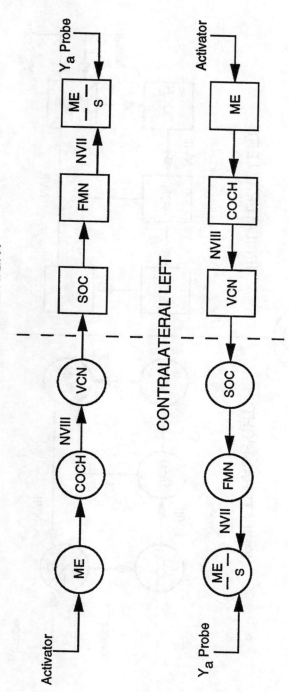

FIGURE 6–6. A block diagram showing the primary neuronal pathways for ipsilateral (uncrossed) and contralateral (crossed) acoustic reflexes. Separate diagrams of both ipsilateral and contralateral pathways are included for the right and left ears. Circles are used to indicate structures for the right ear and squares represent companion structures for the left ear. The key for abbreviations is as follows: COCH: cochlea, ME: middle ear, VCN: ventral cochlear nucleus, SOC: superior olivary complex, FMN: facial motor nucleus, NVIII: cranial nerve eight (auditory), NVII: cranial nerve seven (facial), S: stapedius muscle. The solid and dotted vertical lines indicate the division and crossover point for structures on the right and left sides of the head.

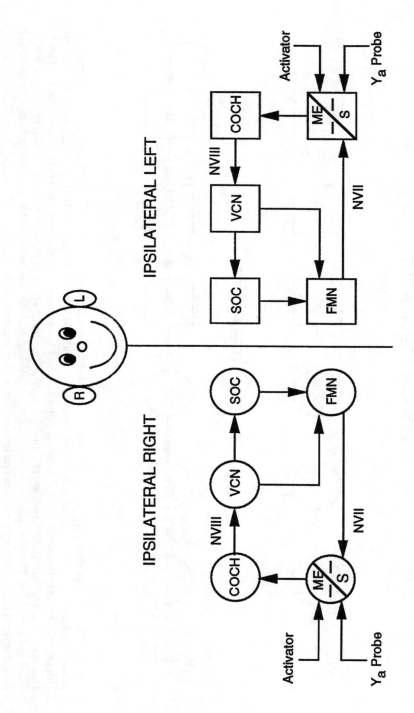

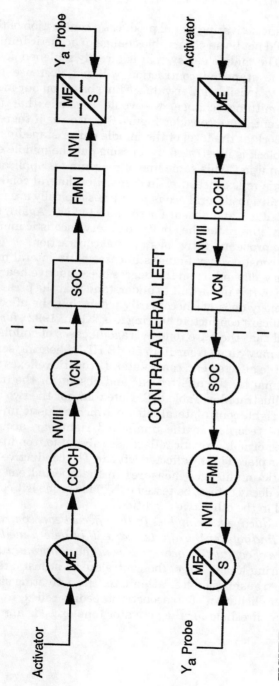

FIGURE 6–7. A block diagram showing the neuronal pathways for ipsilateral (uncrossed) and contralateral (crossed) acoustic reflexes that are affected in the case of bilateral otitis media with effusion. Separate diagrams of both ipsilateral and contralateral pathways are included for the right and left ears. Circles are used to indicate structures for the right ear and squares represent companion structures for the left ear. The key for abbreviations is as follows: COCH: cochlea, ME: middle ear, VCN: ventral cochlear nucleus, SOC: superior olivary complex, FMN: facial motor nucleus, NVIII: cranial nerve eight (auditory), NVII: cranial nerve seven (facial), S: stapedius muscle. The solid and dotted vertical lines indicate the division and crossover point for structures on the right and left sides of the head. The affected portions of the neuronal pathways (both middle ears) are indicated with a diagonal line drawn through the affected structures.

95

sentation of an acoustic activating signal produces a contraction of the stapedius, there would not be an observable change in acoustic immittance at the probe. The middle ear system is already stiffened sufficiently such that the stapedial contraction will not decrease the acoustic admittance to a visibly lower value. Thus, based on our measure of acoustic immittance change, we would conclude that the acoustic reflex is absent. If we consider Figure 6–7, it is as if there is an interruption or block at the level of the middle ear or stapedius in the probe ear. This block is illustrated by crossing out the middle ear in each probe ear condition. This same line of reasoning is applicable for ipsilateral acoustic reflex measures in cases of unilateral conductive lesions. Specifically, ipsilateral acoustic reflexes typically are normal for the unaffected ear and absent for the affected ear. Again, the middle ear pathology eliminates the ability to observe acoustic immittance changes at the probe indicative of stapedial contraction.

Contralateral acoustic reflex findings in cases of unilateral middle ear disorders vary, depending on the degree of conductive hearing loss in the affected ear. It is important to understand that the presence of middle ear pathology does not necessarily mean that the affected ear will have a significant conductive hearing loss. Klein (1992), for example, has reported that the pure tone average in cases of childhood middle-ear effusion may range from 10 to 50 dB HL. If hearing sensitivity is normal for the affected ear, contralateral acoustic reflexes will be present and normal for the affected ear and absent for the unaffected ear. This is illustrated in Table 6–2. Note that, for the two conditions (ipsilateral right, contralateral left) in which acoustic immittance measures are recorded in the unaffected right ear, acoustic reflex measures are normal. Acoustic reflexes are absent for conditions in which the probe is placed in the affected left ear. The conductive disorder blocks acoustic immittance measures in the affected ear (see Figure 6–8). Reflex decay cannot be tested (CNT) for probe left conditions and is normal in the other two conditions.

If there is a conductive hearing loss in the affected ear, contralateral acoustic reflex findings for the affected ear will be determined primarily by the degree of conductive hearing loss in the abnormal ear. If the conductive hearing loss is large, the contralateral acoustic reflex will be absent. The transmission loss attenuates the activating signal to a level too low for elicitation of an acoustic stapedius reflex. In general, if the auditory threshold for the activator tone exceeds approxi-

Table 6–2. Acoustic reflex findings in a case of unilateral conductive disorder with normal hearing in the affected left ear. In this case example, the right ear presents with normal hearing and normal middle ear function.

Acoustic Reflex Thresholds (dB HL)

Frequency	Ipsilateral R	Ipsilateral L	Contralateral R	Contralateral L
500 Hz	Normal	Absent	Absent	Normal
1000 Hz	Normal	Absent	Absent	Normal
2000 Hz	Normal	Absent	Absent	Normal
4000 Hz	Normal	Absent	Absent	Normal
Reflex Decay @ 500 and/or 1000Hz	Normal	CNT	CNT	Normal

mately 35 dB HL, contralateral acoustic reflexes will be absent. If audiometric thresholds for the activator tone are less than 35 dB HL, the contralateral acoustic reflex may be present, but the reflex threshold will be elevated in proportion to the degree of conductive hearing loss. In general, the elevation in acoustic reflex threshold will correspond to the degree of conductive hearing loss.

There is at least one noteworthy exception to the general findings noted above. In selected cases of unilateral ossicular discontinuity, acoustic reflexes may be present with the probe in the affected ear. Specifically, if the unilateral ossicular discontinuity is proximal to the stapes (e.g., the stapes crura are fractured or interrupted), contralateral acoustic reflexes may be present for the condition in which the activator is presented to the opposite ear and acoustic immittance changes are recorded in the affected ear. The remaining continuity between the stapedial tendon and the rest of the ossicular chain in the affected ear provides sufficient connection for observation of acoustic reflexes. Indeed, because the stapes footplate no longer anchors the middle ear system in such cases, the amplitude of acoustic immittance changes indicative of acoustic reflexes may be larger than normal for the affected ear.

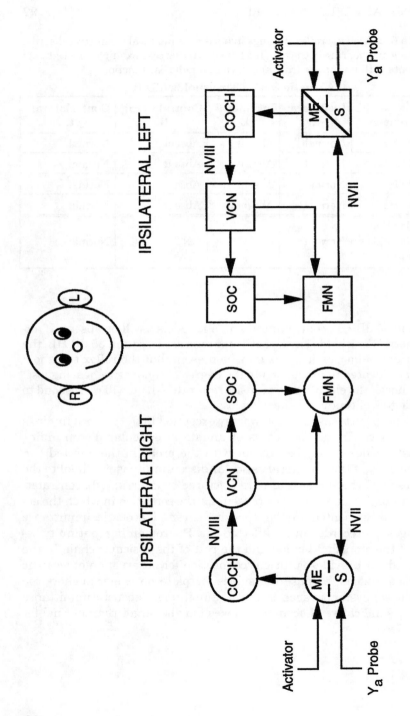

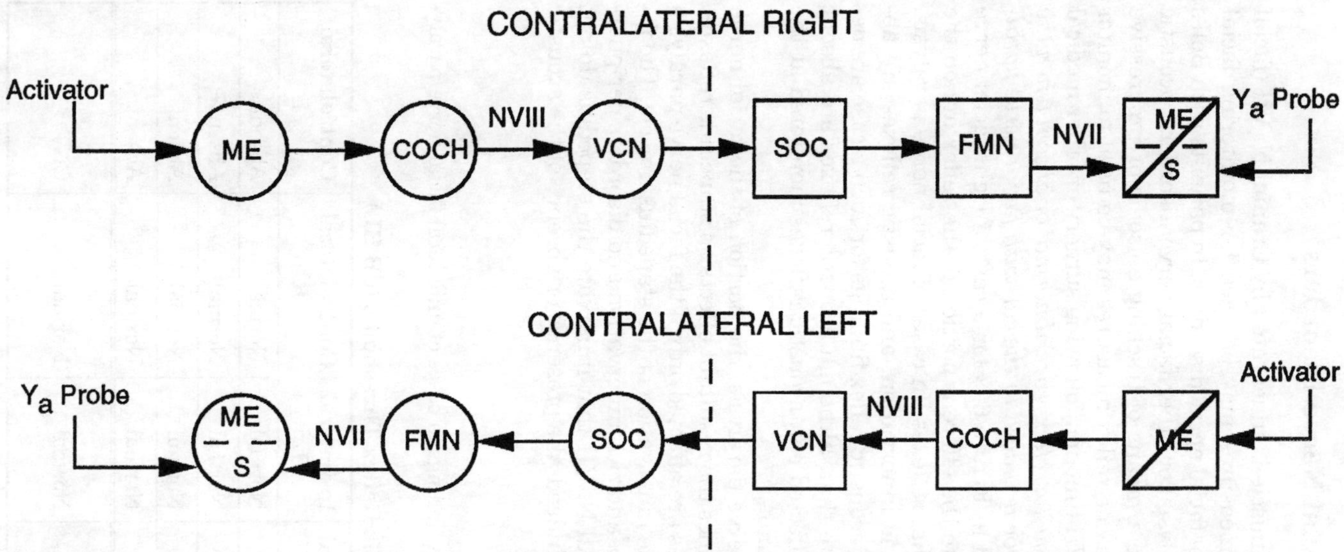

FIGURE 6–8. A block diagram showing the neuronal pathways for ipsilateral (uncrossed) and contralateral (crossed) acoustic reflexes that are affected in a case of a unilateral conductive disorder with normal hearing in the affected left ear. In this example, the right ear presents with normal hearing and normal middle ear function. Separate diagrams of both ipsilateral and contralateral pathways are included for the right and left ears. Circles are used to indicate structures for the right ear and squares represent companion structures for the left ear. The key for abbreviations is as follows: COCH: cochlea, ME: middle ear, VCN: ventral cochlear nucleus, SOC: superior olivary complex, FMN: facial motor nucleus, NVII: cranial nerve eight (auditory), NVII: cranial nerve seven (facial), S: stapedius muscle. The solid and dotted vertical lines indicate the division and crossover point for structures on the right and left sides of the head. The affected portion of the neuronal pathways (left middle ear) is indicated with a diagonal line drawn through the affected structure.

Facial Nerve Disorders

Because the stapedius muscle is innervated by Cranial N. VII (facial nerve), acoustic reflex measures may be used for monitoring facial nerve function in cases of facial nerve disorders. In patients with Bell's palsy (facial nerve paralysis) or other facial nerve disorders, acoustic reflex measures provide a means of tracking episodic or progressive disease processes. The same reflex measures may be used to monitor recovery of Cranial N. VII function following surgery or other medical treatment. *Typically, acoustic reflexes are abnormal or absent when the acoustic immittance probe is placed in the ear with facial nerve paralysis*. This is exemplified in Figure 6–9 for a case of right facial nerve paralysis. Here, insult to the efferent portion of the reflex arc on the right side blocks stapedial reflexes. In cases of facial nerve paralysis, the stapedius receives no innervation, and acoustic reflexes are absent. The full pattern of acoustic reflex findings for such a case are detailed in Table 6–3. Note that, although acoustic reflexes are absent with the probe in the affected ear, acoustic reflexes monitored at the unaffected side are normal.

In cases of facial nerve paralysis, the portion of the facial nerve that is involved determines the resultant effects on stapedius reflexes. Acoustic reflex responses are affected only if the facial nerve paralysis or insult is central to the innervation of the stapedius muscle. The facial nerve has a complex and rich innervation and disorders peripheral to branches of Cranial N. VII that innervate the stapedius do not alter acoustic reflexes. Indeed, the presence or absence of the acoustic

Table 6–3. Acoustic reflex findings in cases of unilateral facial nerve paralysis on the right side.

Acoustic Reflex Thresholds (dB HL)

Frequency	Ipsilateral R	Ipsilateral L	Contralateral R	Contralateral L
500 Hz	Absent	Normal	Normal	Absent
1000 Hz	Absent	Normal	Normal	Absent
2000 Hz	Absent	Normal	Normal	Absent
4000 Hz	Absent	Normal	Normal	Absent
Reflex Decay @ 500 and/or 1000Hz	CNT	Normal	Normal	CNT

stapedius reflex may be useful in determining the site of facial nerve insult.

Cochlear Disorders

Acoustic reflex thresholds in ears with cochlear disorders are determined primarily by the degree of the presenting sensorineural hearing loss. As noted earlier, if auditory thresholds for the stimulus (activator) ear are below 50 or 55 dB HL, acoustic reflex thresholds usually are normal. On the other end, if audiometric hearing levels exceed 80 dB HL, the likelihood of acoustic reflexes being observed is low. For audiometric thresholds between 50 and 80 dB HL, the acoustic reflex thresholds will be elevated in direct proportion to the elevation in hearing (audiometric) thresholds. Specifically, higher auditory thresholds in dB HL are associated with higher acoustic reflex thresholds.

In cases of cochlear disorders for which acoustic reflex decay can be measured, reflex adaptation *may or may not* be observed. It is not unusual to observe acoustic reflex decay in patients with disorders of cochlear origin. Further, it is hard to predict the presence and characteristics of reflex decay from the threshold audiogram. *Generally, if reflex decay is present for patients with cochlear disorders, (a) the amount of reflex decay will be less than that observed for patients with eighth nerve lesions, and (b) the rate of reflex decay will be slower in cochlear disorders than in cases of eighth nerve disorders* (Cartwright & Lilly, 1976).

In patients with severe sensorineural hearing loss, it may be difficult to distinguish diagnostically disorders of cochlear and eighth nerve origin strictly on the basis of acoustic reflex findings. This dilemma will be clarified in the next section. Here, we simply note that acoustic reflex responses in both cases may be absent or there may be elevated acoustic reflex thresholds and abnormal reflex decay (Olsen et al., 1975).

Table 6–4 presents acoustic reflex measures in an exemplary case of bilateral cochlear disorder. In this particular example, there is a sensorineural hearing loss of similar degree in both ears, with the pure tone average for both ears being 70 dB HL. As indicated in Figure 6–10, both cochleas are abnormal. Effectively, the cochlear disorder results in less transmission of neural impulses to higher reflex centers on both sides. Acoustic reflex thresholds are elevated (higher than normal) for all activator frequencies, consistent with the cochlear disorder and associated sensorineural hearing loss. Also noted in Table 6–4, abnormal acoustic reflex decay may or may not be observed in such cases.

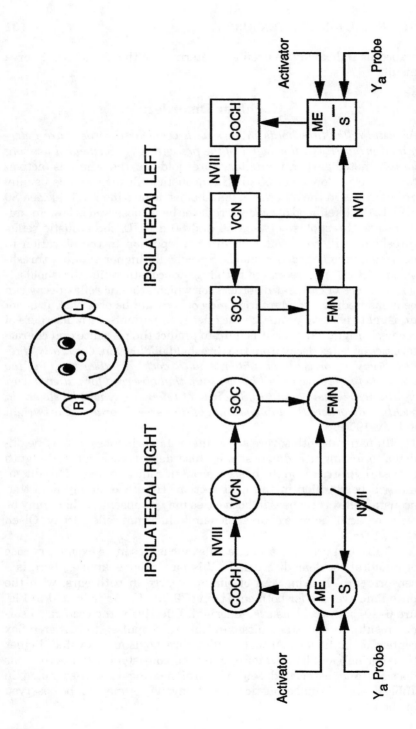

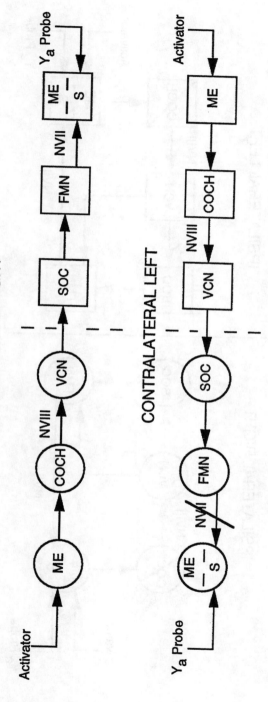

Figure 6-9. A block diagram showing the neuronal pathways for ipsilateral (uncrossed) and contralateral (crossed) acoustic reflexes that are affected in a case of unilateral facial nerve paralysis on the right side. Separate diagrams of both ipsilateral and contralateral pathways are included for the right and left ears. Circles are used to indicate structures for the left ear and squares represent companion structures for the right ear. The key for abbreviations is as follows: COCH: cochlea, ME: middle ear, VCN: ventral cochlear nucleus, SOC: superior olivary complex, FMN: facial motor nucleus, NVIII: cranial nerve eight (auditory), NVII: cranial nerve seven (facial), S: stapedius muscle. The solid and dotted vertical lines indicate the division and crossover point for structures on the right and left sides of the head. The affected portion of the neuronal pathways (right facial nerve, NVII) is indicated with a diagonal line drawn through the affected structure.

103

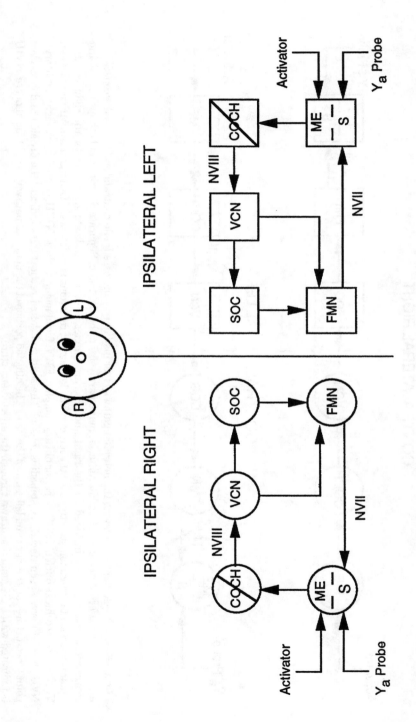

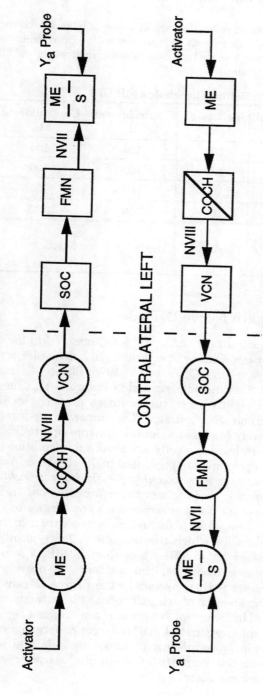

Figure 6–10. A block diagram showing the neuronal pathways for ipsilateral (uncrossed) and contralateral (crossed) acoustic reflexes that are affected in a case of a bilateral cochlear disorder. Separate diagrams of both ipsilateral and contralateral pathways are included for the right and left ears. Circles are used to indicate structures for the right ear and squares represent companion structures for the left ear. The key for abbreviations is as follows: COCH: cochlea, ME: middle ear, VCN: ventral cochlear nucleus, SOC: superior olivary complex, FMN: facial motor nucleus, NVIII: cranial nerve eight (auditory), NVII: cranial nerve seven (facial), S: stapedius muscle. The solid and dotted vertical lines indicate the division and crossover point for structures on the right and left sides of the head. The affected portions of the neuronal pathways (both cochleas) are indicated with a diagonal line drawn through the affected structures.

Table 6–4. Exemplary acoustic reflex findings in a case of bilateral cochlear disorder. Audiometric thresholds in both ears present with a pure tone average of 70 dB HL. The hearing loss for both ears is sensorineural and middle ear function is normal bilaterally.

Acoustic Reflex Thresholds (dB HL)

Frequency	Ipsilateral R	Ipsilateral L	Contralateral R	Contralateral L
500 Hz	100	100	100	100
1000 Hz	100	100	100	100
2000 Hz	100	100	100	100
4000 Hz	100	100	100	100
Reflex Decay @ 500 and/or 1000Hz	Maybe	Maybe	Maybe	Maybe

Eighth Nerve Disorders

An absent acoustic reflex with activating signals presented to the affected ear is the most typical finding in eighth-nerve lesions (Jerger et al., 1974; Jerger & Hayes, 1980; Olsen et al., 1975; Sheehy & Inzer, 1976). The basis for this finding is illustrated in Figure 6–11. The example shown is for an eighth nerve tumor (more properly termed *vestibular schwannoma*) on the right side. The tumor at the level of the eighth nerve effectively blocks any neural transmission to higher centers. Thus, acoustic reflexes typically are absent for conditions in which acoustic activating signals are presented to the right ear. *A cardinal diagnostic sign that separates acoustic reflex findings in cochlear and eighth nerve disorders is that the acoustic reflex commonly is absent in cases of eighth nerve disorders regardless of the degree of presenting sensorineural hearing loss.* This finding is in contrast to findings in cochlear disorders for which the acoustic reflex typically is present for hearing losses having HLs less than 80 dB. For both cochlear and eighth nerve disorders, the incidence of observable acoustic reflexes decreases with increases in the degree of sensorineural hearing loss. The absence of acoustic reflexes in patients with little or no sensorineural hearing loss, however, is a significant sign for eighth-nerve involvement (Jerger et al., 1974; Jerger & Jerger, 1981). This finding is particularly significant in cases of unilateral sensorineural hearing loss; the majority of vestibular schwannomas (eighth nerve tumors) are unilateral.

In cases of eighth nerve lesions for which the acoustic reflex is present, acoustic reflex thresholds typically are elevated compared to those for normals and abnormal acoustic reflex decay is usually always observed . Again, in contrast to findings in cochlear disorders, acoustic reflex thresholds in cases of eighth nerve disorders typically are elevated irrespective of the degree of sensorineural hearing loss. In patients with a unilateral sensorineural hearing loss and audiometric thresholds that are better (less) than 50–55 dB HL, for example, acoustic reflexes will be absent or reflex thresholds will be elevated in cases of eighth nerve disorders. If the same presenting hearing loss is cochlear in origin, the acoustic reflex thresholds typically will be normal.

If acoustic reflexes are present and the acoustic reflex threshold is low enough to permit measurement of acoustic reflex decay, *rapid reflex decay typically is observed in cases of eighth nerve disorders*. Reflex half lives less than 5 seconds for 500 and 1000 Hz tonal activators are often observed. In contrast, if acoustic reflex decay is observed in cases of cochlear disorders, the rate of reflex decay typically is much slower than that observed for cases of eighth nerve involvement. These differences in reflex decay patterns are illustrated in Figure 6–12 taken from the work of Cartwright and Lilly (1976). Cartwright and Lilly reported that the incidence of abnormal acoustic reflex decay was much higher for patients having eighth nerve disorders than for patients having cochlear disorders. As illustrated in Figure 6–12, they also observed that the rate of acoustic reflex decay was considerably more rapid in cases of eighth nerve disorder than for patients with a cochlear disorder (Ménière's disease).

Acoustic reflex findings in an exemplary case of a right vestibular schwannoma are displayed in Table 6–5. Audiometric thresholds in the same patient also are provided. These findings are taken from the report of Wiley and Block (1984). As expected, acoustic reflex findings are normal for conditions in which the activating signal is presented to the normal left ear (ipsilateral left and contralateral left). In contrast, only one condition in which an activator was presented to the right ear resulted in an acoustic reflex. Even in this one condition (contralateral right at 500 Hz), the observed acoustic reflex threshold was elevated relative to expected levels for patients with cochlear disorders and the same degree of sensorineural hearing loss. Given the audiometric threshold of 45 dB HL at 500 Hz, the elevated acoustic reflex threshold is significant for eighth nerve involvement. If the disorder had been cochlear in origin, a normal acoustic reflex threshold would have been expected given the audiometric threshold. Overall, the pattern of absent acoustic reflexes for most activator conditions and an elevated

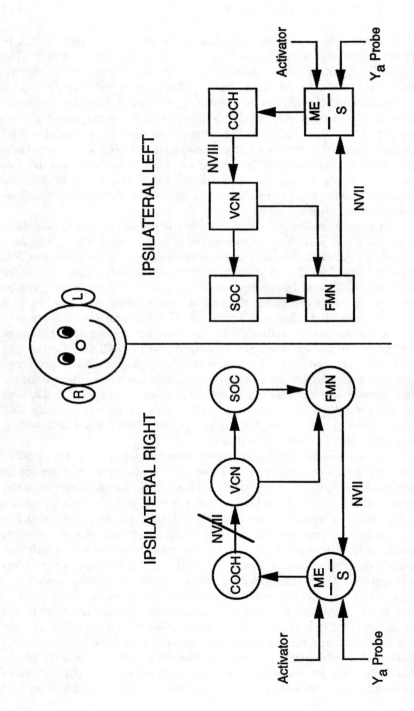

IPSILATERAL LEFT

IPSILATERAL RIGHT

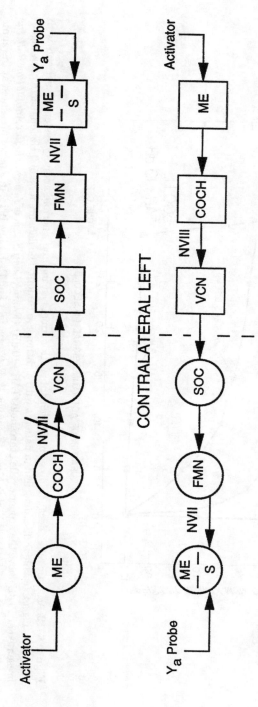

Figure 6–11. A block diagram showing the neuronal pathways for ipsilateral (uncrossed) and contralateral (crossed) acoustic reflexes that are affected in a case of a vestibular schwannoma (eighth nerve tumor) on the right side. Separate diagrams of both ipsilateral and contralateral pathways are included for the right and left ears. Circles are used to indicate structures for the right ear and squares represent companion structures for the left ear. The key for abbreviations is as follows: COCH: cochlea, ME: middle ear, VCN: ventral cochlear nucleus, SOC: superior olivary nucleus, FMN: facial motor nucleus, NVIII: cranial nerve eight (auditory), NVII: cranial nerve seven (facial), S: stapedius muscle. The solid and dotted vertical lines indicate the division and crossover point for structures on the right and left sides of the head. The affected portion of the neuronal pathways (right eighth nerve, N VIII) is indicated with a diagonal line drawn through the affected structure.

109

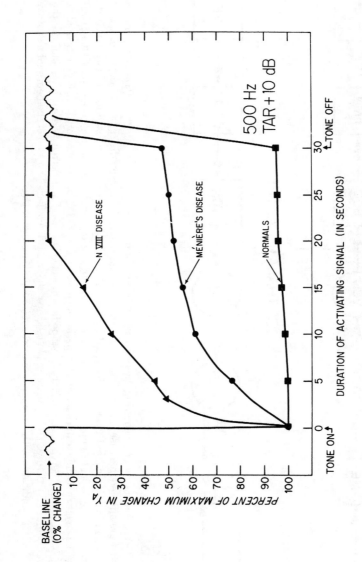

Figure 6-12. Acoustic reflex decay findings in participants with normal hearing and a normal auditory system, in patients with Ménière's disease (cochlear disorder), and in patients with eighth nerve tumors. The data are for a 500 Hz tonal activating signal presented at 10 dB above the acoustic reflex threshold (TAR +10 dB). (From *A Comparison of Acoustic Reflex Adaptation Patterns for Patients with Cochlear and Eighth Nerve Disease* by W. R. Cartwright and D. J. Lilly, 1976, in a paper presented at the annual convention of the American Speech-Language-Hearing Association. Reprinted with the authors' permission.)

Table 6–5. Audiometric thresholds and acoustic reflex findings in a case of right vestibular schwannoma. The hearing loss for the right ear was sensorineural. The case presented is taken from the report of Wiley and Block (1984).

Air Conduction Auditory (Hearing) Thresholds (dB HL)

Frequency	Right Ear	Left Ear
500 Hz	45	10
1000 Hz	65	10
2000 Hz	65	5
4000 Hz	55	20

Acoustic Reflex Thresholds (dB HL)

Frequency	Ipsilateral R	Ipsilateral L	Contralateral R	Contralateral L
500 Hz	Absent	Normal	110	Normal
1000 Hz	Absent	Normal	Absent	Normal
2000 Hz	Absent	Normal	Absent	Normal
Reflex Decay @ 500 and/or 1000Hz	CNT	Normal	CNT	Normal

acoustic reflex at 500 Hz relative to the obtained audiometric threshold support the surgically confirmed diagnosis of a right vestibular schwannoma. In particular, the absence of acoustic reflexes and elevated acoustic reflex threshold are noteworthy given the degree of sensorineural hearing loss for the right ear. If the disorder had been cochlear in origin, one would have expected acoustic reflexes to be present at all activator frequencies, and the acoustic reflex threshold at 500 Hz should have approximated normal levels.

An important diagnostic goal in cases of unilateral sensorineural hearing loss is the differentiation of cochlear and eighth nerve disorders. In general, acoustic reflex findings that are significant for eighth nerve disorder are (a) absent acoustic reflexes in the presence of little or no sensorineural hearing loss, (b) acoustic reflex thresholds disproportionately elevated relative to audiometric thresholds for the same signals, and (c) substantial and rapid acoustic reflex decay. The increased *rate* of acoustic reflex decay in cases of eighth nerve disorders relative to that observed in cochlear disorders is an important diagnostic sign with regard to reflex decay measures.

Central (Brainstem) Disorders

Portions of the neuronal pathways of the acoustic stapedius reflex involve lower parts of the *central* auditory nervous system. The input to the cochlear nucleus is often defined as the inferior border of the central auditory pathways. The collective structures inferior to the cochlear nucleus are referred to as the *peripheral* auditory system. Central auditory pathologies that are proximal to the brainstem may manifest themselves in abnormal acoustic reflex patterns. Evaluation of audiometric and acoustic reflex measures in patients with suspected central disorders may enable diagnostic differentiation of central and peripheral disorders. At the outset of this discussion, however, it is important to note that acoustic reflex measures are restricted to the brainstem portion of the central auditory nervous system. Central disorders above the brainstem have no effect on acoustic stapedius function. Patients with cortical lesions, for example, typically present with normal acoustic reflex measures.

As a general pattern of findings, *patients with brainstem disorders often demonstrate normal ipsilateral acoustic reflexes and some abnormality in contralateral acoustic reflex measures.* The crossed portions of the reflex arc at the level of the superior olivary complex are primarily affected (see Figure 6–6). The secondary ipsilateral pathway from the ventral cochlear nucleus to the facial motor nucleus means that a patient with a lesion to portions of the ventral cochlear nucleus and superior olivary complex may demonstrate normal ipsilateral acoustic reflexes on both sides. Only the crossed, contralateral acoustic reflex may be abnormal.

The generality of these findings and the exact pattern of acoustic reflex results for ipsilateral and contralateral activating signals, however, may vary greatly depending on the exact site and size of brainstem disorder. A larger tumor originating in the brainstem, for example, may impinge on more peripheral structures (e.g., eighth nerve) and may then influence ipsilateral acoustic reflexes as well as contralateral reflexes. Thus, larger or more diffuse brainstem disorders may offer acoustic reflex patterns that resemble those for more peripheral disorders. Further, there are reported cases of combined lesions or insult to both peripheral and central portions of the auditory system. In these cases, the general rule of abnormal crossed or contralateral acoustic reflexes will not hold, and there is the potential for numerous combinations of outcomes for ipsilateral and contralateral acoustic reflex measures.

As a general rule, a brainstem lesion may be suspected when contralateral acoustic reflexes are absent in the presence of normal hearing sensitivity and normal middle ear function. Given the complexities in the neuronal structure of the central auditory nervous system and the possibilities for multiple lesion sites or multiple functional influences of a single lesion, however, further evaluation typically is warranted. In addition to neurologic and radiologic studies, further audiologic studies (e.g., evoked potential measures) sensitive to both eighth nerve disorders and central auditory disorders are performed. In the identification of a central site of pathology, the diagnostic process often is one of attempting to rule out a peripheral site

DISCUSSION ITEMS FOR SELF-STUDY

1. Describe the arrangement of probe and activating signals in each ear for ipsilateral and contralateral acoustic reflex measures. What is meant by stimulus and probe ear in the case of contralateral reflex measures?
2. Why are acoustic reflex decay measures typically performed only at 500 and 1000 Hz in clinical practice?
3. For each of the following clinical cases, describe the expected profile of present and absent acoustic reflexes (both ipsilateral and contralateral) for a 1000 Hz tonal activator:

   bilateral serous otitis media

   left facial nerve paralysis

   right vestibular schwannoma

SUGGESTED EXERCISES FOR SELF-STUDY

1. Commit the ipsilateral and contralateral acoustic reflex pathways to memory (see Figures 6–2 and 6–3). As a self-study test, sketch the ipsilateral and contralateral pathways for one ear. Compare your sketch with Figures 6–2 and 6–3 for accuracy.
2. Measure contralateral acoustic reflex thresholds for tonal activators. Select a participant (e.g., a colleague) who reportedly has normal hearing and normal middle ear function. The acoustic-immittance probe unit should be placed in the left ear and the reflex

activating signals will be presented in the right ear. Set the pressure in the external auditory meatus at 0 daPa. Beginning at 65 dB HL at 1000 Hz, use an ascending technique (in 5 dB steps) to determine the reflex threshold. *Do not exceed an activator level of 105 dB HL.* Repeat the procedure for reflex activators of 500, 2000, and 4000 Hz. Compare your reflex thresholds with those presented in Table 6–1 for young adults with normal hearing and normal middle-ear function.

3. In the same participant as for Exercise 2, measure acoustic reflex decay for a 500 and a 2000 Hz tone at 10 dB above acoustic reflex threshold. *Do not exceed an activator level of 105 dB HL.* Use a 226-Hz probe signal and a contralateral reflex mode. The acoustic immittance probe unit should be placed in the left ear and the reflex activating signals will be presented in the right ear. Set the pressure in the external auditory meatus at 0 daPa. Record reflex decay for a period of 30 seconds. Compute (if possible) reflex half life for your reflex tracing and compare it with data for subjects with a normal auditory system and with data for subjects with cochlear and eighth nerve lesions. (See data from Cartwright & Lilly, Figure 6–12.).

7

Screening Applications

The high prevalence of otitis media in young children has led to the development of screening protocols that include middle ear function as a target of the screening assessment. As noted in the topic overview (Chapter 1), acoustic immittance measures offer a more sensitive index of middle ear function than audiometry or other clinical assessment devices. Our purpose here is to review the bases for middle ear screening and the use of acoustic immittance measures in screening for middle ear disorders. The emphasis is on middle ear screening in preschool and school-age children because middle ear disorders are most prevalent in these age groups. The principles of middle ear screening and some of the specific screening measures discussed, however, are relevant to middle ear screening in all age groups. Screening for middle ear function and hearing impairment in newborns presents a number of unique concerns and is treated as an independent section at the end of the chapter.

RATIONALE FOR MIDDLE EAR SCREENING

Otitis media is a prevalent disorder of childhood and is the most common ear disorder in preschool children (Bluestone, 1978; Klein, 1978).

The greatest prevalence of childhood otitis media is found in children under 5 years of age (Schappert, 1992). Although there is some disagreement about the justification for universal middle ear screening, most sources agree that the potential complications and possible sequelae of otitis media represent significant health problems if the disorder is not detected and treated in developing children. Further, otitis media with associated hearing loss may result in significant auditory, linguistic, educational, and psychosocial complications for affected children. In particular, undetected and untreated otitis media may lead to long-standing deficits in speech production, language development, and learning for selected children. In summary, the high prevalence of otitis media in children and the potential medical, auditory, and developmental complications of the disorder warrant identification of potentially affected children as early as possible. Cases identified early in the disease process may be treated medically, and the potential adverse complications may be avoided. The rationale for middle ear screening in children also is based, in part, on the fact that, in early stages of the disease process, many cases of otitis media offer few, if any, clinical symptoms. Thus, without screening programs, these cases would go undetected and untreated. Accordingly, many communities, clinics, and public schools have developed screening programs for the early detection of middle ear disorders.

RATIONALE FOR ACOUSTIC IMMITTANCE MEASURES IN MIDDLE EAR SCREENING

The sensitivity of acoustic immittance measures in screening for middle ear disorders forms the basic rationale for the use of such measures in screening protocols. In contrast, audiometry is relatively ineffective in identifying children with middle ear disease. As an historical example, the Pittsburgh study in the 1960s demonstrated that a majority of children with active middle ear disease had little or no hearing loss (see Eagles, 1972). Over the past 25 years or so, numerous research reports have documented the increased efficacy of tympanometry and associated acoustic immittance measures in screening for middle ear disorders (Brooks, 1973, 1978a, 1978b, 1978c; Liden & Renvall, 1980; Paradise, Smith, & Bluestone, 1976). These findings have led to the use of both audiometry and acoustic immittance measures in screening programs designed to identify children with hearing loss and middle ear disorders, respectively.

ACOUSTIC IMMITTANCE
MEASURES IN SCREENING

Several tympanometric measures have been used in middle ear screening protocols, including peak compensated static acoustic susceptance (B_{tm}) peak compensated static acoustic admittance (Y_{tm}), tympanogram width (TW), equivalent ear canal volume (V_{ea}), tympanogram peak pressure (TPP), tympanometric gradient, and tympanogram shape (ASHA, 1979, 1990; Brooks, 1978b; Holmberg, Axelsson, Hansson, & Renvall, 1986; Liden & Renvall, 1978; Paradise et al., 1976; Roush & Tait, 1985). These measures were defined and described in Chapter 4. Based on laboratory research and on field studies in children with middle ear disorders, only selected tympanometric measures have proven effective in screening programs, and current protocols are typically restricted to these few measures.

As noted earlier in the section on tympanometry (Chapter 4), ambiguity in the interpretation of tympanograms based on various shape classification systems is a notable limitation in the clinical application of tympanometric measures. Certainly, the significance of a flat tympanogram is still relevant. Other than this particular tympanogram type, however, shape classifications alone are no longer recommended as a basis for decision making in middle ear screening. A primary problem with the use of tympanogram shapes is that the tympanograms were expressed in arbitrary units that compromise direct comparisons across clinics and data sets (Wiley & Block, 1979; Wiley, Oviatt, & Block, 1987). More recent studies and contemporary screening protocols have incorporated measures expressed in standard variables and units that can be compared from clinic to clinic.

Other measures also are no longer recommended in middle ear screening protocols. The computation of tympanogram gradient basically provides essentially the same information as that derived from compensated static acoustic immittance measures. Thus, compensated measures based on normative data have displaced tympanogram gradient in contemporary screening protocols. Tympanogram peak pressure (TPP) is still used in selected diagnostic applications (e.g., Eustachian tube function), but the extreme variability in the measure and the substantial overlap in the measure for normal and pathologic ears has resulted in the omission of the measure in screening protocols (ASHA, 1990, 1997). Most commercially available screening instruments now provide only a single component measure, typically acoustic admittance. Thus, component screening measures (e.g., B_{tm}) are not used in most current screening protocols.

Current protocols for middle ear screening generally are based on some combination of the three following basic measures: (1) compensated static acoustic admittance, (2) equivalent ear canal volume, and (3) tympanogram width. These measures are derived from an acoustic admittance tympanogram for a low-frequency (typically 226 Hz) probe tone. These basic measures formed the middle ear screening protocol recommended in the 1990 ASHA screening guidelines and also are basic to the 1997 ASHA recommendations for middle ear screening in children. Research findings for these basic measures were recently reviewed by Wiley and Smith (1995). The new ASHA (1997) Guidelines for Audiologic Screening also provide useful background on the rationale for using these measures in screening programs.

Compensated Static Acoustic Admittance

Most screening protocols are aimed at the identification of middle ear disorders that produce an abnormally low compensated static acoustic admittance (Y_{tm}) The reason for this emphasis is that *otitis media is the most common middle ear disorder in children and the most common effect of the disorder is a dampening or stiffening of the middle ear system. Thus, the most likely finding is a reduced Y_{tm}.* An abnormally high Y_{tm} also may be important diagnostically, such as in the diagnosis of ossicular discontinuity, but such disorders are much less common and are not a primary focus of the screening protocol. In the case of Y_{tm} measures in screening, then, the examiner is looking for an abnormally low Y_{tm} value that may be significant for middle ear disorder. As a part of the 1997 ASHA Guidelines for Screening Infants and Children for Outer and Middle Ear Disorders, normal criteria values for Y_{tm} are provided for different age groups. If the measured Y_{tm} value for a particular child falls below the lower limit of normal, middle ear disorder is suspected and the child may need to be referred medically for further evaluation. In the case of Y_{tm} and other measures, the ASHA guidelines offer specific recommendations regarding what criteria should be used in making a decision regarding a medical referral.

Equivalent Ear Canal Volume

As noted in the earlier section on tympanometry, equivalent ear canal volume is represented by the admittance value at the tympanogram tail. Typically, the acoustic admittance value at 200 daPa is taken as the clinical estimate of equivalent ear canal volume. In the case of equivalent ear canal volume, the estimate is expressed in cm^3. A measure of equivalent ear canal volume is valuable clinically in the detection of tympanic membrane perforations and in evaluating the patency of tympanostomy (ventilation) tubes that may have been surgically placed in the tympanic membrane of children with otitis media. The use of equivalent ear canal volume in screening for tympanic membrane perforations is useful because marginal and small perforations are often difficult to view otoscopically in young children. Shanks et al. (1992) reported pre- and postoperative equivalent ear canal volumes in a large clinical sample of children who underwent otic surgery consisting of myringotomy and tympanostomy tube insertion. Based on their database, Shanks et al. provided normative equivalent ear canal volumes that can be used for the detection of tympanic membrane perforations in children and for the determination of tympanostomy tube patency. Specifically *an equivalent ear canal volume greater than 1.0 cm^3 for a child is most likely indicative of a perforated tympanic membrane or patent tympanostomy tube*. The normative data and diagnostic criteria suggested by Shanks et al. (1992) have been recommended by ASHA (1997) for use in middle ear screening programs.

Tympanogram Width

The rationale for using tympanogram width (TW) measures in screening is based on the finding that *TW is often widened in cases of middle ear effusion* (liquid in the middle ear usually resulting from otitis media). Thus, based on normative findings in children of different ages, normal limits have been established for TW values. Children presenting TW values wider than the normal range are suspect for middle ear effusion and may require medical referral. The ASHA (1997) Guidelines provide normal TW limits for different age groups and recommended screening cutoffs for TW. The TW criteria are coupled with Y_{tm} findings in the medical referral process recommended by ASHA.

ACOUSTIC REFLEX MEASURES AND MIDDLE EAR SCREENING

The efficacy of acoustic reflex measures in screening for middle ear disorders has a mixed history. (See Wiley and Smith [1995] for a recent review on the topic.) Dating back to the work of Brooks in the 1970s, there has been evidence documenting the high sensitivity of acoustic reflex measures in the identification of middle ear disorders (see Brooks, 1978b). Based on these findings, an acoustic reflex measure was included as a part of the recommended protocol in the original ASHA Guidelines for Acoustic Immittance Screening for Middle-Ear Function (1979). Subsequent experience with acoustic reflex measures in middle ear screening, however, revealed that the measure presented poor specificity in screening applications. So, although the acoustic reflex measure was sensitive in the identification of children with middle ear disorders, the use of the measure in screening programs resulted in an excessive number of overreferrals (see ASHA, 1990). Based on this reportedly high false positive rate, acoustic reflex measures were excluded from the 1990 and 1997 ASHA guidelines for middle ear screening.

More recent studies suggest that acoustic reflex measures may be both sensitive and specific for the identification of middle ear disorders, particularly when acoustic reflex measures are combined with selected tympanometric measures (Hirsch, Margolis, & Rykken, 1992; Marchant et al., 1986; Silman, Silverman, & Arick, 1992; Smith, Wiley, & Pyle, 1992, 1993). Presently, then, there are contrasting opinions regarding the efficacy of acoustic reflex measures in middle ear screening. One of the primary factors contributing to the uncertainty of using acoustic reflex measures in screening is the limited published research on the efficacy of acoustic reflex measures based on surgical confirmation. Further, past investigations on the topic have differed considerably in terms of the activator signal used, the activator level used as an index of reflex presence or absence, and the criteria used for pass/fail in the screening process (Wiley & Smith, 1995). Additional clinical research is needed to resolve the issue. Dependent on the outcome of such research, acoustic reflex measures may or may not become an integral part of future middle ear screening protocols.

NEWBORN SCREENING AND
MIDDLE EAR FUNCTION

In 1993, the National Institutes of Health (1993) issued a Consensus Statement calling for the universal screening of infants for the purpose of early identification of hearing loss. The intent was to encourage the identification of permanent, congenital hearing loss in order to institute habilitation before the loss caused a signficant delay in the development of speech and language. The NIH statement recommended an initial screen with otoacoustic emissions (OAE) and a follow-up screen with an auditory brainstem response (ABR) test in all infants who failed the OAE screen. Some audiologists (Bess & Paradise, 1994) considered this statement premature for a number of reasons, including the fact that the data on the efficacy of this screening protocol are not yet established. Our concern here is the potential confounding effect that disorders of the middle ear have, predominantly on the OAE measures, but also on the ABR measures.

Tympanometry and Acoustic Reflexes

The identification of middle ear disorders in newborns is difficult, with few data available on the best strategy to use. Tympanometry and acoustic reflexes, however, can be useful. Tympanograms have more complex shapes in newborns than they have in adults, as discussed in Chapter 4. As a result, few data are available on the criteria that should be used to determine if a tympanogram in a given infant is normal. The ASHA (1997) guidelines, for example, do not provide norms for infants under the age of 7 months. Nevertheless, Sprague et al. (1985) tested a series of 53 normal neonates under the age of 130 hours and found that no infant had a flat tympanogram at 220 Hz (Sprague et al., 1985). A flat tympanogram in an infant, therefore, is cause for further concern that a middle ear disorder exists. We need more studies on infants with normal middle ears and on infants with confirmed middle ear disorders in order to identify with confidence abnormalities in their tympanograms. Until then, however, tympanometry is viable option for assessing the middle ear function of infants prior to hearing screening with OAE and ABR measures.

Acoustic reflexes also can be recorded in newborns, as discussed in Chapter 6. In newborns, the acoustic reflex is more likely to be present with a 660 Hz probe than with a 220 Hz probe (McMillan, Bennett, Marchant, & Shurin, 1985; Sprague et al., 1985). In both studies, acoustic reflexes were recorded in up to 80% of the infants with the 660 Hz probe, whereas acoustic reflexes were recorded in under 50% of the infants with a 220 Hz probe. Because the reflex cannot be elicited in all infants, its absence cannot be interpreted as signifying a hearing loss. On the other hand, the presence of the reflex is a strong indication that the infant's peripheral sensitivity is not worse than the level of the reflex activating signal. Further, the presence of the acoustic reflex, and in particular the ipsilateral reflex, is a strong indication that there is not a significant conductive component present.

As part of a screening program, therefore, the recording of tympanometry and acoustic reflexes can provide additional information that is useful in interpreting results from the other screening tools, such as otoacoustic emissions and auditory brainstem responses. It is clear, however, that additional studies are necessary to develop the appropriate normative data, as well as to define the effects of different types of middle ear pathology. Completion of these studies will improve our use of immittance measures in neonates and should also improve the efficacy of our screening programs.

Otoacoustic Emissions

Otoacoustic emissions, originally described by Kemp (1978), are low-level acoustic responses from the outer hair cells that are recorded with a sensitive miniature microphone placed in the ear canal. The emissions are generated by an active process in the normal cochlea (Brownell, 1990). The active process is disrupted by the same agents that cause damage to the outer hair cells. The result is a concomitant cochlear hearing loss and reduction or loss of the OAE. This property makes the OAE useful for identifying cochlear hearing loss.

Two types of emissions, transient and distortion product (Lonsbury-Martin, Whitehead, & Martin, 1991), are gaining increasing favor in hearing screening programs. *Transient evoked otoacoustic emissions* (TEOAE) are elicited using a brief stimulus, most commonly a click, to stimulate the cochlea and record the returning waveform. The response is analyzed in frequency bands to provide an estimate of cochlear function at different frequencies. The *distortion product otoacoustic emission* (DPOAE) is elicited with a pair of stimuli, and the response is actually a third tone, the distortion product, that is produced by the interaction of the stimulus tones. Different combinations of the two tones are used to elicit different distortion products which are used to estimate cochlear function at different frequencies.

The OAEs are attractive responses for newborn screening programs because they are present in ears with normal or near-normal cochlear function and do not require active participation from the patient. The process of recording the emissions requires that a signal is delivered though the ear canal and middle ear to the cochlea where it travels along the basilar membrane to the appropriate place of stimulation. Once the emission is generated, the emission must travel backwards along the basilar membrane and then out through the middle ear and into the external ear canal where it is recorded. Despite the cochlear origin of the responses, the middle ear is traversed twice in the process—once as the stimulus travels to the cochlea and once as the response exits the cochlea. The successful recording of the emissions, therefore, requires an intact middle ear system.

A middle ear disorder can disrupt the recording of the emissions in two ways. First, a conductive hearing loss will decrease the amplitude of the stimulus to the cochlea, possibly enough that the emission cannot be generated. Second, as the emission travels back through the middle ear, the amplitude of the emission may be attenuated by the presence of any middle ear pathology. The condition of the middle ear as measured with tympanometry can provide clues as to the likelihood of an emission being recorded and the reason for the absence of an emission. For example, the application of negative or positive ear canal pressure will decrease the amplitude of the emission for the frequencies below 2000 Hz (Kemp, Ryan, & Bray, 1990; Naeve, Margolis, Levine, & Founier, 1992). Tympanograms indicating negative middle ear pressure, therefore, are associated with the reduction of emission amplitudes in the low frequencies. *Flat tympanograms with large ear canal volumes, consistent with patent PE tubes, are associated with recordable emissions if the middle ear is otherwise healthy* (Prieve, 1992). In contrast, *flat tympanograms with normal middle ear volume, consistent with liquid-filled middle ears, are associated with reduced amplitudes of emissions, and possibly absence of emissions* (Glattke, Pafitis, Commiskey, & Herer, 1995; Prieve, 1992). Even when emissions are present, the presence of the middle ear disorder may alter the frequency characteristics of the stimulus, resulting in emissions that reflect the altered stimulus characteristics (Kemp et al. 1990; Prieve, 1992).

The Auditory Brainstem Response (ABR)

The auditory brainstem response (ABR) (Jewett, 1970; Sohmer & Feinmesser, 1967) is the second objective test that is used in newborn screening (Jacobson & Hall, 1994). The ABR is a sequence of five electrical potentials, labeled with Roman numerals from I to V, that are elicited from the eighth nerve and auditory brainstem with brief signals such as clicks and tone pips. Because these potentials are quite small and are buried in the ongoing electroencephalographic activity, they must be averaged over many sweeps to increase the signal-to-noise ratio so that they can be observed. The recording is noninvasive and requires no active participation from the patient. Electrodes are attached to the scalp and stimuli are presented through earphones. The patient must be quiet during the test, and may be sleeping.

The two main uses for the ABR are to identify lesions along the neural pathways of the auditory system and to estimate auditory thresholds. For identification of neural lesions, waves I–V are used. For estimation of auditory thresholds, only wave V is used because it is robust and is present down to levels near the threshold of hearing. The predominant use of the ABR in newborn screening programs is the estimation of hearing sensitivity. For this purpose, the ABR is elicited at a high stimulus level to identify the sequence of waves, and then the stimulus is dropped to the chosen screening level to determine if wave V is still present. If wave V is present, the peripheral hearing sensitivity is considered adequate; if wave V is absent, the loss exceeds the screening level. As a follow-up measure to screening, ABR can be used to determine actual thresholds by tracing wave V to the visual detection threshold. A disadvantage of the ABR, however, is that when click stimuli are used, only high frequency peripheral sensitivity is tested; no information is provided on low frequency peripheral sensitivity.

In screening programs, the first aim is simply to identify the presence of a hearing loss. The underlying goal, however, is to identify a permanent sensorineural hearing loss rather than a transient conductive loss. Because either type of loss will cause an elevation of wave V thresholds, further testing may be necessary to determine the cause of the loss. Acoustic immittance measures, including both tympanometry and acoustic reflexes, can provide important diagnostic information that will help identify the appropriate cause of the loss. For example, the presence of a normal tympanogram with acoustic reflexes would suggest the problem is more likely to be cochlear, whereas the presence of a flat tympanogram with a normal ear canal volume would suggest a significant middle ear effusion. Once the middle ear disorder is cleared, a repeat of the screen can provide information on the cochlear component of the loss.

The ABR also may be used to determine the cause of the hearing loss if an entire stimulus level function is recorded. This procedure requires measuring the latencies of waves I and V, and their relative latency differences, and comparing them to age-appropriate norms. Cochlear and conductive pathologies may yield different patterns (Fowler & Durrant, 1994) that may help determine the cause of the hearing loss. There is still room for ambiguity with many ABR functions, and additional information such as acoustic immittance measures, may help resolve the cause of the loss. For example, if wave V has an elevated threshold and a delayed latency, a flat tympanogram with normal volume and absent acoustic reflexes may suggest the presence of middle ear effusion. On the other hand, if the tympanogram is not flat and acoustic reflexes are present in the low frequencies, one is more likely to suspect a high frequency cochlear pathology.

Summary

In summary, the effect of the status of the middle ear must be considered for the proper interpretation of OAE and ABR results. OAEs are more critically dependent on middle ear function than are the ABRs, but both responses are altered in the presence of middle ear disorders. If OAEs are absent, the cause may be either middle ear or cochlear in origin, and the distinction must be made for appropriate clinical management. If the ABR screen is failed, the contribution of a conductive component must be considered. Conductive and sensorineural hearing losses require different medical management plans and different habilitative strategies, and they have different prognoses for speech and language development. Evaluation of middle ear function with acoustic immittance measures can greatly enhance the reliability and validity of both OAE and ABR measures in the infant population.

DISCUSSION ITEMS FOR SELF-STUDY

1. Why is it important to screen for the presence of middle ear disorders in preschool children?
2. Why are *both* audiometry and tympanometry important in screening for hearing loss and for middle ear disorders in young children?

SUGGESTED EXERCISE FOR SELF-STUDY

Obtain an acoustic admittance tympanogram for a 226-Hz probe tone in one ear of one participant (e.g., a colleague or family member). Run the tympanogram in measurement plane mode using a positive-to-negative direction of pressure change and a pump speed of 200 daPa/sec. Using your single tympanogram, determine values of *tympanogram width, peak-compensated static acoustic admittance, and equivalent ear-canal volume*. Use 200 daPa as your ear canal referent for all measures. Compare your three resultant measures with ASHA (1997) norms, taking into account the age of your participant. Determine whether the measures for your one ear are within normal limits according to the ASHA guidelines.

8

Conclusion

In the preceding chapters, we have attempted to acquaint readers with the fundamental concepts important for understanding the application of acoustic immittance measures in diagnostic audiology. Throughout the text, we have aimed our treatment at a basic introductory level. Our goal was to provide essential basic knowledge for any reader interested in understanding the basis, rationale, and principles of clinical acoustic-immittance measures. Hopefully, readers will be prepared for further study in the area and will be better versed in the principles and issues underlying current clinical measurement protocols.

The topic of acoustic immittance measures has expanded dramatically over the past 30 years. During the 1960s, acoustic immittance measures were used in research applications but were used in only a few selected audiology clinics. In those early clinical applications, acoustic immittance measures typically were restricted to selected clinical cases. Presently, acoustic immittance measures are used routinely by almost all audiologists in clinical practice. Current clinical applications of the measures encompass the range of audiologic applications from screening to specialized diagnostic procedures in otoneurology. The manual tympanometers of the 1960s have been succeeded by computer-based measurement systems that accommodate a full range of acoustic immittance procedures and permit digital storage and representation of measures for later retrieval and manipulation. Surely, these technologic advances will enable refinement and improvement in clinical applications of acoustic immittance measures during the next 30 years.

In this regard, it should be clear to the reader that future study of developments in the area will be necessary. Certainly, clinical measures will change. At the same time, the need for a basic understanding of (a) the anatomy and physiology of the auditory system inherent in acoustic immittance measures, (b) the basis and rationale for clinical acoustic-immittance measures, and (c) the basic physics of acoustic impedance and acoustic admittance measures will remain essential. Hopefully, this text has provided the necessary basic information that will serve as a solid foundation for further study in the area.

References

Anderson, H., Barr, B., & Wedenberg, E. (1969). Intra-aural reflexes in retrocochlear lesions. In C. A. Hamberger & J. Wersäll (Eds.), *Disorders of the skull base region* (pp. 49–55). Nobel symposium 10. Stockholm: Almqvist and Wiksell.

ANSI. (1987). *Specifications for instruments to measure aural acoustic impedance and admittance (aural acoustic immittance). ANSI S3.39-1987.* New York: American National Standards Institute.

ANSI. (1996). *Specification for audiometers. ANSI S3.6-1996.* New York: American National Standards Institute.

ASHA. (1979). Guidelines for acoustic immittance screening for middle-ear function. *Asha, 21*, 283–288.

ASHA. (1990). Guidelines for screening for hearing impairment and middle-ear disorders. *Asha, 32*(Suppl. 2), 17–24.

ASHA. (1991). Acoustic-immittance measures: A bibliography. *Asha, 33*(Suppl. 4), 1–44.

ASHA. (1997). *Guidelines for audiologic screening.* Rockville, MD: American Speech-Language-Hearing Association.

Beranek, L. L. (1949). *Acoustic measurements.* New York: John Wiley & Sons.

Beranek, L. L. (1954). *Acoustics.* New York: McGraw-Hill.

Bess, F. H., & Paradise, J. L. (1994). Universal screening for hearing impairment: Not simple, not risk-free, not necessarily beneficial, and not presently justified. *Pediatrics, 93,* 330–334.

Bluestone, C. D. (1975). Assessment of Eustachian tube function. In J. Jerger (Ed.), *Handbook of clinical impedance audiometry* (pp. 127–148). Dobbs Ferry, NY: American Electromedics.

Bluestone, C. D. (1978). Morbidity, complications, and sequelae of otitis media. In E. R. Harford, F. H. Bess, C. D. Bluestone, & J. O. Klein (Eds.), *Impedance screening for middle ear disease in children* (pp. 17–22). New York: Grune and Stratton.

Bluestone, C. D., & Cantekin, E. (1981). Panel on experiences with Eustachian tube function tests. *Annals of Otology, Rhinology, and Laryngology, 90,* 552–562.

Borg, E. (1973). On the neuronal organization of the acoustic middle era reflex. A physiological and anatomical study. *Brain Research, 49,* 101–123.

Borg, E. (1976). Neurophysiology of the acoustic stapedius reflex. *Proceedings of the Third International Symposium on Impedance Audiometry* (pp. 6–11). Acton, MA: American Electromedics Corp.

Brooks, D. (1969). The use of the electro-impedance bridge in the assessment of middle ear function. *International Audiology, 7,* 280–286.

Brooks, D. (1973). Hearing screening: A comparative study of an impedance method and pure tone screening. *Scandinavian Audiology, 2,* 67–76.

Brooks, D. (1978a). Acoustic impedance testing for screening auditory function in school children. Part I. *Maico Audiological Library Series, 15*(Report 8), 1–3.

Brooks, D. (1978b). Acoustic impedance testing for screening auditory function in school children. Part II. *Maico Audiological Library Series, 15*(Report 9), 1–4.

Brooks. D. (1978c). Impedance screening for school children. State of the art. In E. R. Harford, F. H. Bess, C. D. Bluestone, & J. O. Klein (Eds.), *Impedance screening for middle ear disease in children* (pp. 173–180). New York: Grune and Stratton.

Brownell, W. E. (1990). Outer hair cell electromotility and otoacoustic emissions. *Ear and Hearing, 11,* 82–92.

Cartwright, W. R., & Lilly, D. J. (1976, November). *A comparison of acoustic-reflex adaptation patterns for patients with cochlear and eighth-nerve disease.* Paper presented at the meeting of the American Speech-Language-Hearing Association, Houston, TX.

Causse, J. R., Causse, J. B., & Bel, J. (1983). Tympanometry and fistula test. *Audiology, 22*(5), 451–462.

Chesnutt, B., Stream, R. W., Love, J. T., & McLarey, D. C. (1975). Otoadmittance measurements in cases of dual ossicular disorders. *Archives of Otolaryngology, 101,*109–113.

Dallos, P. (1973). *The auditory periphery.* New York: Academic Press.

Daspit, C. P., Churchill, D., & Linthicum, F. H. (1980). Diagnosis of perilymph fistula using ENG and impedance. *Laryngoscope, 90*(2), 217–223.

deJonge, R. (1986). Normal tympanometric gradient: A comparison of three methods. *Audiology, 25,* 299–308.

Eagles, E. L. (1972). Selected findings from the Pittsburgh study. *Transactions of the American Academy of Ophthalmology and Otolaryngology, 76,* 343–348.

Eliachar, I., & Northern, J. L. (1974). Studies in tympanometry: Validation of the present technique for determining intra-tympanic pressures through the intact eardrum. *Laryngoscope, 84,* 247–255.

Falk, B. (1982). Sniff-induced negative middle ear pressure: Study of a consecutive series of children with otitis media with effusion. *American Journal of Otolaryngology, 3*(3), 155–162.

Falk, B., & Magnuson, B. (1984). Evacuation of the middle ear by sniffing: A cause of high negative pressure and development of middle ear disease. *Otolaryngology—Head and Neck Surgery, 92*(3), 312–318.

Firestone, F. A. (1956). Twixt earth and sky with rod and tube; the mobility and classical impedance analogies. *Journal of the Acoustical Society of America, 28,* 1117–1153.

Fowler, C. G., & Durrant, J. D. (1994). The effects of peripheral hearing loss on the auditory brainstem response. In J. Jacobson (Ed.), *Principles and applications in auditory evoked potentials* (pp. 237–250). Needham Heights, MA: Allyn & Bacon.

Fowler, C. G., & Wilson, R. H. (1984). Adaptation of the acoustic reflex. *Ear and Hearing, 5,* 281–288.

Givens, G. D., & Seidemann, M. F. (1984). Acoustic immittance testing of the Eustachian tube. *Ear and Hearing, 5,* 297–299.

Glattke, T. J., Pafitis, I. A., Commiskey, C., & Herer, G. R. (1995). Identification of hearing loss in children and young adults using measures of transient emission reproducibility. *American Journal of Audiology, 4,* 71–86.

Hirsch, J. E., Margolis, R. H., & Rykken, J. R. (1992). A comparison of acoustic reflex and auditory brain stem response screening of high-risk infants. *Ear and Hearing, 13,* 181–186.

Holmberg, K., Axelsson, A., Hansson, P., & Renvall, U. (1986). Comparison of tympanometry and otomicroscopy during healing of otitis media. *Scandinavian Audiology, 15,* 3–8.

Holmquist, J., & Bergstrom, B. (1977). Eustachian tube function and size of the mastoid air cell system in middle ear surgery. *Scandinavian Audiology, 6,* 87–89.

Holmquist, J., & Bergstrom, B. (1978). The mastoid air cell system in ear surgery. *Archives of Otolaryngology, 104,* 127–129.

Holte, L., Margolis, R. H., & Cavanaugh, R. M. (1991). Developmental changes in multifrequency tympanograms. *Audiology, 30,* 1–24.

Ivey, R. (1975). Tympanometric curves and otosclerosis. *Journal of Speech and Hearing Research, 18,* 554–558.

Jacobson, J. T., & Hall, J. W. (1994). Newborn and infant auditory brainstem response applications. In J. Jacobson (Ed.), *Principles and applications in auditory evoked potentials* (pp. 313–344). Needham Heights, MA: Allyn & Bacon.

Jerger, J. (1970). Clinical experience with impedance audiometry. *Archives of Otolaryngology, 92,* 311–324.

Jerger, J., Hartford, E., Clemis, J., & Alford, B. (1974). The acoustic reflex in eighth nerve disorders. *Archives of Otolaryngology, 99,* 409–413.

Jerger, J., & Hayes, D. (1980). Diagnostic applications of impedance audiometry: Middle ear disorder; sensorineural disorder. In J. Jerger & J. L. Northern (Eds.), *Clinical impedance audiometry* (2nd ed., pp. 109–127). Acton, MA: American Electromedics.

Jerger, J., Jerger, S. J., & Mauldin, L. (1972). Studies in impedance audiometry: I. Normal and sensorineural ears. *Archives of Otolaryngology, 96,* 513–523.

Jerger, S. (1980). Diagnostic application of impedance audiometry in central auditory disorders. In J. Jerger & J. L. Northern (Eds.), *Clinical impedance audiometry* (2nd ed., pp. 128–140). Acton, MA: American Electromedics.

Jerger, S., & Jerger, J. (1981). *Auditory disorders: A manual for clinical evaluation.* Austin, TX: PRO-ED.

Jewett, D. L. (1970). Volume conducted potentials in response to auditory stimuli as detected by averaging in the cat. *Electroencepalography and Clinical Neurophysiology, 28,* 609–618.

Kemp, D. T. (1978). Stimulated acoustic emission from the human auditory system. *Journal of the Acoustical Society of America, 64,* 1386–1391.

Kemp, D. T., Ryan, S., & Bray, P. (1990). A guide to the effective use of otoacoustic emissions. *Ear and Hearing, 11,* 93–105.

Klein, J. O. (1978). Epidemiology of otitis media. In E. R. Harford, F. H. Bess, C. D. Bluestone, & J. O. Klein (Eds.), *Impedance screening for middle ear disease in children* (pp. 11–16). New York: Grune and Stratton.

Klein, J. O. (1992). Hearing loss and otitis media: Epidemiology, etiology, and pathogenesis. In *Hearing loss in childhood: A primer* (pp. 41–45). Report of the 102nd Ross Conference on Pediatric Research. Columbus, OH: Ross Laboratories.

Koebsell, K. A., & Margolis, R. H. (1986). Tympanometric gradient measured from normal preschool children. *Audiology, 25,* 149–157.

Liden, G. (1969). Tests for stapes fixation. *Archives of Otolaryngology, 89,* 215–219.

Liden, G., & Renvall, U. (1978). Impedance audiometry for screening for middle ear disease in school children. In E. R. Harford, F. H. Bess, C. D. Bluestone, & J. O. Klein (Eds.), *Impedance screening for middle ear disease in children* (pp. 197–206). New York: Grune and Stratton.

Liden, G., & Renvall, U. (1980). Impedance and tone screening of school children. *Scandinavian Audiology, 9,* 121–126.

Lildholt, T. (1980). Negative middle ear pressure. Variations by season and sex. *Annals of Otology, Rhinology, and Laryngology, 89*(Suppl. 68), 67–70.

Lilly, D. J. (1972). Acoustic impedance at the tympanic membrane: A review of basic concepts. In D. Rose & L.W. Keating (Eds.), *Impedance symposium* (pp. 1–25). Rochester, MN: Mayo Clinic-Mayo Foundation.

Lilly, D. J. (1973). Measurement of acoustic impedance at the tympanic membrane. In J. Jerger (Ed.), *Modern developments in audiology* (2nd ed., pp. 345–406). New York: Academic Press.

Lilly, D. J. (1984). Evaluation of the response time of acoustic-immittance instruments. In S. Silman (Ed.), *The acoustic reflex: Basic principles and clinical applications* (pp. 101–135). New York: Academic Press.

Lilly, D. J., & Shanks, J. E. (1981). Acoustic immittance of an enclosed volume of air. In G. R. Popelka (Ed.), *Hearing assessment with the acoustic reflex* (pp. 145–160). New York: Grune & Stratton.

Lonsbury-Martin, B., Whitehead, M. L., & Martin, G. K. (1991). Clinical applications of otoacoustic emissions. *Journal of Speech and Hearing Research, 34,* 964–981.

Lyon, M. J. (1978). The central location of the motor neurons to the stapedius muscle in the cat. *Brain Research, 143,* 437–444.

Magnuson, B. (1981). On the origin of the high negative pressure in the middle ear space. *American Journal of Otolaryngology, 2*(1), 1–12.

Marchant, C. D., McMillan, P. M., Shurin, P. A., Johnson, C. E., Turczyk, V. A., Feinstein, J. C., & Panek, M. (1986). Objective diagnosis of otitis media in early infancy by tympanometry and ipsilateral acoustic reflex thresholds. *Journal of Pediatrics, 109*(4), 590–595.

Margolis, R. H., & Heller, J. W. (1987). Screening tympanometry: Criteria for medical referral. *Audiology, 26,* 197–208.

Margolis, R. H., & Shanks, J. E. (1985). Tympanometry. In J. Katz (Ed.), *Handbook of clinical audiology* (3rd ed., pp. 438–475). Baltimore: Williams & Wilkins.

McMillan, P., Bennett, M. J., Marchant, C. D., & Shurin, P. A. (1985). Ipsilateral and contralateral acoustic reflexes in neonates. *Ear and Hearing, 6,* 320–324.

Melnick, W. (1991). Instrument calibration. In W. Rintelmann (Ed.), *Hearing assessment* (2nd ed., pp. 805–837). Austin, TX: PRO-ED.

Naeve, S. L., Margolis, R. H., Levine, S. C., & Fournier, E. M. (1992). Effect of ear canal pressure on evoked otoacoustic emissions. *Journal of the Acoustical Society of America, 91,* 2091–2095.

NIH. (1993). Early identification of hearing impairment in infants and young children. *NIH Consensus Statement 1993 Mar 1–3, 11*(1), 1–24.

Nozza, R. J., Bluestone, C. D., Kardatze, D., & Bachman, R. (1992). Towards the validation of aural acoustic immitance measures for diagnosis of middle ear effusion in children. *Ear and Hearing, 13,* 442–453.

Nozza, R. J., Bluestone, C. D., Kardatzke, D., & Bachman, R. (1994). Identification of middle ear effusion by aural acoustic admittance and otoscopy. *Ear and Hearing, 15,* 310–323.

Olsen, W. O., Noffsinger, D., & Kurdziel, S. A. (1975). Acoustic reflex and reflex decay: Occurrence with cochlear and eighth nerve lesions. *Archives of Otolaryngology, 101,* 622–625.

Paradise, J., Smith, C., & Bluestone, C. (1976). Tympanometric detection of middle ear effusion in infants and young children. *Pediatrics, 58,* 198–210.

Popelka, G. R. (Ed.). (1981). *Hearing assessment with the acoustic reflex.* New York: Grune and Stratton.

Prieve, B. A. (1992). Otoacoustic emissions in infants and children: Basic characteristics and clinical application. *Seminars in Hearing, 13*(1), 37–52.

Riedel, C. L., Wiley, T. L., & Block, M. G. (1987). Tympanometric measures of Eustachian tube function. *Journal of Speech and Hearing Research, 30,* 207–214.

Robinette, M. S., Barry, S. J., Dybka, M. E., Bruger, B., Popelka, G. R., Wiley, T. L., Williams, P. S., & Resnick, S. (1982) *Calibration of pure-tone air-conducted signals delivered via earphones.* Rockville, MD: American Speech-Language-Hearing Association.

Roush, J., & Tait, C. A. (1985). Pure-tone and acoustic immitance screening of preschool-aged children: An examination of referral criteria. *Ear and Hearing, 6,* 245–249.

Roush, J., Bryant, K., Mundy, M., Zeisel, S., & Roberts, J. (1995). Developmental changes in static admittance and tympanometric width in infants and toddlers. *Journal of the American Academy of Audiology, 6*, 334–338.

Schappert, S. M. (1992). Office visits for otitis media: United States, 1975–1990. Advance data from vital and health statistics, No. 214, Hyattsville, MD: National Center for Health Statistics.

Schuknecht, H. (1993). *Pathology of the ear* (2nd ed.). Baltimore: Williams & Wilkins.

Shanks, J. E. (1984). Tympanometry. *Ear and Hearing, 5*, 268–280.

Shanks, J. E., & Lilly, D. (1981). An evaluation of tympanometric estimates of ear canal volume. *Journal of Speech and Hearing Research, 24*, 557–566.

Shanks, J. E., Lilly, D., Margolis, R. H., Wiley, T. L., & Wilson, R. H. (1988). Tympanometry. *Journal of Speech and Hearing Disorders, 53*, 354–377.

Shanks, J., & Shelton, C. (1991). Basic principles and clinical applications of tympanometry. *Otolaryngologic Clinics of North America, 24*, 299–328.

Shanks, J. E., Stelmachowicz, P. G., Beauchaine, K. L., & Schulte, L. (1992). Equivalent ear canal volumes in children pre- and post-tympanostomy tube insertion. *Journal of Speech and Hearing Research, 35*, 936–941.

Shanks, J. E., Wilson, R. H., & Cambron, N. K. (1993). Multiple frequency tympanometry: Effects of ear canal volume compensation on static acoustic admittance and estimates of middle ear resonance. *Journal of Speech and Hearing Research, 36*, 178–185.

Sheehy, J. L., & Inzer, B. E. (1976). Acoustic reflex test in neuro-otologic diagnosis. *Archives of Otolaryngology, 102*, 647–658.

Silman, S. (Ed.). (1984). *The acoustic reflex: Basic principles and clinical applications.* New York: Academic Press.

Silman, S., Gelfand, S. A., Piper, N., Silverman, C. A., & van Frank, L. (1984). Prediction of hearing loss from the acoustic reflex threshold. In S. Silman (Ed.), *The acoustic reflex: Basic principles and clinical applications* (pp. 187–223). New York: Academic Press.

Silman, S., Silverman, C. A., & Arick, D. S. (1992). Acoustic-immittance screening for detection of middle-ear effusion in children. *Journal of the American Academy of Audiology, 3*, 262–268.

Smith, P. S. Utech, Wiley, T. L., & Pyle, M. G. (1992). Screening for middle-ear effusion in children. *Asha, 34*(10), 154.

Smith, P. S. Utech, Wiley, T. L., & Pyle, M. G. (1993). Efficacy of ASHA guidelines for screening middle-ear function. *Asha, 35*(10), 114.

Sohmer, H., & Feinmesser, M. (1967). Cochlear action potentials recorded from the external ear in man. *Annals of Otology, Rhinology, and Laryngology, 76*, 427–438.

Sprague, B. H., Wiley, T. L., & Goldstein, R. (1985). Tympanometric and acoustic-reflex studies in neonates. *Journal of Speech and Hearing Research, 28*, 265–272.

Strangerup, S. E., Sederberg-Olsen, J., & Balle, V. (1992). Autoinflation as a treatment of secretory otitis media: A randomized controlled study. *Archives of Otolaryngology—Head and Neck Surgery, 118*, 149–152.

Susskind, C. (1962a). Heaviside, Oliver (1850–1925). In C. Susskind (Ed.), *The encyclopedia of electronics* (p. 354). New York: Reinhold Publishing Corporation.

Susskind, C. (1962b). Steinmetz, Charles Proteus (1865–1923). In C. Susskind (Ed.), *The encyclopedia of electronics* (pp. 786–787). New York: Reinhold Publishing Corporation.

Van Camp, K. J., Creten, W. L., Vanpeperstraete, P. M., & Van de Heyning, P. H. (1980). Tympanometry: Detection of middle ear pathologies. *Acta Otorhinolaryngologica (Belgium), 34*, 574–583.

Van Camp, K. J., Shanks, J. E., & Margolis, R. H. (1986). Simulation of pathological high impedance tympanograms. *Journal of Speech and Hearing Research, 29*, 505–514.

Van de Heyning, P. H., Van Camp, K. J., Creten, W. L., & Vanpeperstraete, P. M. (1982). Incudo-stapedial joint pathology: A tympanometric approach. *Journal of Speech and Hearing Research, 25*, 611–618.

Vanhuyse, V. J., Creten, W. L., & Van Camp, K. J. (1975). On the w-notching of tympanograms. *Scandinavian Audiology, 4,* 45–50.

Webster, A. G. (1919). Acoustical impedance, and the theory of horns and of the phonograph. *Proceedings of the National Academy of Science, 5*, 275–282.

Wiley, T. L., & Barrett, K. A. (1991). Test-retest reliability in tympanometry. *Journal of Speech and Hearing Research, 34*, 1197–1206.

Wiley, T. L., & Block, M. G. (1979). Static acoustic-immittance measurements. *Journal of Speech and Hearing Research, 22*, 677–696.

Wiley, T. L., & Block, M. G. (1984). Acoustic and nonacoustic reflex patterns in audiologic diagnosis. In S. Silman (Ed.). *The acoustic reflex: Basic principles and clinical applications* (pp. 387–411). New York: Academic Press.

Wiley, T. L., Cruickshanks, K. J., Nondahl, D. M., Tweed, T. S., Klein, R., & Klein, B. E. K. (1996). Tympanometric measures in older adults. *Journal of the Academy of Audiology, 7*, 260–268.

Wiley, T. L., Oviatt, D. L., & Block, M. G. (1987). Acoustic-immittance measures in normal ears. *Journal of Speech and Hearing Research, 30,* 161–170.

Wiley, T. L., & Smith, P. S. U. (1995). Acoustic-immittance measures and middle-ear screening. *Seminars in Hearing, 16*(1), 60–79.

Wilson, R. H., Shanks, J. E., & Kaplan, S. K. (1984). Tympanometric changes at 226 Hz and 678 Hz across 10 trials and for two directions of ear canal pressure change. *Journal of Speech and Hearing Research, 27,* 257–266.

Wilson, R. H., Shanks, J. E., & Lilly, D. J. (1984). Acoustic reflex adaptation. In S. Silman (Ed.), *The acoustic reflex: Basic principles and clinical applications* (pp. 329–387). New York: Academic Press.

Zemlin, W. R. (1988). *Speech and hearing science: Anatomy and physiology.* Englewood Cliffs, NJ: Prentice-Hall.

Zwislocki, J. (1963). An acoustic method for clinical examination of the ear. *Journal of Speech and Hearing Research, 6,* 303–314.

Zwislocki, J. (1976). The acoustic middle ear function. In A. Feldman & L. Wilbur (Eds.), *Acoustic impedance and admittance: The measurement of middle ear function* (pp. 66–77). Baltimore: Williams & Wilkins.

Zwislocki, J., & Feldman, A. S. (1970). *Acoustic impedance of pathological ears.* Monograph No. 15. Rockville, MD: American Speech-Language-Hearing Association.

APPENDIX

Glossary of Selected Terms[1]

5.13   **probe:** a coupling device that is used to connect the acoustic-immittance instrument to the external auditory meatus.

5.14   **probe tip:** a cuff that is used to seal the probe into the external auditory meatus.

5.15   **probe signal:** an acoustic signal that is emitted through the probe into the external auditory meatus. This signal is used to measure acoustic immittance.

5.16   **probe ear:** an ear into which a probe is inserted and in which an acoustic-immittance measurement is made.

5.17   **measurement plane:** a plane located at the frontal surface of the probe perpendicular to the volume-velocity vector.

5.18   **static acoustic immittance:** measured in the external auditory meatus at a constant, specified air pressure, and in the absence of a middle-ear muscle reflex-activating signal.

---

[1]From ANSI. (1987). *Specifications for instruments to measure aural acoustic imped-ance and admittance (aural acoustic immittance)*. ANSI S3.39-1987, pp. 3–4. New York: American National Standards Institute.

5.19   **compensated static acoustic immittance:** static acoustic immittance that has been compensated (or corrected) for the acoustic immittance of the external auditory meatus. This value represents an estimate of the acoustic immittance at the lateral surface of the tympanic membrane and may be indicated by replacing the "a" subscript with a "tm" subscript when using the symbols in Table 2–1. (For example, "Z_{tm}" indicates compensated static acoustic impedance at the tympanic membrane.) The method used for determining the acoustic immittance of the external auditory meatus must be specified.

5.19.1   ambient compensated static acoustic immittance: the static acoustic immittance obtained with ambient air pressure in the external auditory meatus. (For example, "ambient Z_{tm}" indicates compensated static acoustic impedance at ambient air pressure.)

5.19.2   peak compensated static acoustic immittance: the static acoustic immittance obtained with air pressure in the external auditory meatus adjusted to produce an extremum in the measured acoustic immittance. This value usually is obtained from a centrally located extremum in the tympanogram (see definition 5.22). (For example, "peak Z_{tm}" indicates compensated static acoustic impedance at the extremum in the tympanogram.) When the tympanogram is characterized by multiple extrema, or no extremum over the specified range of air pressures, the extremum or reference selected for this measurement shall be specified. (For example, "$-400Y_{tm}$" indicates compensated static acoustic admittance measured with an air pressure of –400 daPa in the external auditory meatus.)

5.21   **tympanometry:** the measurement of acoustic immittance in the external auditory meatus as a function of air pressure within the external auditory meatus.

5.21.1   measurement-plane tympanometry: a measurement of acoustic immittance in the measurement plane. This measurement comprises the combined acoustic immittance of the external auditory meatus and the middle ear.

5.21.2   compensated tympanometry: a measurement of acoustic immittance that has been compensated (or corrected) for the acoustic immittance of the external auditory meatus (or other specified values of acoustic immittance).

5.22   **tympanogram:** a graphic display of tympanometry data.

5.23   **middle-ear muscle reflex:** a change in the tonus of muscles of the middle ear in response to a stimulus. These contractions may be monitored as a change in the acoustic immittance within the external auditory meatus.

5.23.1   acoustic reflex: a middle-ear muscle reflex elicited by an acoustic stimulus.

5.23.2   nonacoustic reflex: a middle-ear muscle reflex elicited by a nonacoustic stimulus

5.24   **acoustic-reflex activating stimulus:** an acoustic signal that is used to elicit an acoustic reflex.

5.25   **nonacoustic reflex activating stimulus:** may be electrical, tactile, pneumatic, photic, or any other nonacoustic signal that is used to elicit a middle-ear muscle reflex.

5.26   **stimulus ear:** the ear to which the acoustic-reflex activating signal is presented in order to elicit a middle-ear muscle reflex. The middle-ear muscle reflex elicited is identified with respect to the stimulus ear.

NOTE: If a bone vibrator or a loudspeaker is used to deliver the acoustic-reflex activating signal, it may not be possible to define the stimulus ear.

5.27   **ipsilateral reflex:** the middle-ear muscle reflex that is elicited in the stimulus ear. This reflex also is referred to as the uncrossed reflex.

5.28   **contralateral reflex:** the middle-ear muscle reflex that is elicited in the ear contralateral to the stimulus ear. This reflex also is referred to as the crossed reflex.

APPENDIX

Acoustic-Immittance Measures: A Biblography[1]

Terry L. Wiley, PhD

and

Committee on Audiologic Evaluation
Sandra M. Gordon-Salant, PhD [Chair]
S. Joseph Barry, PhD
Evelyn Cherow, M.A., ex officio
John D. Durrant, PhD
Gregg D. Givens, PhD
Susan W. Jerger, PhD
Sharon A. Lesner, PhD
Laura Ann Wilber, PhD
Monitoring Vice President
Teris K. Schery, PhD
American Speech-Language-Hearing Association

[1]Reprinted from American Speech-Language-Hearing Association (1991). Acoustic-Immittance Measures: A Bibliography. *Asha, 33*(Suppl. 4), 1–44. (Reprinted with the permission of the American Speech-Language-Hearing Association.)

PREFACE

This bibliography on acoustic-immittance measures has evolved over the past several years. It has been used primarily as a teaching and research resource in the Department of Communicative Disorders, University of Wisconsin-Madison. Subsequently, through the efforts of the American Speech-Language-Hearing Association Committee on Audiologic Evaluation, it has been prepared as an ASHA product in the interest of providing a resource to the ASHA membership.

The Committee on Audiologic Evaluation members includes: S. Joseph Barry; Evelyn Cherow (ex officio); John Durrant; Gregg Givens; Sandra Gordon-Salant (Chair); Susan Jerger; Sharon Lesner; and Laura Ann Wilber. Teris K. Schery, Vice President for Clinical Affairs (1988–1990), was the monitoring vice president. The contribution of Jo Williams is also acknowledged.

In the interests of simplicity, the topic outline is brief and limited to major areas. Cross-listing of references is limited; this may necessitate a review of different sections for the reader interested in very specific subtopics. New students of the area are advised to begin with the tutorial references listed under 1.0 and the source material provided under 10.0. Readers already familiar with the general topic area can skip from section to section depending on their topic interests. The bibliography is not a complete compilation of references for the topic area; only published manuscripts are listed.

ACKNOWLEDGMENTS

The lead author wishes to thank the Department of Communicative Disorders and the University of Wisconsin-Madison for the support and secretarial services critical to the compilation of the bibliography. Dana Oviatt provided substantive assistance in the early reference compilation. Numerous Wisconsin graduate students in audiology and selected colleagues in the area have added to the bibliography over the past several years. Nancy Duren and Sharon Ruch were primarily responsible for the lengthy and tedious task of entering the references into our word processor and for editing reference citations throughout the bibliography. Tinney Kees, Jay Edgar, Monica Maso, and Ellen Todd provided crucial assistance in the reference compilation and in proofreading the document.

TABLE OF CONTENTS

1.0 TUTORIALS

Alberti, P. W., & Kristensen, R. (1970). The clinical application of impedance audiometry. *Laryngoscope, 80*, 735–746.

Berlin, C. I., & Cullen, J. K., Jr. (1975). The physical basis of impedance measurement. In J. F. Jerger (Ed.), *Handbook of clinical impedance audiometry* (pp. 1–20). Dobbs Ferry, NY: American Electromedics.

Bluestone, C. D. (1975). Assessment of Eustachian function. In J. F. Jerger (Ed.), *Handbook of clinical impedance audiometry* (pp. 127–148). Dobbs Ferry, NY: American Electromedics.

Bluestone, C. D. (1980). Assessment of Eustachian tube function. In J. Jerger & J. Northern (Eds.), *Clinical impedance audiometry* (2nd ed., pp. 83–108). Acton, MA: American Electromedics.

Dempsey, C. (1975). Static compliance. In J. F. Jerger (Ed.), *Handbook of clinical impedance audiometry* (pp. 71–84). Dobbs Ferry, NY: American Electromedics.

Djupesland, G. (1976). Nonacoustic reflex measurement. Procedures, interpretations and variables. In A. S. Feldman & L. A. Wilber (Eds.), *Acoustic impedance and admittance: The measurement of middle ear function* (pp. 217–235). Baltimore: Williams & Wilkins.

Feldman, A. S. (1971). Impedance measurement and the middle ear. Part I *Maico Audiological Library Series, 9*, Report 7.

Feldman, A. S. (1971). Impedance measurement and the middle ear. Part II *Maico Audiological Library Series, 9*, Report 8.

Feldman, A. S. (1975). Acoustic impedance/admittance measurement. In L. Bradford (Ed.), *Physiologic measures of the audio-vestibular system* (pp. 87–145). New York: Academic Press.

Feldman, A. S. (1976). Tympanometry: Application and interpretation. *Annals of Otology, Rhinology and Laryngology, 85*, 202–208.

Goodall, L. M., Bradford, P. J., Bulteau V., & Upfold, L. J. (1980). What is impedance audiometry? *Medical Journal of Autism, 2*, 545–548.

Greenberg, H. J. (1977). Fundamentals of acoustic impedance and admittance measurements—A tutorial presentation. *Asha, 17*, 729–732.

Hall, J. W. (Guest Ed.). (1987). Immittance audiometry. *Seminars in Hearing, 8* (4).

Hannley, M. (1986). Clinical applications of acoustic immitance. In M. Hannley (Ed.), *Basic principles of auditory assessment* (pp. 51–88). San Diego: College-Hill.

Harford, E. R. (1975). Tympanometry. In J. F. Jerger (Ed.), *Handbook of clinical impedance audiometry* (pp. 47–70). Dobbs Ferry, NY: American Electromedics.

Harper, A. R. (1961). Acoustic impedance as an aid to diagnosis in otology. *Journal of Laryngology and Otology, 75*, 614–620.

Holmquist, J. (1976). Eustachian tube evaluation. In A. S. Feldman & L. A. Wilber (Eds.), *Acoustic impedance and admittance: The measurement of middle ear function*. Baltimore: Williams & Wilkins.

Jerger, J. (1975). Diagnostic use of impedance measures. In J. Jerger (Ed.), *Handbook of clinical impedance audiometry* (pp. 149–174). Dobbs Ferry, NY: American Electromedics.

Jerger, J., & Hayes, D. (1980). Diagnostic applications of impedance audiometry: Middle ear disorder: Sensorineural disorders. In J. Jerger & J. L. Northern (Eds.), *Clinical impedance audiometry* (2nd ed., pp. 109–127). Acton, MA: American Electromedics.

Keating, L. W., & Olsen, W. O. (1978). Practical considerations and applications of middle-ear impedance measurements. In D. E. Rose (Ed.), *Audiological assessment* (2nd ed., pp. 336–367). Englewood Cliffs, NJ: Prentice-Hall.

Lamb, L. E. (1971). Impedance measurements and the middle ear. *Maico Audiological Library Series, 9*, Report 9.

Lamb, L. E., & Norris, T. W. (1969). Acoustic impedance measurement. In R. T. Fulton & L. L. Lloyd (Eds.), *Audiometry for the retarded* (pp. 164–209). Baltimore: Williams & Wilkins.

Lilly, D. J. (1972). Acoustic impedance at the tympanic membrane. In J. Katz (Ed.), *Handbook of clinical audiology* (pp. 434–469). Baltimore: Williams & Wilkins.

Lilly, D. J. (1973). Measurement of acoustic impedance at the tympanic membrane. In J. Jerger (Ed.), *Modern developments in audiology* (2nd ed., pp. 345–406). New York: Academic Press.

Margolis, R. H. (1981). Fundamentals of acoustic immittance. In G. R. Popelka (Ed.), *Hearing assessment with the acoustic reflex* (pp. 117–143). New York: Grune & Stratton

Margolis, R. H., & Shanks, J. E. (1985). Tympanometry. In J. Katz (Ed.), *Handbook of clinical audiology* (3rd ed., pp. 438–475). Baltimore: Williams & Wilkins.

McCandless, G.A. (1979). Impedance measures. In W. F. Rintelmann, (Ed.), *Hearing assessment* (pp. 281–320). Baltimore: University Park Press.

Northern, J. L. (1971). Clinical application of acoustic impedance measurements. *Otolaryngology Clinics of North America, Symposium on Congenital Deafness, 4*, 359–368.

Northern, J. L. (1976). Clinical implications of impedance audiometry. In J. L. Northern (Ed.), *Hearing disorders* (pp. 20–36). Boston: Little, Brown.

Northern, J. L. (1977). Acoustic impedance in the pediatric population. In F. H. Bess (Ed.), *Childhood deafness: Causation, assessment, and management* (pp. 135–152). New York: Grune & Stratton.

Northern, J. L. (1984). Impedance audiometry. In J. L. Northern (Ed.), *Hearing disorders* (pp. 41–56). Boston: Little, Brown & Co.

Northern, J. L., Gabbard, S. A., & Kinder, D. L. (1985). The acoustic reflex. In J. Katz (Ed.), *Handbook of clinical audiology* (3rd ed., pp. 476–495). Baltimore: Williams & Wilkins.

Popelka, G. R. (1983). Basic acoustic immittance measures. *Audiology, 8*, 1–16.

Popelka, G. R. (1984). Acoustic immittance measures: Terminology and instrumentation. *Ear and Hearing, 5*, 262–267.

Rock, E. H. (1972). Electroacoustic impedance measurements in clinical otology. *Impedance Newsletter, 1*(3), 1–45.

Sanders, J. W. (1975). Impedance measurement. *Otolaryngologic Clinics of North America, 8*, 109–124.

Shanks, J. E. (1984). Tympanometry. *Ear and Hearing, 5*, 268–280.

Shanks, J. E., Lilly, D. J., Margolis, R. H., Wiley, T. L., & Wilson, R. H. (1988). Tympanometry. *Journal of Speech and Hearing Disorders, 53*, 354–377.

Sheehy, J. L., & Hughes, R. L. (1974). The ABC's of impedance audiometry. *Laryngoscope, 84*, 1935–1949.

Van Camp, K. J., & Creten, W. L. (1976). Principles of acoustic impedance and admittance. In A. S. Feldman & L. A. Wilber (Eds.), *Acoustic impedance and admittance: The measurement of middle ear function* (pp. 300–334). Baltimore: Williams & Wilkins.

Van Camp, K. J., Margolis, R. H., Wilson, R. H., Creten, W. L., & Shanks, J. E. (1986). *Principles of tympanometry*, (Monograph No. 24). Rockville, MD: American Speech–Language-Hearing Association.

Wiley, T. L. (1986). Acoustic-immittance measures. In *Encyclopedia of deaf people and deafness* (Vol. 1, pp. 51–54). New York: McGraw-Hill.

Wiley, T. L., & Block, M. G. (1979). Tutorial: Static acoustic-immittance measurements. *Journal of Speech and Hearing Research, 22*, 677–696.

Wiley, T. L., & Block, M. G. (1984). Acoustic and nonacoustic reflex patterns in audiologic diagnosis. In S. Silman (Ed.), *The acoustic reflex: Basic principles and clinical applications* (pp. 387–411). New York: Academic Press.

Wiley, T. L., & Block, M. G. (1985). Overview and basic principles of acoustic-immittance measurements. In J. Katz (Ed.), *Handbook of clinical audiology* (3rd ed., pp. 423–437). Baltimore: Williams & Wilkins.

Zwislocki, J. J. (1976). The acoustic middle ear function. In A. S. Feldman and L. A. Wilber (Eds.), *Acoustic impedance and admittance: The measurement of middle ear function* (pp. 66–77). Baltimore: Williams & Wilkins.

2.0 ANATOMY AND PHYSIOLOGY OF THE MIDDLE EAR

Akaan-Penttila, E. (1982). Middle ear mucosa in newborn infants. A topographical and microanatomical study. *Acta Otolaryngologica, 93*, 251–259.

Albin, N. (1984). The anatomy of the Eustachian tube. *Acta Otolaryngologica* (Stockholm), (Suppl. 414), 34–37.

Anderson, H., Jepsen, O., & Ratjen, E. (1962). Ossicular-chain defects. *Acta Otolaryngologica, 54*, 393–402.

Andreasson, L. (1977). Correlation of tubal function and volume of mastoid and middle ear space as related to otitis media. *Acta Otolaryngologica, 83*, 29–33.

Andreasson, L., & Mortensson, W. (1975). Comparison between the area and the volume of the air filled ear space. *Acta Radiologica, 16*, 347–352.

Anson, B. J., & Donaldson, J. A. (1981). *The surgical anatomy of the temporal bone and ear*. Philadelphia: W. B. Saunders.

Ars, B. (1981). The tympanic cavity: Tomographic anatomy. *Clinical Otolaryngology, 6*, 311–315.

Bentler, R. A. (1989). External ear resonance characteristics in children. *Journal of Speech and Hearing Disorders, 54*, 264–268.

Blevins, C. E. (1967). Innervation patterns of the human stapedius muscle. *Archives of Otolaryngology, 86*, 136–142.

Blevins, C. E. (1968). Motor units in the stapedius muscle. *Archives of Otolaryngology, 87*, 249–254.

Blevins, C. E., & Noble, B. (1965). Innervation of human fetal and neonatal stapedius muscle. *Anatomy Record, 151*, 325–326.

Bluestone, C., Beery, Q., & Andrus, W. (1974). Mechanics of the Eustachian tube as it influences susceptibility to and persistence of middle ear effusion in children. *Annals of Otology, Rhinology and Laryngology, 83* (Suppl. 11), 27–34.

Borg, E. (1968). A quantitative study of the effect of the acoustic stapedius reflex on sound transmission through the middle ear of man. *Acta Otolaryngologica* (Stockholm), *66*, 461–472.

Borg, E. (1972). Acoustic middle ear reflexes: A sensory-control system. *Acta Otolaryngologica* (Stockholm), (Suppl. 304), 1–34.

Borg, E. (1973). Nonlinear dynamic properties of a somatomotor reflex system. A model study. *Acta Physiologica* (Scandinavia), *87*, 15–26.

Borg, E. (1973). On the neuronal organization of the acoustic middle ear reflex. A physiological and anatomical study. *Brain Research, 49*, 101–123.

Borg, E. (1976). Neurophysiology of the acoustic stapedius reflex. In J. Jerger & J. Northern (Eds.), *Proceedings of the Third International Symposium on Impedance Audiometry* (pp. 6–11). Dobbs Ferry, NY: American Electromedics.

Borg, E., & Counter, S. A. (1989, August). The middle-ear muscles. *Scientific American*, 74–80.

Bosatra, A. (1977). Pathology of the nervous arc of the acoustic reflexes. *Audiology, 16*, 307–315.

Candiollo, L. (1967). The control mechanism of the middle ear transmission system: The middle ear muscles in the morphology and function of auditory input control. *Translations of the Beltone Institute for Hearing Research, 20*, 13–41.

Chitore, D. S., Saxena, S. C., & Mukhopadhyay, P. (1983). Electronic model of the middle ear. *Medical and Biological Engineering and Computing, 21*, 176–178.

Counter, S. A., & Borg, E. (1970). Physiological activation of the stapedius muscle in Gallus gallus. *Acta Otolaryngologica* (Stockholm), *88*, 13–19.

Counter, S. A., & Borg, E. (1982). The avian stapedius muscle: Influence on auditory sensitivity and sound transmission. *Acta Otolaryngologica, 94*, 267–274.

Dallos, P. (1973). *The auditory periphery*. Englewood Cliffs, NJ: Prentice-Hall.

Daniel, H. J., Brinn, J. E., Fulghum, R. S., & Barrett, K. A. (1982). Comparative anatomy of Eustachian tube and middle ear cavity in animal models for otitis media. *Annals of Otology, Rhinology and Laryngology, 91*, 82–89.

Dickson, D. R. (1976). Anatomy of the normal and cleft palate Eustachian tube. *Annals of Otology, Rhinology and Laryngology, 85*, 25–29.

Elisassen, S., & Gisselson, L. (1955). Electromyographic studies of the middle ear muscles of the cat. *Neurophysiology, 7*, 399–406.

Elner, A., Ingelstedt, S., & Ivarsson, A. (1971). The elastic properties of the tympanic membrane. *Acta Otolaryngologica, 72*, 397–403.

Erulkar, S. D., Shelanski, M. L., Whitsel, B. L., & Ogle, P. (1964). Studies of muscle fibers of the tensor tympani of the cat. *Anatomy Record, 149*, 279–297.

Fisch, U., & von Schulthess, G. (1963). Electromyographic studies on the human stapedial muscle. *Acta Otolaryngologica, 56*, 287–297.

Galambos, R., & Rubert, A. (1959). Action of the middle ear muscles in normal cats. *Journal of the Acoustical Society of America, 31*, 349–355.

Giacomelli, F., & Mozzo, W. (1965). An experimental and clinical study on the influence of the brainstem reticular formation on the stapedial reflex. *International Audiology, 9*, 42–44.

Glattke, T. J. (1981). The middle ear: Anatomy and physiology. In F. N. Martin (Ed.), *Medical audiology* (pp. 87–108). Englewood Cliffs, NJ: Prentice-Hall.

Guindi, G. M. (1981). Nasopharyngeal mechanoreceptors and their role in auto-regulation of endotympanic pressure. *Journal of Otorhinolaryngology and Related Specialties, 43*, 56–60.

Harty, M. (1953). Elastic tissue in the middle ear cavity. *Journal of Laryngology and Otology, 67*, 723–729.

Henson, O. W., Jr. (1965). The activity and function of the middle-ear muscles in echo-locating bats. *Journal of Physiology* (London), *180*, 871–887.

Hergils, M., & Magnuson, B. (1985). Morning pressure in the middle ear. *Archives of Otolaryngology, 111*, 86–89.

Holst, H., Ingelstedt, S., & Ortegner, V. (1962). Eardrum movements following stimulation of the middle ear muscles. *Acta Otolaryngologica*, (Suppl. 182), 73–83.

Hugelin, A., Dumont, S., & Paillas, N. (1960). Tympanic muscles and control of auditory input during arousal. *Science, 131*, 1371–1372.

Ingelstedt, S. (1976). Physiology of the Eustachian tube. *Annals of Otology, Rhinology and Laryngology, 85*, 156–160.

Ingelstedt, S., Ivarsson, A., & Jonson, B. (1969). Mechanics of the human middle ear. *Acta Otolaryngologica*, (Suppl. 228), 1–58.

Itoh, K., Nomura, S., Konishi, A., Yasui, Y., Sugimoto, T., & Muzino, N. (1986). A morphological evidence of direct connections from the cochlear nuclei to tensor tympani motor neurons in the cat: A possible afferent limb of the acoustic middle ear reflex pathways. *Brain Research, 375*, 214–219.

Kamerer, D. B., & Rood, S. R. (1978). The tensor tympani, stapedius, and tensor veli palatini muscles—An electromyographic study. *Otolaryngology*, *86*, 416–421.

Klinke, R., & Hartman, R. (1983). Hearing—Physiological bases and psychophysics. In *Proceedings of the Sixth International Symposium on Hearing*. Berlin: Springer-Verlag, Berlin Hudelberg.

Klockhoff, I., & Anderson, H. (1960). Reflex activity in the tensor tympanic muscle recorded in man: A preliminary report. *Acta Otolaryngologica*, *51*, 184–189.

Kobrak, H. G. (1959). *The middle ear*. Chicago: University of Chicago Press.

Kruger, B. (1987). An update on the external ear resonance in infants and young children. *Ear and Hearing*, *8*, 333–336.

Kruger, B., & Ruben, R. J. (1987). The acoustic properties of the infant ear: A preliminary report. *Acta Otolaryngologica* (Stockholm), *103*, 578–585.

Lawrence, M. (1965). The double innervation of the tensor tympani. *Annals of Otology, Rhinology and Laryngology*, *82*, 478–482.

Lim, D. J. (1976). Functional morphology of the mucosa of the middle ear and Eustachian tube. *Annals of Otology, Rhinology and Laryngology*, *85*, 36–43.

Lim, D. J. (1979). Anatomy and functional morphology of the middle ear and Eustachian tube: A review. In R. J. Wiet & S. W. Coulthard (Eds.), *Proceedings of the Second National Conference of Otitis Media* (pp. 35–39). Columbus, OH: Ross Laboratories.

Lim, D. J. (1984). Functional morphology of the tubotympanum. *Acta Otolaryngologica* (Stockholm), (Suppl. 414), 13–18.

Lipscomb, D. M. (1984). Mechanisms of the middle ear. In J. Northern (Ed.), *Hearing disorders* (2nd ed., pp. 241–251). Boston: Little, Brown.

Lorente de No, R. (1935). The function of the central acoustic nuclei examined by means of the acoustic reflexes. *Laryngoscope*, *45*, 573–594.

Lupin, A. L. (1969). The relationship of the tensor tympani and the tensor palatini muscles. *Annals of Otology, Rhinology and Laryngology*, *70*, 792–795.

Lyon, M. J. (1978). The central location of the motor neurons to the stapedius muscle in the cat. *Brain Research*, *143*, 437–444.

Lyon, M. J., & Malmgren, L. T. (1982). Histochemical characterization of muscle fiber types in the middle ear muscles of the cat. 1. The stapedius muscle. *Acta Otolaryngologica* (Stockholm), *94*, 99–109.

Malmsfors, T., & Wersall, J. (1960). Innervation of the middle ear muscles in the rabbit with special reference to nerve caliber and motor unit. I—Musculus tensor tympani. *Acta Morphologica Neurologica* (Scandinavia), *3*, 163–169.

McRobert, H. (1968). The response of the tympanic muscles in human ears. *Sound*, *2*, 71–76.

McRobert, H. (1972). The physiology and normal responses of the acoustic reflex. In D. Rose & L. Keating (Eds.), *Proceedings of the Mayo Impedance Symposium* (pp. 203–210). Rochester, MN: Mayo Foundation.

McRobert, H., Bryan, M. E., & Tempest, W. (1968). The acoustic stimulation of the middle ear muscles. *Sound and Vibration, 7,* 129–142.

Miller, J. M., & Holmquist, J. (1974). An animal model for study of Eustachian tube and middle ear function. *Scandinavian Audiology, 3,* 63–72.

Moller, A. R. (1961). Network model of the middle ear. *Journal of the Acoustical Society of America, 33,* 168–176.

Moller, A. R. (1963). Transfer function of the middle ear. *Journal of the Acoustical Society of America, 35,* 1526–1534.

Moller, A. R. (1965). An experimental study of the acoustic impedance of the middle ear and its transmission properties. *Acta Otolaryngologica, 60,* 129–149.

Moller, A. R. (1972). The middle ear. In J. Tobias (Ed.), *Foundations of modern auditory theory* (pp. 133–194). New York: Academic Press.

Moller, A. R. (1983). *Auditory physiology.* New York: Academic Press.

Moller, A. R. (1984). Neurophysiological basis of the acoustic middle ear reflex. In S. Silman (Ed.), *The acoustic reflex* (pp. 9–34). Orlando, FL: Academic Press.

Molvaer, O., Vallersnes, F., & Kringlebotn, M. (1978). The size of the middle ear and the mastoid air cell. *Acta Otolaryngologica, 85,* 24–32.

Neergaard, E. B., Anderson, H. C., Hansen, C. C., & Jepsen, O. (1963). Experimental studies on sound transmission in the human ear: Influence of the stapedius and tensor tympani muscles. *Acta Otolaryngologica,* (Suppl. 188), 280–286.

Nolan, M. N., Lyon, J., & Mok, C. L. L. (1985). Air pressure changes in the external auditory meatus (the influence on pure tone bone conduction thresholds). *Journal of Laryngology and Otology, 99,* 315–326.

Onchi, Y. (1961). Mechanism of the middle ear. *Journal of the Acoustical Society of America, 33,* 794–805.

Pickles, J. O. (1982). *An introduction to the physiology of hearing.* New York: Academic Press.

Pohlman, A. G., & Kranz, F. W. (1925). The problem of middle ear mechanics. *Annals of Otology, Rhinology and Laryngology, 34,* 1224–1238.

Politzer, A. (1869). *The membrana tympani.* New York: William Wood.

Potter, A. B. (1936). Function of the stapedius muscle. *Annals of Otology, Rhinology and Laryngology, 45,* 639–643.

Rossi, G., & Solero, P. (1984). Dynamic parameters of the stapedius muscle reflex in response to stimuli of varying duration but with the same energy content. *Acta Otolaryngologica* (Stockholm), *97,* 460–466.

Russolo, M., & Semeraro, A. (1977). Value of the isolated tensor tympani reflex elicited by electric lingual stimulation. *Audiology, 16,* 373–379.

Salomon, G. (1966). Middle ear muscle activity. *Proceedings of the Royal Society of Medicine, 59,* 966–971.

Salomon, G., & Starr, A. (1963). Electromyography of middle ear muscles in man during motor activities. *Acta Neurologica* (Scandinavia), *39,* 161–168.

Salomon, G., & Starr. A. (1965). Electromyographic study of click evoked middle ear muscle activity in cats. *International Audiology, 4,* 31–33.

Sato, R., & Ono, Y. (1969). The displacement of the stapes by the reflex of the human stapedius muscle. *Acta Otolaryngologica, 68,* 509–513.

Simmons, F. B. (1964). Perceptual theories of middle ear muscle function. *Annals of Otology, Rhinology and Laryngology, 73,* 724–739.

Smith, H. D. (1943). Audiometric effects of voluntary contraction of the tensor tympani muscle. *Archives of Otolaryngology, 38,* 369–372.

Stirneman, A. (1981). A network model of the middle ear and its applications. In R. Penna & P. Pizarro (Eds.), *Proceedings of the Fourth International Symposium on Acoustic Impedance Measurements* (pp. 495–504). Lisbon, Portugal: Universidade Nova de Lisboa.

Terkildsen, K. (1957). Movements of the eardrum following inter-aural muscle reflexes. *Archives of Otolaryngology, 66,* 484–488.

Terkildsen, K. (1960). Acoustic reflexes of the human musculus tensor tympani. *Acta Otolaryngologica,* (Suppl. 158), 230–238.

Terkildsen, K. (1961). Conduction of sound in the middle ear. *Archives of Otolaryngology, 73,* 69–79.

Torvik, A. (1956). Afferent connections to the sensory trigeminal nuclei, the nucleus of the solitary tract and adjacent structures. An experimental study in the rat. *Journal of Comparative Neurology, 106,* 51–141.

Tos, M. (1984). Anatomy and histology of the middle ear. *Clinical Reviews in Allergy, 2,* 267–284.

Webster, D. B., Packer, D. J., & Webster, M. (1985). Functional anatomy of the external and middle ear. *Ear, Nose and Throat Journal, 64,* 275–281.

Wersall, R. (1958). The tympanic muscles and their reflexes. *Acta Otolaryngologica,* (Suppl. 139), 1–112.

Wever, E. G., & Bray, C. W. (1937). The tensor tympani muscle and its relation to sound conduction. *Annals of Otology, Rhinology and Laryngology, 46,* 947–961.

Wever, E. G., & Bray, C. W. (1942). The stapedius muscle in relation to sound conduction. *Journal of Experimental Psychology, 31,* 35–43.

Wever, E. G., & Vernon, J. A. (1955). The effects of the tympanic muscle reflexes upon sound transmission. *Acta Otolaryngologica, 45,* 433–439.

Wever, E. G., & Vernon, J. A. (1956). The control of sound transmission by the middle ear muscles. *Annals of Otology, Rhinology and Laryngology, 65,* 5–14.

Wiggers, H. C. (1937). The functions of the intra-aural muscles. *American Journal of Physiology, 120,* 771–780.

Wong, M. (1983). Embryology and developmental anatomy of the ear. In C. Bluestone & S. Stool (Eds.), *Pediatric otolaryngology* (pp. 90–92). Philadelphia: W. B. Saunders.

3.0 PRINCIPLES OF MEASUREMENT

Anderson, H., Holmgren, L., & Holst, H. E. (1956). Experiments with an objective method of testing the middle ear function. *Acta Otolaryngologica, 46,* 381–383.

Brooks, D. N. (1968). Clinical use of the acoustic impedance meter. *Sound*, *2*, 40–43.

Burke, K. S., Herer, G. R., & McPherson, D. L. (1970). Middle ear impedance measurement: Acoustic and electro–acoustic comparisons. *Acta Otolaryngologica*, *70*, 29–34.

Burke, K. S., Nilges, T. C., & Henry, G. B. (1970). Middle ear impedance measurements. *Journal of Speech and Hearing Research*, *13*, 317–325.

Eliachar, I., Danino, Y., Braun, S., Meged, D., Joachime, H., & Frank, A. (1983). Verification of impedance measurements by a volumetric and electromechanical model. *Scandinavian Audiology*, (Suppl. 17), 21–26.

Elner, A., Ingelstedt, S., & Ivarsson, A. (1971). A method for studies of the middle ear mechanics. *Acta Otolaryngologica*, *72*, 191–200.

Feldman, A. S., Djupesland, G., & Grimes, C. T. (1971). A comparison of impedance measurements. *Archives of Otolaryngology*, *93*, 416–418.

Hudde, H. (1983). Measurement of the eardrum impedance of human ears. *Journal of the Acoustical Society of America*, *73*, 242–247.

Ithell, A. H. (1963). The measurement of acoustical input impedance of human ears. *Acoustica*, *13*, 140–145.

Kennelly, A., & Kurokawa, K. (1921). Acoustic impedance and its measurement. *American Academy of Arts and Sciences Proceedings*, *56*, 1–42.

Lawton, B., & Stinson, M. (1986). Standing wave patterns in the human ear canal used for estimation of acoustic energy reflectance at the eardrum. *Journal of the Acoustical Society of America*, *79*, 1003–1009.

Lilly, D. J. (1972). Acoustic impedance at the tympanic membrane: A review of basic concepts. In D. Rose & L. Keating (Eds.), *Proceedings of the Mayo Impedance Symposium* (pp. 1–34). Rochester, MN: Mayo Foundation.

Lilly, D. J. (1972). Acoustic impedance at the tympanic membrane: An overview of clinical applications. In D. Rose & L. Keating (Eds.), *Proceedings of the Mayo Impedance Symposium* (pp. 51–74). Rochester, MN: Mayo Foundation.

Lilly, D. J., & Shanks, J. E. (1981). Acoustic immittance of an enclosed volume of air. In G. R. Popelka (Ed.), *Hearing assessment with the acoustic reflex* (pp. 145–160). New York: Grune & Stratton.

Lindeman, P., & Holmquist, J. (1981). Measurement of middle ear volume using the impedance audiometer. *American Journal of Otolaryngology*, *2*, 301–303.

Macrae, J. H. (1974). Body inversion and the acoustic immittance of the ear. *Journal of Speech and Hearing Research*, *17*, 310–320.

Margolis, R. H. (1981). Fundamentals of acoustic immittance. In G. R. Popelka (Ed.), *Hearing assessment with the acoustic reflex* (pp. 117–143). New York: Grune & Stratton.

Marwardi, O. K. (1949). Measurement of acoustic impedance. *Journal of the Acoustical Society of America*, *21*, 84–91.

Mendelson, E. S. (1957). A sensitive method for registration of human intratympanic muscle reflex. *Journal of Applied Physiology*, *11*, 499–502.

Metz, O. (1946). The acoustic impedance measured on normal and pathological ears. *Acta Otolaryngologica*, (Suppl. 63), 1–245.

Moller, A. (1960). Improved technique for detailed measurement of the middle ear impedance. *Journal of the Acoustical Society of America, 32*, 250–257.

Moller, A. (1965). An experimental study of the acoustic impedance of the middle ear and its transmission properties. *Acta Otolaryngologica, 60*, 129–149.

Osguthorpe, J. D., & Lam, C. (1981). Methodologic aspects of tympanometry in cats. *Otolaryngology Head and Neck Surgery, 89*, 1037–1040.

Painton, S. W. (1989). Automatic immittance audiometry on children with transtympanic ventilation tubes. *Ear and Hearing, 10*, 209–210.

Porter, T. A., & Winston, M. E. (1975). Methodological aspects of admittance measurements of the middle ear. In *The reflex*. Concord, MA: Grason-Stadler.

Shaw, E. (1974). Transformation of sound pressure level from the free field to the eardrum in the horizontal plane. *Journal of the Acoustical Society of America, 56*, 1848–1861.

Sivian, L. (1935). Acoustic impedance of small orifices. *Journal of the Acoustical Society of America, 7*, 94.

Stinson, M. R., Shaw, E. A. G., & Lawton, B. W. (1982). Estimation of acoustical energy reflectance at the eardrum from measurements of pressure distribution in the human ear canal. *Journal of the Acoustical Society of America, 72*, 766–773.

Terkildsen, K. (1964). Clinical application of impedance measurements with a fixed frequency technique. *International Audiology, 3*, 147–155.

Webster, A. G. (1919). Acoustical impedance, and the theory of horns and of the phonograph. *Proceedings of the National Academy of Science, 5*, 275–282.

West, W. (1928). Measurement of the acoustical impedance of human ears. *Post Office Electrical Engineers Journal, 21*, 293–300.

Wheatstone, C. (1843). An account of several new instruments and processes for determining the constants of a Voltaic circuit. *Philosophical Transactions of the Royal Society of London, 133*, 303–328.

Wiener, F., & Ross, D. (1946). The pressure distribution in the auditory canal in a progressive sound field. *Journal of the Acoustical Society of America, 18*, 401–408.

Wiley, T. L., & Block, M. (1979). Tutorial: Static acoustic-immittance measurements. *Journal of Speech and Hearing Research, 22*, 677–696.

Van Camp, K. J., Vanhuyse, V. J., Creten, W. L., & Vanpeperstraete, P. M. (1978). Impedance and admittance tympanometry. II. Mathematical approach. *Audiology, 17*, 108–119.

Zwislocki, J. (1961). Acoustic measurement of the middle ear function. *Annals of Otology, Rhinology and Laryngology, 70*, 599–606.

Zwislocki, J. (1963). An acoustic method for clinical examination of the ear. *Journal of Speech and Hearing, 6*, 303–314.

Zwislocki, J. (1982). Normal function of the middle ear and its measurement. *Audiology*, *11*, 4–14.

3.1 Variables and Units

Berlin, C. I., & Cullen, J. K., Jr. (1975). The physical basis of impedance measurement. In J. F. Jerger (Ed.), *Handbook of clinical impedance audiometry* (pp. 1–20). Dobbs Ferry, NY: American Electromedics.

Burke, K. S. (1972). An impedance conversion table (G and B to Z). *Asha*, *14*, 655–657.

Fay, R. D., & White, J. E. (1948). Acoustic impedance from motional impedance diagrams. *Journal of the Acoustical Society of America*, *20*, 98–107.

Feldman, A. S., Djupesland, G., & Grimes, C. (1971). A comparison of impedance measurements. *Archives of Otolaryngology*, *93*, 416–418.

Jerger, J. (1972). Suggested nomenclature for impedance audiometry. *Archives of Otolaryngology*, *96*, 1–3.

Popelka, G. (1984). Acoustic immittance measures: Terminology and instrumentation. *Ear and Hearing*, *5*, 262–267.

Sivian, L. (1935). Acoustic impedance of small orifices. *Journal of the Acoustical Society of America*, *7*, 94.

Van Camp, K. J., Margolis, R. H., Wilson, R. H., Creten, W. L., & Shanks, J. E. (1986). *Principles of tympanometry* (Monograph No. 24). Rockville, MD: American Speech–Language-Hearing Association.

3.2 Instrumentation

Bicknell, M., & Morgan, N. (1968). A clinical evaluation of the Zwislocki acoustic bridge [Letter]. *Journal of Laryngology and Otology*, *82*, 673–691.

Burke, K. S., & Herer, G. R. (1973). Impedance and admittance bridge differences in middle ear study. *Journal of Auditory Research*, *13*, 251–256.

Burke, K. S., Herer, G. R., & McPherson, D. L. (1970). Middle ear impedance measurement: Acoustic and electro-acoustic comparisons. *Acta Otolaryngologica*, *70*, 29–34.

Burke, K. S., Schultz, R. E., & Milo, A. P. (1967). On the Zwislocki acoustic bridge [Letter]. *Journal of the Acoustical Society of America*, *41*, 1364.

Cooper, J. C., Jr., Gates, G. A., Owen, J. H., & Dickson, H. D. (1975). An abbreviated impedance bridge for school screening. *Journal of Speech and Hearing Disorders*, *40*, 260–269.

Feldman, A. S. (1972). Mechanical acoustic bridge in normal and pathological ears. In D. Rose, & L. Keating (Eds.), *Proceedings of the Mayo Impedance Symposium* (pp. 147–158). Rochester, MN: Mayo Foundation.

Fria, T. J., Cantekin, E. I., & Probst, G. (1980). Validation of an automatic otoadmittance middle ear analyzer. *Annals of Otology, Rhinology and Laryngology*, *89*, 253–256.

Grason, R. L. (1972). Otoadmittance meter: An instrument for measuring the acoustic admittance of the ear. In D. Rose, & L. Keating (Eds.), *Proceedings of the Mayo Impedance Symposium* (pp. 95–102). Rochester, MN: Mayo Foundation.

Haughton, P. M. (1976). Impedance meters: Some basic considerations. *British Journal of Audiology, 10*, 115–116.

International Electrotechnical Commission (1986). *Measuring devices, aural impedance/admittance instruments* (IEC SC29C) [Draft]. Geneva, Switzerland: Author.

Ivarsson, A., Tjernstrom, O., Bylander, A., & Bennrup, S. (1983). High speed tympanometry and ipsilateral middle ear reflex measurements using a computerized impedance meter. *Scandinavian Audiology, 12*(3), 157–163.

Jacobson, J. T., Kimmel, B. L., & Fausti, S. A. (1975). Clinical application of the Grason-Stadler otoadmittance meter. *Asha, 17*, 11–16.

Jerger, J., Oliver, T. A., & Stach, B. (1986). Problems in the clinical measurement of acoustic reflex latency. *Scandinavian Audiology, 15*, 31–40.

Kennelly, A. E. (1925). The measurement of acoustic impedance with the aid of the telephone receiver. *Journal of the Franklin Institute, 200*, 467–488.

Klar, I. (1972). Madsen impedance measurement system. In D. E. Rose & L. Keating (Eds.), *Proceedings of the Mayo Impedance Symposium* (pp. 75–94). Rochester, MN: Mayo Foundation.

Leis, B. R., & Lutman, M. E. (1979). Calibration of ipsilateral acoustic reflex stimuli. A comparison of loudness balance and equal reflex response methods. *Scandinavian Audiology, 8*, 93–99.

Liden, G., Bjorkman, G., & Peterson, J. L. (1972). Clinical equipment for measurement of middle-ear muscle reflexes and tympanometry. *Journal of Speech and Hearing Disorders, 37*, 100–112.

Lilly, D. J. (1972). Instrumentation for clinical acoustic impedance equipment. In D. E. Rose & L. Keating (Eds.), *Proceedings of the Mayo Impedance Symposium* (pp. 103–108). Rochester, MN: Mayo Foundation.

Lilly, D. J. (1984). Evaluation of the response time of acoustic-immittance instruments. In S. Silman, (Ed.) *The acoustic reflex* (pp. 101–135). New York: Academic Press.

Lutman, M. E. (1980). Note on identification and rectification of the "overshoot" observed with the Grason-Stadler otoadmittance meter during acoustic reflex measurements. *Acta Otolaryngologica* (Stockholm), *89*, 63–65.

Lutman, M. E. (1980). Real-ear calibration of ipsilateral acoustic reflex stimuli from five types of impedance meter. *Scandinavian Audiology, 9*, 137–145.

Margolis, R. H., & Silman, S. (1977). Methods for measuring the temporal characteristics and filter response of electroacoustic impedance instruments. *Journal of Speech and Hearing Research, 20*, 409–414.

Mowry, H. J., & Naughton, R. F. (1973). On the use of an inflatable probe assembly in electroacoustic impedance bridges. *Journal of Speech and Hearing Research, 38*, 354–358.

Neergaard, E. B., Rasmussen, P. E., & Jepsen, O. (1965). Measurement of acoustic impedance by a new principle: Cross-coupling. *Audiology, 4*, 20–24.

Nilges, T. C., Northern, J. L., & Burke, K. (1969). Zwislocki acoustic bridge: Clinical correlations. *Archives of Otolaryngology*, *89*, 69–86.

Niswander, P. S., & Ruth, R. A. (1979). A discussion of some temporal characteristics of electroacoustic impedance bridges. *Journal of the American Auditory Society*, *5*, 151–155.

Pinto, L. H., & Dallos, P. J. (1968). An acoustic bridge for measuring the static and dynamic impedance of the eardrum. *I. E. E. E. Transactions Biomedical Engineering BME-15*, 10–16.

Richards, G. B., & Kartye, J. P. (1973). Comparison of three types of ear tips used for impedance audiometry. *Archives of Otolaryngology*, *97*, 437–440.

Robinette, L. N., & Thompson, D. J. (1986). Digital instrument for measurement of aural acoustic immittance: A preliminary report. *Journal of Rehabilitation Research and Development*, *23*(2), 34–47.

Robinson, D. O., & Brey, R. H. (1978). A study on the calibration characteristics of twenty impedance bridges in clinical use. *Asha*, *20*, 7–14.

Robinson, N. W. (1937). An acoustic impedance bridge. *London, Edinburgh and Dublin Philosophical Magazine and Journal of Science*, (Suppl. 23, Ser. 7), 665–681.

Shanks, J. E., Wilson, R. H., & Jones, H. C. (1985). Earphone-coupling technique for measuring the temporal characteristics of aural acoustic-immittance devices. *Journal of Speech and Hearing Research*, *28*, 305–308.

Sheehy, J. L., & Hughes, R. L. (1974). The ABC's of impedance audiometry. *Laryngoscope*, *84*, 1935–1949.

Terkildsen, K., & Scott-Nielsen, S. (1960). An electroacoustic impedance bridge for clinical use. *Archives of Otolaryngology*, *72*, 339–346.

Thomson, L. R. (1982). Understanding tympanometry. *Pediatric Nursing*, *8*, 193–197.

Van Camp, K. J., Margolis, R. H., Wilson, R. H., Creten, W. L., & Shanks, J. E. (1986). *Principles of tympanometry* (Monograph No. 24). Rockville, MD: American Speech-Language-Hearing Association.

3.3 Standards and Guidelines

American National Standards Institute. (1987). *Specifications for instruments to measure aural acoustic impedance and admittance (Aural Acoustic Immittance)* (ANSI S3. 39-1987). New York: Author.

American Speech-Language-Hearing Association. (1979). Guidelines for acoustic immittance screening of middle-ear function. *Asha*, *21*, 283–298.

American Speech-Language-Hearing Association. (1985). Guidelines for identification audiometry. *Asha*, *27*, 49–52.

American Speech-Language-Hearing Association. (1990). Guidelines for audiometric symbols. *Asha*, *32*(Suppl. 2), 25–30.

American Speech-Language-Hearing Association. (1990). Guidelines for screening for hearing impairment and middle-ear disorders. *Asha*, *32*(Suppl. 2), 17–24.

Ewertsen, H. W. (1973). Audiogram interpretation: Standardization of symbols for stapedial reflexes. *Scandinavian Audiology*, *1*, 61–63.

Feldman, A. S. (1976). Impedance terminology. *Archives of Otolaryngology*, *102*, 251–252.

International Electrotechnical Commission. (1986). *Measuring devices, aural impedance/admittance instruments.* (IEC SC29C) [Draft]. Geneva, Switzerland: Author.

Jerger, J. F. (1972). Suggested nomenclature for impedance audiometry. *Archives of Otolaryngology*, *96*, 1–3.

Jerger, J. F. (1975). Impedance terminology. *Archives of Otolaryngology*, *101*, 589–590.

Schow, R. L., Pedersen, J. K., Nerbonne, M. A., & Boe, R. (1981). Comparison of ASHA's immittance guidelines and standard medical diagnostic procedures. *Ear and Hearing*, *2*, 251–255.

Shanks, J. (1987). Aural acoustic immittance standards. *Seminars in Hearing*, *8*, 307–318.

4.0 STATIC MEASURES

Alberti, P. W., & Kristensen, R. (1972). The compliance of the middle ear: Its accuracy in routine clinical practice. In D. E. Rose & L. Keating (Eds.), *Proceedings of the Mayo Impedance Symposium* (pp. 159–168). Rochester, MN: Mayo Foundation.

Ashby, J. K., Pope, G.D., & Barron, S. J. (1980). A reliability study of the electro-acoustic impedance bridge in private pediatric practice. *American Journal of Otology*, *1*, 168–170.

Beattie, R., & Leamy, D. (1975). Otoadmittance normative values, procedural variables, and reliability. *Journal of the American Auditory Society*, *1*, 21–27.

Bel, J., Causse, J., & Michaux, P. (1975). Paradoxical compliances in otosclerosis. *Audiology*, *14*, 118–129.

Bicknell, M., & Morgan, N. A. (1968). Clinical evaluation of the Zwislocki acoustic bridge. *Journal of Laryngology and Otology*, *82*, 673–691.

Blood, I. M., & Greenberg, H. J. (1977). Acoustic admittance of the ear in the geriatric person. *Journal of the American Auditory Society*, *2*, 185–187.

Brooks, D. N. (1968). Clinical use of the acoustic impedance meter. *Sound*, *2*, 40–43.

Brooks, D. N. (1971). Electro-acoustic impedance bridge studies on normal ears of children. *Journal of Speech and Hearing Research*, *14*, 247–253.

Brooks, D. N. (1982). Acoustic impedance studies on otitis media with effusion. *International Journal of Pediatric Otorhinolaryngology*, *4*, 89–94.

Burke, K. S. (1972). An impedance conversion table (G and B to Z). *Asha*, *14*, 655–656.

Burke, K., & Nilges, T. (1970). A comparison of three middle ear impedance norms as predictors of otosclerosis. *Journal of Auditory Research*, *10*, 52–58.

Creten, W. L., Van de Heyning, P. H., & Van Camp, K. J. (1985). Immittance audiometry. *Scandinavian Audiology*, *14*, 115–121.

Cunningham, D. (1976). Admittance values associated with the acoustic reflex and reflex decay. *Journal of the American Auditory Society*, *l*, 197–205.

de Jonge, R. R., & Valente, M. (1979). Interpreting ear differences in static compliance measurements. *Journal of Speech and Hearing Disorders*, *44*, 209–213.

Dempsey, C. (1975). Static compliance. In J. F. Jerger (Ed.), *Handbook of clinical impedance audiometry* (pp. 71–84). Dobbs Ferry, NY: American Electromedics.

Djupesland, G. (1964). Mechanical component to deafness in Meniere's disease. *Acta Otolaryngologica*, (Suppl. 188), 206–208.

Djupesland, G. (1969). Use of impedance indicator in diagnosis of middle ear pathology. *Audiology*, *8*, 570–579.

Djupesland, G., & Kvernvold, H. (1973). A comparison between absolute and "relative" impedance measurement as a method of distinguishing between otosclerosis and ossicular chain discontinuity. *Scandinavian Audiology*, *2*, 93–97.

Farrant, R. H., & Skurr, B. (1966). Measuring the acoustic impedance of severely deaf ears to test for conductive component. *Journal of Otolaryngological Society of Australia*, *2*, 49–53.

Feldman, A. S. (1963). Impedance measurements at the eardrum as an aid to diagnosis. *Journal of Speech and Hearing Research*, *6*, 315–327.

Feldman, A. S. (1964). Acoustic impedance measurements as a clinical procedure. *Audiology*, *3*, 1–11.

Feldman, A. S. (1967). Acoustic impedance studies of the normal ear. *Journal of Speech and Hearing Research*, *10*, 165–176.

Feldman, A. S. (1969). Acoustic impedance measurements of post-stapedectomized ears. *Laryngoscope*, *79*, 1132–1155.

Feldman, A. S. (1972). Mechanical acoustic bridge in normal and pathological ears. In D. Rose & L. Keating (Eds.), *Proceedings of the Mayo Impedance Symposium* (pp. 147–158). Rochester, MN: Mayo Foundation.

Feldman, A. S. (1974). Eardrum abnormality and the measurement of middle ear function. *Archives of Otolaryngology*, *99*, 211–217.

Fria, T. J., Cantekin, E. I., & Probst, G. (1980). Validation of an automatic otoadmittance middle ear analyzer. *Annals of Otology, Rhinology and Laryngology*, *89*, 253–256.

Gersdorff, M. C. (1977). Comparative study between the normally hearing child and the hard of hearing child, by acoustic impedance measurements of the ear. *Archives of Otorhinolaryngology*, *217*, 13–31.

Hall, J. W. (1979). Effects of age and sex on static compliance. *Archives of Otolaryngology*, *105*, 153–156.

Hall, M., & Hughes, R. (1975). Maximum compliance and the symptom of fullness in Meniere's disease. *Archives of Otolaryngology*, *4*, 227–228.

Herman, L. E. (1977). Static compliance of the eardrum in Meniere's disease. *Archives of Otolaryngology*, *103*, 84–86.

Hopkinson, N., Schramm, V., Bosse, B., & Leggett, S. (1978). A comparison of results: Acoustic susceptance and otolaryngology. *Journal of the American Auditory Society*, *3*, 191–199.

Hudde, H. (1983). Measurement of the eardrum impedance of human ears. *Journal of the Acoustical Society of America*, *73*, 242–247.

Ithell, A. H. (1963). The measurement of acoustical input impedance of human ears. *Acoustica*, *13*, 140–145.

Ivey, R. (1975). Tympanometric curves and otosclerosis. *Journal of Speech and Hearing Research*, *18*, 554–558.

Jacobson, J. T., & Mahoney, T. M. (1977). Admittance tympanometry in otosclerotic ears. *Journal of the American Auditory Society*, *3*, 91–98.

Jerger, J. (1970). Clinical experience with impedance audiometry. *Archives of Otolaryngology*, *92*, 311–324.

Jerger, J., Anthony, L., Jerger, S., & Mauldin, L. (1974). Studies in impedance audiometry: III. Middle-ear disorders. *Archives of Otolaryngology*, *99*, 165–171.

Jerger, J., Jerger, S., & Maudlin, L. (1972). Studies in impedance audiometry: Normal and sensorineural ears. *Archives of Otolaryngology*, *99*, 513–523.

Jerger, J., & Keith, W. (1980). Inter- versus intrasubject variability in acoustic immittance. *Ear and Hearing*, *1*, 338–340.

Jerger, S., Jerger, J., Mauldin, L., & Segal, P. (1974). Studies in impedance audiometry: II. Children less than six-years old. *Archives of Otolaryngology*, *99*, 1–9.

Lindeman, P., & Holmquist, J. (1981). Measurement of middle ear volume using the impedance audiometer. *American Journal of Otolaryngology*, *2*, 301–303.

Lindeman, P., & Holmquist J. (1982). Volume measurement of middle ear and mastoid air cell system with impedance audiometry on patients with eardrum perforations. *American Journal of Otolaryngology*, *4*, 46–51.

Macrae, J. H. (1972). A theoretical investigation of cochlear effects on the acoustic impedance of the ear. *Journal of Auditory Research*, *12*, 265–270.

Margolis, R. H., & Popelka, G. R. (1975). Static and dynamic acoustic impedance measurements in infant ears. *Journal of Speech and Hearing Research*, *18*, 435–443.

Marston, L. E., Sterret, M. L., & Clennan, R. O. (1980). Effect of cigarette smoking on tympanic membrane admittance characteristics. *Ear and Hearing*, *1*, 267–270.

Marwardi, O. K. (1949). Measurement of acoustic impedance. *Journal of the Acoustical Society of America*, *21*, 84–91.

Moffat, D. A., Ramsden, R. T., Rosenberg, J. N., Booth, J. B., & Gibson, W. P. (1977). Otoadmittance measurements in patients with rheumatoid arthritis. *Journal of Laryngology and Otology*, *91*, 917–927.

Moller, A. R. (1964). The acoustic impedance in experimental studies on the middle ear. *Audiology*, *2*, 123–134.

Nerbonne, M., Bliss, A., & Schow, R. (1978). Acoustic impedance values in the elderly. *Journal of the American Auditory Society*, *4*, 57–59.

Nilges, T. C., Northern, J. L., & Burke, K. (1969). Zwislocki acoustic bridge: Clinical correlations. *Archives of Otolaryngology*, *89*, 69–86.

Nixon, J. C., & Glorig, A. (1964). Reliability of acoustic impedance measures of the eardrum. *Journal of Auditory Research*, *4*, 261–276.

Parson, I., Kunov, H., Abel, S. M., & Alberti, P. W. (1984). The acoustic impedance locus for normal human ears. *Scandinavian Audiology*, (Suppl. 22), 1–14.

Porter, T. (1972). Normal otoadmittance values for three populations. *Journal of Auditory Research*, *12*, 53–58.

Porter, T. A., & Winston, M. E. (1973). Reliability of measures obtained with the otoadmittance meter. *Journal of Auditory Research*, *13*, 142–146.

Porter, T., & Winston, M. (1975). Methodological aspects of admittance measurements of the middle ear. *Journal of Auditory Research*, *13*, 172–177.

Priede, V. M. (1970). Acoustic impedance in two cases of ossicular discontinuity. *International Audiology*, *9*, 127–136.

Rabinowitz, W. M. (1981). Measurement of the acoustic input immittance of the human ear. *Journal of the Acoustical Society of America*, *70*, 1025–1035.

Roberto, M., & Zito, F. (1983). Acoustic admittance measures in human temporal bones. *Audiology*, *22*, 438–450.

Shanks, J. E., & Lilly, D. J. (1981). An evaluation of tympanometric estimates of ear canal volume. *Journal of Speech and Hearing Research*, *24*, 557–566.

Stewart, G. W. (1927). Direct absolute measurement of acoustic impedance. *Physiology Review*, *28*, 1038–1047.

Terkildsen, K., Osterhammel, P., & Wielsen, S. (1970). Impedance measurements, probe-tone intensity, and middle ear reflexes. *Acta Otolaryngologica*, (Suppl. 263), 205–207.

Terkildsen, K., & Thomsen, K. A. (1959). The influence of pressure variations on the impedance of the human eardrum. *Laryngoscope*, *73*, 409–418.

Thompson, D., Sills, J., Recke, K., & Bui, D. (1979). Acoustic admittance and the aging ear. *Journal of Speech and Hearing Research*, *22*, 29–36.

Tillman, T., Dallos, P., & Kuruvilla, T. (1964). Reliability of measures obtained with the Zwislocki acoustic bridge. *Journal of the Acoustical Society of America*, *36*, 582–588.

West, W. (1928). Measurement of the acoustical impedance of human ears. *Post Office Electrical Engineers Journal*, *21*, 293–300.

Wilber, L. (1972). Use of absolute and relative impedance in defining the nature of middle ear lesions in children. In D. Rose & L. Keating (Eds.), *Proceedings of the Mayo Impedance Symposium* (pp. 109–126). Rochester, MN: Mayo Foundation.

Wiley, T. L. (1989). Static acoustic-admittance measures in normal ears: A combined analysis for ears with and without notched tympanograms. *Journal of Speech and Hearing Research*, *32*, 688.

Wiley, T. L., & Block, M. G. (1979). Tutorial: Static acoustic-immittance measurements. *Journal of Speech and Hearing Research*, *22*, 677–696.

Wiley, T. L., Oviatt, D. L., & Block, M. G. (1987). Acoustic-immittance measures in normal ears. *Journal of Speech and Hearing Research*, *30*, 161–170.

Wilson, R. H., Shanks, J. E., & Velde, T. M. (1981). Aural acoustic-immittance measurements: Inter-aural differences. *Journal of Speech and Hearing Disorders*, *46*, 413–421.

Woodford, C. M., Henderson, D., Hamernik, R. P., & Feldman, A. S. (1975). Static acoustic impedance of the chinchilla middle ear: Awake and sedated. *Journal of the Acoustical Society of America, 58*, 1100–1103.

Zwislocki, J. (1957). Some impedance measurements of normal and pathological ears. *Journal of the Acoustical Society of America, 29*, 1312–1317.

Zwislocki, J. (1957). Some measurements of the impedance at the eardrum. *Journal of the Acoustical Society of America, 29*, 349–356.

Zwislocki, J. (1961). Acoustic measurement of the middle ear function. *Annals of Otology, Rhinology and Laryngology, 70*, 599–606.

Zwislocki, J. (1962). Analysis of the middle ear function—Part I: Input impedance. *Journal of the Acoustical Society of America, 34*, 1514–1523.

Zwislocki, J. (1963). An acoustic method for clinical examination of the ear. *Journal of Speech and Hearing Research, 6*, 303–314.

Zwislocki, J. (1982). Normal function of the middle ear and its measurement. *Audiology, 21*, 4–14.

Zwislocki, J., & Feldman, A. S. (1963). Post-mortem acoustic impedance of human ears. *Journal of the Acoustical Society of America, 35*, 104–105.

Zwislocki, J., & Feldman, A. S. (1970). Acoustic impedance of pathological ears. (Monograph No. 15). Rockville, MD: American Speech-Language-Hearing Association.

5.0 TYMPANOMETRY

Brooks, D. N. (1968). Clinical use of the acoustic impedance meter. *Sound, 2*, 40–43.

Creten, W. L., & Van Camp, K. J. (1974). Transient and quasi-static tympanometry. *Scandinavian Audiology, 3*, 39–42.

Feldman, A. (1976). Tympanometry: Application and interpretation. *Annals of Otology, Rhinology and Laryngology, 85*, 202–208.

Fria, T. J., Cantekin, E. I., & Probst, G. (1980). Validation of an automatic otoadmittance middle ear analyzer. *Annals of Otology, Rhinology and Laryngology, 89*, 253–256.

Harford, E. R. (1975). Tympanometry. In J. F. Jerger (Ed.), *Handbook of clinical impedance audiometry* (pp. 47–70). Dobbs Ferry, NY: American Electromedics.

Horning, J. (1975, April). Tympanometry and hearing aid selection. *Hearing Aid Journal, 28*, 8, 50.

Keating, L., Rose, D., Facer, G., Whicker, J., & Schreurs, K. (1972, June). Acoustic-impedance measurements in the deaf. In D. Rose & L. Keating (Eds.), *Proceedings of the Mayo Impedance Symposium* (pp. 177–186). Rochester, MN: Mayo Foundation.

Liden G., Peterson, J. L., & Bjorkman, G. (1970). Tympanometry: A method for analysis of middle ear function. *Acta Otolaryngologica*, (Suppl. 263), 218–224.

Lindeman, P., Holmquist, J., & Aberg, B. (1984). Ear drum mobility and middle ear volume measured with tympanometry. *Scandinavian Audiology, 13*, 147–150.

Lopes, O., Granato, L., & Elisabestky, M. (1972). The early diagnosis of a glomic tumor in the middle ear by means of acoustic impedance. *Impedance Newsletter*, *1*(5). Dobbs Ferry, NY: American Electromedics.

Macrae, J. H., & Bulteau, V. G. (1976). Cochlear effects in tympanometry. *Journal of Auditory Research*, *16*, 102–113.

Morgenstern, N., & Jones-Crymes, B. (1979). Analysis of tympanometry of a severe to profound hearing-impaired population of school-age children. *Journal of Speech and Hearing Disorders*, *44*, 230–235.

Paradise, J. L. (1982). Editorial retrospective: Tympanometry. *New England Journal of Medicine*, *307*, 1074–1076.

Peterson, J. L., & Liden, G. (1970). Tympanometry in human temporal bones. *Archives of Otolaryngology*, *92*, 258–266.

Plath, P. (1983). The importance of tympanometry in cases of sensorineural hearing loss. *Scandinavian Audiology*, (Suppl. 17), 18–20.

Renvall, U., Liden, G., & Bjorkman, G. (1975). Experimental tympanometry in human temporal bones. *Scandinavian Audiology*, *4*, 135–144.

Roberto, M., & Zito, F. (1983). Acoustic admittance measures in human temporal bones. *Audiology*, *22*, 438–450.

Shanks, J. E. (1984). Tympanometry. *Ear and Hearing*, *5*, 268–280.

Shanks, J. E., Lilly, D. J., Margolis, R. H., Wiley, T. L., & Wilson, R. H. (1988). Tympanometry. *Journal of Speech and Hearing Disorders*, *53*, 354–377.

Thomson, L. R. (1982). Understanding tympanometry. *Pediatric Nursing*, *8*, 193–197.

Vanpeperstraete, P. M., Creten, W. L., & Van Camp, K. J. (1979). On the asymmetry of susceptance tympanograms. *Scandinavian Audiology*, *8*, 173–179.

5.1 Measurement Techniques

Alberti, P. W., & Jerger, J. F. (1974). Probe-tone frequency and the diagnostic value of tympanometry. *Archives of Otolaryngology*, *99*, 206–210.

Belal, A., Jr., & Forquer, B. D. (1980). Experimental tympanometry. *Journal of Laryngology and Otology*, *94*, 595–605.

Brooks, D. N. (1983). Comment on "Normal tympanometric shape." *Ear and Hearing*, *4*, 114.

Brooks, D. N. (1985). Acoustic impedance measurement as screening procedure in children: Discussion paper. *Journal of the Royal Society of Medicine*, *78*, 119–121.

Causse, J. R. (1983). Tympanometry and fistula test. *Audiology*, *22*, 451–462.

Cooper, J. C., Jr., Hearne, E. M., & Gates, G. A. (1982). Normal tympanometric shape. *Ear and Hearing*, *3*, 241–245.

Creten, W. L., & Van Camp, K. J. (1974). Transient and quasi-static tympanometry. *Scandinavian Audiology*, *3*, 39–42.

Creten, W. L. Vanpeperstraete, P. M., & Van Camp, K. J. (1978). Impedance and admittance tympanometry. I. Experimental approach. *Audiology*, *17*, 97–107.

Decraemer, W. F., Creten, W. L., & Van Camp, K. J. (1984). Tympanometric middle ear pressure determination with two component admittance meters. *Scandinavian Audiology, 13*, 165–172.

Eliachar, I., Danino, Y., Braun, S., Meged, D., Joachims, H., & Frank, A. (1983). Verification of impedance measurements by a volumetric and electromechanical model. *Scandinavian Audiology*, (Suppl. 17), 21–26.

Eliachar, I., & Northern, J. (1974). Studies in tympanometry: Validation of the present technique for determining intra-tympanic pressures through the intact eardrum. *Laryngoscope, 84*, 247–255.

Eliachar, I., Sando, I., & Northern, J. L. (1974). Measurement of middle ear pressure in guinea pigs. *Archives of Otolaryngology, 99*, 172–176.

Feldman, A. S. (1976). Tympanometry procedures, interpretations and variables. In A. S. Feldman & L. A. Wilber (Eds.), *Acoustic impedance and admittance: The measurement of middle ear function* (pp. 282–284). Baltimore: Williams & Wilkins.

Funasaka, S., Fuani, H., & Kumakawa, K. (1984). Sweep frequency tympanometry: Its development and diagnostic value. *Audiology, 23*, 366–379.

Gates, G. A. (1986). Differential otomanometry. *American Journal of Otolaryngology, 7*, 147–150.

Iandola, A., Marciano, E., & Saulino, C. (1983). Mathematical description of tympanometric data. *Revue de Laryngologie, Otologie, Rhinologie* (Bordeaux), *104*, 263–265.

Karlsson, K., & Hagerman, B. (1984). A clinical comparison between a laboratory and a commercial impedance audiometer. *Scandinavian Audiology, 13*, 199–203.

Liden, G., Harford, E., & Hallen, O. (1974). Automatic tympanometry in clinical practice. *Audiology, 13*, 126–139.

Lindeman, P., Holmquist, J., & Aberg, B. (1984). Ear drum mobility and middle ear volume measured with tympanometry. *Scandinavian Audiology, 13*, 147–150.

Nomura, Y., Harada, T., & Fukaya, T. (1979). Dynamic tympanometry. *Journal of the American Auditory Society, 4*, 190–194.

Osguthorpe, J. D., & Lam, C. (1981). Methodologic aspects of tympanometry in cats. *Otolaryngology, Head and Neck Surgery, 89*, 1037–1040.

Pepper, M. G., & Baxter, J. S. (1981). Measurement of middle ear pressure with a single transducer and a half-wavelength acoustic transmission line. *Medical and Biological and Engineering Computing, 19*, 179–184.

Terkildsen, K. (1964). Clinical application of impedance measurements with a fixed frequency technique. *Audiology, 3*, 147–153.

Thomsen, K. A. (1960). Objective determination of middle ear pressure. *Acta Otolaryngologica*, (Suppl. 158), 212–216.

Thomson, L. R. (1982). Understanding tympanometry. *Pediatric Nursing, 8*, 193–197.

Van Camp, K. J., Vanhuyse, V. J., Creten, W. L. & Vanpeperstraete, P. M. (1978). Impedance and admittance tympanometry. II. Mathematical approach. *Audiology, 17*, 108–119.

Wiley, T. L., & Block, M. G. (1979). Tutorial: Static acoustic-immittance measurements. *Journal of Speech and Hearing Research, 22*, 677–696.

5.1.1 Sources of Variability

Alberti, P., & Jerger, J. (1974). Probe-tone frequency and the diagnostic value of tympanometry. *Archives of Otolaryngology, 99*, 206–210.

Ashby, J. K., Pope, G. D., & Baron, S. J. (1980). A reliability study of the electro-acoustic impedance bridge in private pediatric practice. *American Journal of Otology, 1*, 168–170.

Berry, R. A., & Roman, T. (1982). The middle ear in long term dialysis. *Southern Medical Journal, 75*, 1227–1228, 1231.

Brey, R. H., Robinson, D. O., Ahroon, W. A., & Frazer, G. J. (1980). Hysteresis resulting from two tympanometric recording procedures. *Michigan Speech-Language-Hearing Association Journal, 16*(1), 13–29.

Brooks, D. N. (1979). Tympanometry: Between ear symmetry and normative values. *Journal of the American Auditory Society, 5*, 112–117.

Drake-Lee, A. B., & Casey, W. F. (1983). Anaesthesia and tympanometry. *International Journal of Pediatric Otorhinolaryngology, 6*(2), 171–178.

Feldman, A. S. (1974). Eardrum abnormality and the measurement of middle ear function. *Archives of Otolaryngology, 99*, 211–217.

Feldman, A. S., & Williams, P. S. (1976). Tympanometric measurement of the transmission characteristics of the ear with and without the acoustic reflex. *Scandinavian Audiology, 5*, 43–47.

Feldman, R. M., Fria, T. J., Palfrey, C. C., & Dellecker, C. M. (1984). Effects of rate of air pressure change on tympanometry. *Ear and Hearing, 5*, 91–95.

Flisberg, K., Hallgarde, U., & Paulsson, B. (1982). Tympanometry before and during nitrous oxide anasthesia with middle ear effusion. *American Journal of Otolaryngology, 3*, 344–348.

Jerger, J., & Keith, W. (1980). Inter- versus intrasubject variability in acoustic immittance. *Ear and Hearing, 1*, 338–340.

Lildholdt, T. (1980). Negative middle ear pressure. Variations by season and sex. *Annals of Otology, Rhinology and Laryngology*, (Suppl. 89), 67–70.

Macrae, J. H. (1974). Body inversion and the acoustic immitance of the ear. *Journal of Speech and Hearing Research, 17*, 310–320.

Margolis, C. Z., Porter, B., Barnoon, S., & Pilpel, D. (1979). Reliability of the middle ear examination. *Israel Journal of Medical Science, 15*, 23–28.

Margolis, R. H., & Popelka, G. R. (1977). Interactions among tympanometric variables. *Journal of Speech and Hearing Research, 20*, 447–462.

Margolis, R. H., & Smith, P. (1977). Tympanometric asymmetry. *Journal of Speech and Hearing Research, 20*, 437–446.

Marston, L. E., Sterret, M. L., & Clennan, R. O. (1980). Effect of cigarette smoking on tympanic membrane admittance characteristics. *Ear and Hearing, 1*, 267–270.

Osguthorpe, J. D., & Lam, C. (1981). Methodologic aspects of tympanometry in cats. *Otolaryngology, Head and Neck Surgery, 89*, 1037–1040.

Pearlman, R. C., & Graber, D. J. (1978). The significant asymmetrical tympanogram [Letter]. *Journal of Speech and Hearing Research, 21,* 606–607.

Robinette, M. S., Rhoads, D. P., & Marion, M. W. (1975). Effects of secobarbital on impedance audiometry. *Archives of Otolaryngology, 100,* 351–354.

Shanks, J. E., & Lilly, D. J. (1981). An evaluation of tympanometric estimates of ear canal volume. *Journal of Speech and Hearing Research, 24,* 557–566.

Shanks, J. E., & Wilson, R. H. (1986). Effects of duration and rate of ear canal pressure changes on tympanometric measures. *Journal of Speech and Hearing Research, 29,* 11–19.

Smith, C. G., Paradise, J. L., & Young T. I. (1982). Modified schema for classifying positive-pressure tympanograms. *Pediatrics, 69,* 351–354.

Terkildsen, K., & Thomsen, K. A. (1959). The influence of pressure variations on the impedance of the human eardrum. *Laryngoscope, 73,* 409–418.

Thomsen, K. A., Terkildsen, K., & Arfred, I. (1965). Middle ear pressure variations during anesthesia. *Archives of Otolaryngology, 92,* 609–611.

Van Camp, K. J., Creten, W. L., Vanpeperstraete, P. M., & Van de Heyning, P. H. (1981). Physical parameters influencing tympanometry. In R. Penna & P. Pizarro (Eds.), *Proceedings of the Fourth International Symposium on Acoustic Impedance Measurements* (pp. 309–317). Lisbon, Portugal: Universidade Nova de Lisboa.

Vanpeperstraete, P. M., Creten, W. L., & Van Camp, K. J. (1979). On the asymmetry of susceptance tympanograms. *Scandinavian Audiology, 8,* 173–179.

Wever, E. G., Bray, C. W., & Lawrence, M. (1942). The effect of pressure in the middle ear. *Journal of Experimental Psychology, 30,* 40–52.

Wilson, R. H., Shanks, J. E., & Kaplan, S. K. (1984). Tympanometric changes in 226 Hz and 678 Hz across trials for two directions of ear canal pressure change. *Journal of Speech and Hearing Research, 27,* 257–266.

5.1.2 Multi-Frequency/Phasor Tympanometry

Arslan, E., Canavesio, F., & Cerutti, R. (1979). A new approach to a multi-frequential impedance measurement [Letter]. *Scandinavian Audiology, 8,* 127–128.

Bennett, M. J., & Weatherby, L. A. (1979). Multiple probe frequency acoustic reflex measurements. *Scandinavian Audiology, 8,* 233–239.

Causse, J., Bel, J., & Causse, B. (1977). Multifrequency impedance testing in relation to otospongiotic stapedial fixation and other factors. *Audiology, 16,* 338–354.

Colletti, V. (1975). Methodologic observations on tympanometry with regard to the probe tone frequency. *Acta Otolaryngologica, 80,* 54–60.

Colletti, V. (1976). Tympanometry from 200 to 2000 Hz probe tone. *Audiology, 15,* 106–119.

Colletti, V. (1977). Multifrequency tympanometry. *Audiology, 16,* 278–287.

Creten, W. L., Van Camp, K. J., Maes, M. A., & Vanpeperstraete, P. M. (1981). The diagnostic value of phase-angle tympanograms. *Audiology, 20,* 1–14.

Creten, W. L., Van Camp, K. J., Vanpeperstraete, P. M., & Van de Heyning, P. H. (1981). On phase angle tympanograms and phasor curves. In R. Penna & P. Pizarro (Eds.), *Proceedings of the Fourth International Symposium on Acoustic Impedance Measurements* (pp. 579–588). Lisbon, Portugal: Universidade Nova de Lisboa.

Creten, W. L., Vanpeperstraete, P. M., & Van Camp, K. J. (1978). Impedance and admittance tympanometry. I. Experimental approach. *Audiology, 17,* 97–107.

Funasaka, S., Fuani, H., & Kumakawa, K. (1984). Sweep frequency tympanometry: Its development and diagnostic value. *Audiology, 23,* 366–379.

Gersdorff, M., & Stoquart, T. (1985). Phasor diagram: A comparative study between normal ears and otosclerotic ears. *Audiology, 24,* 167–173.

Liden, G., Peterson, J. L., & Bjorkman, G. (1970). Tympanometry. *Archives of Otolaryngology, 92,* 248–257.

Lilly, D. J. (1984). Multiple frequency, multiple component tympanometry: New approaches to an old diagnostic problem. *Ear and Hearing, 5,* 300–308.

Lutman, M. E. (1984). Phasor admittance measurements of the middle ear. I. Theoretical approach. *Scandinavian Audiology, 13,* 253–264.

Lutman, M. E., McKenzie, H., & Swan, I. R. C. (1984). Phasor admittance measurements of the middle ear. *Scandinavian Audiology, 13,* 265–274.

Margolis, R. H., Van Camp, K. J., Wilson, R. H., & Creten, W. L. (1985). Multifrequency tympanometry in normal ears. *Audiology, 24,* 44–53.

Shanks, J. E., Lilly, D. J., Margolis, R. H., Wiley, T. H., & Wilson, R. H. (1988). Typanometry. *Journal of Speech and Hearing Disorders, 53,* 354–377.

Van Camp, K. J., Creten, W. L., Van de Heyning, P. H., Decraemer, W. F., & Vanpeperstraete, P. M. (1983). A search for the most suitable immittance components and probe tone frequency in tympanometry. *Scandinavian Audiology, 12,* 27–34.

Van Camp, K. J., Decraemer, P. M., Vanpeperstraete, P. M., & Creten, W. L. (1980). The interpretation of multi-extrema tympanograms. In *The reflex.* Concord, MA: Grason-Stadler.

Van Camp, K. J., Raman, E. R., & Creten, W. L. (1976). Two component versus admittance tympanometry. *Audiology, 15,* 120–127.

Van Camp, K. J., Vanhuyse, V. J., Creten, W. L. & Vanpeperstraete, P. M. (1978). Impedance and admittance tympanometry. II. Mathematical approach. *Audiology, 17,* 108–119.

Vanhuyse, V. J., Creten, W. L., & Van Camp, K. J. (1975). On the W-notching of tympanograms. *Scandinavian Audiology, 4,* 45–50.

Wada, H., Kobayashi, T., Suetake, M., & Tachizaki, H. (1989). Dynamic behavior of the middle ear based on sweep frequency tympanometry. *Audiology, 28,* 127–134.

5.2 Studies in Subjects with Normal Middle Ears

Ashby, J. K., Pope, G. D., & Barron, S. J. (1980). A reliability study of the electro-acoustic impedance bridge in private practice. *American Journal of Otolaryngology, 1,* 169–170.

Bennett, M. J. (1975). Acoustic impedance bridge measurements with the neonate. *British Journal of Audiology, 9*, 117–124.

Bennett, M. J. (1976). A longitudinal study of middle ear function in a group of infants after measles immunization. *British Journal of Audiology, 10*, 13–16.

Brooks, D. N. (1971). Electro-acoustic impedance bridge studies on normal ears of children. *Journal of Speech and Hearing Research, 14*, 247–253.

Brooks, D. (1979). Tympanometry: Between ear symmetry and normative values. *Journal of the American Auditory Society, 5*, 112–117.

Cavanaugh, R. M., Jr. (1982). Pneumatic otoscopy in infants and children. *Southern Medical Journal, 75*, 335–338.

Chermak, G. D., & Luchini, A. (1978). Reliability of tympanometric measures obtained with children. *Journal of the American Auditory Society, 4*, 60–63.

Cooper, J. C., Jr., Hearne, E. M., & Gates, G. A. (1982). Normal tympanometric shape. *Ear and Hearing, 3*, 241–245.

Creten, W. L., & Van Camp, K. J. (1974). Transient and quasi-static tympanometry. *Scandinavian Audiology, 3*, 13–19.

Creten, W. L., Van de Heyning, P. H., & Van Camp, K. J. (1985). Immittance audiometry. *Scandinavian Audiology, 14*, 115–121.

Creten, W. L., Vanpeperstraete, P. M., & Van Camp, K. J. (1978). Impedance and admittance tympanometry. I. Experimental approach. *Audiology, 17*, 97–107.

Eliachar, I., & Northern, J. L. (1974). Studies in tympanometry: Validation of present technique for determining intra-tympanic pressures through the intact eardrum. *Laryngoscope, 84*, 207–255.

Falk, B. (1981). Negative middle ear pressure induced by sniffing. A tympanometric study in persons with healthy ears. *Journal of Otolaryngology, 10*, 299–305.

Feldman, A. S. (1967). Acoustic impedance studies of the normal ear. *Journal of Speech and Hearing Research, 10*, 165–178.

Feldman, A. S. (1974). Eardrum abnormality and the measurement of middle ear function. *Archives of Otolaryngology, 99*, 211–217.

Feldman, A., & Williams, P. (1976). Tympanometric measurements of the transmission characteristics of the ear with and without the acoustic reflex. *Scandinavian Audiology, 5*, 43–47.

Fiellau-Nikolajsen, M. (1979). Tympanometry in three-year-old children. II. Seasonal influence on tympanometric results in non-selected groups of three-year-old children. *Scandinavian Audiology, 8*, 181–185.

Fiellau-Nikolajsen, M. (1980). Serial tympanometry and middle ear status in 3-year-old children. *O. R. L. Journal of Otorhinolaryngology and Related Specialties, 42*, 220–232.

Fiellau-Nikolajsen, M. (1980). Tympanometry in three-year-old children. Prevalence and spontaneous course of MEE. *Annals of Otology, Rhinology and Laryngology, 89*(Suppl. 68), 223–227.

Fiellau-Nikolajsen, M. (1981). Tympanometry in three-year-old children. The 3-year follow-up of a cohort study. *O. R. L. Journal of Otorhinolaryngology and Related Specialties, 43*, 89–103.

Fiellau-Nikolajsen, M., Falbe-Hansen, J., & Knudstrup, P. (1980). Tympanometry in three-year-old children. III. Correlation between tympanometry and findings at paracentesis in a prospectively followed population of otherwise healthy children aged 3–4 years. *Scandinavian Audiology*, *9*, 49–54.

Fiellau-Nikolajsen, M., & Lous, J. (1979). Prospective tympanometry in 3-year-old children. *Archives of Otolaryngology*, *105*, 461–466.

Fiellau-Nikolajsen, M., & Lous, J. (1982). Long-term prognostic-significance of serial tympanometry. A cohort study of preschool children. *O. R. L. Journal of Otorhinolaryngology and Related Specialties*, *44*, 90–100.

Fiellau-Nikolajsen, M., Lous, J., Vang Pedersen, S., & Schousboe, H. H. (1977). Tympanometry in three-year-old children. I. A regional prevalence study on the distribution of tympanometric results in a non-selected population of 3-year-old children. *Scandinavian Audiology*, *6*, 199–204.

Fulton, R., & Lamb, L. (1970). *Acoustic impedance and tympanometry with the retarded: A normative study* (Report No. 1). Parsons Research Center. Parsons, KS.

Gersdorff, M. C. (1977). Comparative study between the normally hearing child and the hard of hearing child, by acoustic impedance measurements of the ear. *Archives of Otorhinolaryngology* (New York), *217*, 13–31.

Hall, J. W., & Weaver, T. (1979). Impedance audiometry in a young population. The effect of age, sex, and tympanogram abnormalities. *Journal of Otolaryngology*, *8*, 210–222.

Harford, E. R. (1975). Tympanometry. In J. F. Jerger (Ed.), *Handbook of clinical impedance audiometry* (pp. 47–70). Dobbs Ferry, NY: American Electromedics.

Himelfarb, M. Z., Popelka, G. R., & Shanon, E. (1979). Tympanometry in normal neonates. *Journal of Speech and Hearing Research*, *22*, 179–191.

Jerger, J. (1970). Clinical experience with impedance audiometry. *Archives of Otolaryngology*, *92*, 311–324.

Jerger, J., Jerger, S., & Maudlin, L. (1972). Studies in impedance audiometry: Normal and sensorineural ears. *Archives of Otolaryngology*, *99*, 513–523.

Jerger, J., & Keith, W. (1980). Inter- versus intrasubject variability in acoustic immittance. *Ear and Hearing*, *1*, 338–340.

Jerger, S., Jerger, J., Mauldin, L., & Segal, P. (1974). Studies in impedance audiometry: II. Children less than six years old. *Archives of Otolaryngology*, *99*, 1–9.

Keith, R. W. (1973). Impedance audiometry with neonates. *Archives of Otolaryngology*, *97*, 465–467.

Keith, R. W. (1975). Middle ear function in neonates. *Archives of Otolaryngology*, *101*, 376–379.

Liden, G., Bjorkman, G., Nyman, H., & Kunov, H. (1976). Tympanometry and acoustic impedance. In *The reflex*. Concord, MA: Grason-Stadler.

Liden, G., Peterson, J. L., & Bjorkman, G. (1969). Tympanometry. A method for analysis of middle-ear function. *Acta Otolaryngologica* (Stockholm), (Suppl. 263), 218–224.

Liden, G., Peterson, J. L., & Bjorkman, G. (1970). Tympanometry. *Archives of Otolaryngology, 92,* 248–257.

Margolis, R. H., & Heller, J. W. (1987). Screening tympanometry: Criteria for medical referral. *Audiology, 26,* 197–208.

Margolis, R. H., & Popelka, G. R. (1975). Static and dynamic acoustic impedance measurements in infant ears. *Journal of Speech and Hearing Research, 18,* 435–443.

Margolis, R. H., & Popelka, G. R. (1977). Interactions among tympanometric variables. *Journal of Speech and Hearing Research, 20,* 447–462.

Margolis, R. H., & Smith, P. (1977). Tympanometric asymmetry. *Journal of Speech and Hearing Research, 20,* 437–446.

Meistrup-Larsen, K. I., Andersen, M. S., Helweg, J., Deigaard, J., & Peitersen, E. (1981). Variations in tympanograms in children attending group-care during a one-year period. *O. R. L. Journal of Otorhinolaryngology and Related Specialties, 43,* 153–163.

Nerbonne, M. A., Bliss, A. T., & Schow, R. L. (1978). Acoustic impedance values in the elderly. *Journal of the American Auditory Society, 4,* 57–59.

Parson, I., Kunou, H., Abel, S., & Alberti, P. (1984). The acoustic impedance locus for normal hearing ears. *Scandinavian Audiology,* (Suppl. 22).

Porter, T. (1972). Normative otoadmittance values for three populations. *Journal of Auditory Research, 12,* 53–58.

Porter, T., & Winston, M. (1973). Reliability of measures obtained with the otoadmittance meter. *Journal of Auditory Research, 13,* 142–146.

Poulsen, G., & Tos, M. (1978). Screening tympanometry in newborn infants and during the first six months of life. *Scandinavian Audiology, 7,* 159–166.

Robertson, E. O., Peterson, J. L., & Lamb, L. E. (1968). Relative impedance measurements in young children. *Archives of Otolaryngology, 88,* 162–168.

Sly, R. M., Zambie, M. F., Fernandes, D. A., & Frazer, M. (1980). Tympanometry in kindergarten children. *Annals of Allergy, 44,* 1–7.

Sprague, B. H., Wiley, T. L., & Goldstein, R. (1985). Tympanometric and acoustic-reflex studies in neonates. *Journal of Speech and Hearing Research, 28,* 265–272.

Thompson, D. J., Sills, J. A., Recke, K. S., & Bui, P. M. (1979). Acoustic admittance and the aging ear. *Journal of Speech and Hearing Research, 22,* 29–36.

Thomsen, J., Tos, M., Hanke, A. B., & Melchiors, H. (1982). Repetitive tympanometric screenings in children followed from birth to age four. *Acta Otolaryngologica,* (Suppl. 386), 155–157.

Tos, M., Poulsen, G., & Borch, J. (1978). Tympanometry in 2-year-old children. *O. R. L. Journal for Oto-Rhino-Laryngology and Its Borderlands, 40,* 77–85.

Van Camp, K. J., Vanhuyse, V. J., Creten, W. L., & Vanpeperstraete, P. M. (1978) Impedance and admittance tympanometry. II. Mathematical approach. *Audiology, 17,* 108–119.

Wedenberg, E. (1963). Objective auditory tests on non-cooperative children. *Acta Otolaryngologica,* (Suppl. 175), 1–32.

Wilber, L. (1972). Use of absolute and relative impedance in defining the nature of middle ear lesions in children. In D. Rose & L. Keating (Eds.),

Proceedings of the Mayo Impedance Symposium (pp. 109–126). Rochester, MN: Mayo Foundation

Wiley, T. L., Oviatt, D. L., & Block, M. G. (1987). Acoustic-immittance measures in normal ears. *Journal of Speech and Hearing Research, 30,* 161–170.

Zwislocki, J. (1982). Normal function of the middle ear and its measurement. *Audiology, 11,* 4–14.

5.3 Studies in Subjects with Abnormal Middle Ears

Arora, M. M., Sharma, V. L., Gudi, S. P., & Balakrishnan, C. (1979). Acoustic impedance measurements and their importance in cleft palate patients. *Journal of Laryngology and Otology, 93,* 443–445.

Axelson, A., & Lewis, C. (1976). The comparison of otoscopic findings and impedance measurements. *Scandinavian Audiology, 5,* 149–155.

Baddour, H. M., Watson, J., Erwin, B. J., Clark, M. J., Holt, G. R., Steed, D. L., & Tilson, H. B. (1981). Tympanometric changes after total maxillary osteotomy. *Journal of Oral Surgery, 39,* 336–339.

Beery, Q. C., Andrus, W. S., Bluestone, C. D., & Cantekin, E. I. (1975). Tympanometric pattern classification in relation to middle ear effusions. *Annals of Otology, Rhinology and Laryngology, 84,* 56–64.

Bel, J., Causse, J., & Michaux, P. (1975). Paradoxical compliances in otosclerosis. *Audiology, 14,* 118–129.

Ben-David, J., Podoshin, L., & Fradis, M. (1981). Tympanometry and audiometry in diagnosis of middle-ear effusions. *Ear, Nose and Throat Journal, 60,* 120–123.

Bess, F. H., Schwartz, D. M., & Redfield, N. P. (1970). Audiometric impedance, and otoscopic findings in children with cleft palates. *Archives of Otolaryngology, 102,* 405–469.

Bess, F. H., Lewis, H. D., & Cieliczka, D. J. (1975). Acoustic impedance measurements in cleft-palate children. *Journal of Speech and Hearing Disorders, 40,* 13–24.

Black, M. J., Berger, H., Tritt, R. A., & Schloss, M. D. (1979). Impedance audiometry: Its use in the diagnosis of glomus tympanicum tumors. *Journal of Otolaryngology, 8,* 360–367.

Bluestone, C., Beery, Q., & Paradise, J. L. (1974). Audiometry and tympanometry in relation to middle ear effusion in children. *Laryngoscope, 83,* 594–603.

Booth, J. B. (1973). Tympanoplasty: Factors in post-operative assessment. *Journal of Laryngology and Otology, 87,* 27–67.

Brenman, A. K., & Swogger-Rosenberg, J. R. (1977). Infant tympanometry and myringotomy. *Transactions of the Pennsylvania Academy of Ophthalmology and Otolaryngology, 30,* 134–139.

Brooks, D. N. (1968). An objective method of detecting fluid in the middle ear. *International Audiology, 3,* 280–286.

Brooks, D. N. (1982). Acoustic impedance studies on otitis media with effusion. *International Journal of Pediatric Otorhinolaryngology, 4,* 89–94.

Browning, G. G., Swan, I. R. C., & Gatehouse, S. (1985). The doubtful value of tympanometry with diagnosis of otosclerosis. *Journal of Laryngology and Otology, 99*(6), 545–547.

Buckingham, R. A., Farag, A. Z., Patel, M. G., & Geick, M. R. (1980). Correlation between micro-otoscopy, micropneumatoscopy and otoadmittance tympanometry. *Laryngoscope, 90*, 1297–1304.

Cantekin, E. I., Beery, Q. C., & Bluestone, C. D. (1977). Tympanometric patterns found in middle ear effusion. *Annals of Otology, Rhinology and Laryngology, 86*(Suppl. 41), 16–20.

Causse, J., Bel, J., & Causse, B. (1977). Multifrequency impedance testing in relation to otospongiotic stapedial fixation and other factors. *Audiology, 16*, 338–354.

Chesnutt, B., Stream, R. W., Love, J. T., & McLarey, D. C. (1975). Otoadmittance measurements in cases of dual ossicular disorders. *Archives of Otolaryngology, 101*, 109–113.

Diefendorf, A. O., Ferrell, C. J., & McCallen, P. (1986). Diagnostic implications of tympanometry in the presence of patent pressure-equalization tubes. *American Journal of Otology, 7*(1), 44–46.

Dieroff, H. G. (1978). Differential diagnostic value of tympanometry in adhesive processes and otosclerosis. *Audiology, 17*, 77–86.

Djupesland, G. (1964). Mechanical component to deafness in Meniere's disease. *Acta Otolaryngologica*, (Suppl. 188), 206–208.

Djupesland, G. (1969). Use of impedance indicator in diagnosis of middle ear pathology. *Audiology, 8*, 570–579.

Djupesland, G., & Kvernvold, H. (1973). A comparison between absolute and "relative" impedance measurement as a method of distinguishing between otosclerosis and ossicular chain discontinuity. *Scandinavian Audiology, 2*, 93–98.

Farrant, R. H. (1966). Measuring the acoustic impedance of severely deaf ears to test for conductive component. *Journal of the Otolaryngological Society of Australia, 2*, 49–53.

Feldman, A. (1974). Eardrum abnormality and the measurement of middle ear function. *Archives of Otolaryngology, 99*, 211–217.

Feldman, A. S. (1977). Diagnostic application and interpretation of tympanometry and the acoustic reflex. *Audiology, 16*, 294–306.

Fernandes, D., Gupta, S., Sly, R. M., & Frazer, M. (1978). Tympanometry in children with allergic respiratory disease. *Annals of Allergy, 40*, 181–184.

Fiellau-Nikolajsen, M. (1979). Tympanometry in 3-year-old children. Type of care as an epidemiological factor in secretory otitis media and tubal dysfunction in unselected populations of 3-year-old children. *O. R. L. Journal for Oto-Rhino-Laryngology and Its Borderlands, 41*, 193–205.

Fiellau-Nikolajsen, M. (1980). Tympanometry in three-year-old children. Prevalence and spontaneous course of MEE. *Annals of Otology, Rhinology and Laryngology, 89*(Suppl. 68), 223–227.

Fiellau-Nikolajsen, M. (1981). Tympanometry in three-year-old children. The 3-year follow-up of a cohort study. *O. R. L. Journal of Otorhinolaryngology and Related Specialties, 43*, 89–103.

Fiellau-Nikolajsen, M. (1983). Tympanometry and secretory otitis media. Observations on diagnosis, epidemiology, treatment and prevention in prospective cohort studies of three-year-old children. *Acta Otolaryngologica* (Stockholm), (Suppl. 394), 1–73.

Fiellau-Nikolajsen, M., Falbe-Hansen, J., & Knudstrup, P. (1980). Tympanometry in three-year-old children. III. Correlation between tympanometry and findings at paracentesis in a prospectively followed population of otherwise healthy children aged 3-4 years. *Scandinavian Audiology*, 9, 49–54.

Fiellau-Nikolajsen M., & Lous J. (1979). Prospective tympanometry in 3-year-old children. A study of the spontaneous course of tympanometry types in a nonselected population. *Archives of Otolaryngology*, 105, 461–466.

Fiellau-Nikolajsen, M., & Lous, J. (1979). Tympanometry in three-year-old children. A cohort study on the prognostic value of tympanometry and operative findings in middle ear effusion. *O. R. L. Journal for Oto-Rhino-Laryngology and Its Borderlands*, 41, 11–25.

Fiellau-Nikolajsen, M., & Lous, J. (1982). Long-term prognostic-significance of serial tympanometry. A cohort study of preschool children. *O. R. L. Journal of Otorhinolaryngology and Related Specialties*, 44, 90–100.

Fiellau-Nikolajsen, M., Lous, J., Vang Pedersen, S., & Schousboe, H. H. (1977). Tympanometry in three-year-old children. I. A regional prevalence study on the distribution of tympanometric results in a non-selected population of 3-year-old children. *Scandinavian Audiology*, 6, 199–204.

Forquer, B. D., & Linthicum, F. H., Jr. (1980). Middle ear effusions: Relationship of tympanometry and air-bone gap to viscosity. *Ear and Hearing*, 1, 87–90.

Fulton, R., & Lamb, L. (1970). *Acoustic impedance and tympanometry with the retarded: A normative study* (Report No. 1). Parsons Research Center. Parsons, KS.

Gates, G. A., Avery, C. A., Cooper, J. C., Hearne, E. M., & Holt, G. R. (1986). Predictive value of tympanometry in middle ear effusion. *Annals of Otology, Rhinology and Laryngology*, 95, 46–50.

Gersdorff, M. C. (1977). Comparative study between the normally hearing child and the hard of hearing child, by acoustic impedance measurements of the ear. *Archives of Otorhinolaryngology*, 217, 13–31.

Gersdorff, M., & Stoquart, T. (1985). Phasor diagram: A comparative study between normal ears and otosclerotic ears. *Audiology*, 24, 167–173.

Giebink, G. S., & Harford, E. R. (1983). Tympanometry [Letter]. *New England Journal of Medicine*, 308, 526.

Giebink, G. S., Heller, K. A., & Harford, E. R. (1982). Tympanometric configurations and middle ear findings in experimental otitis media. *Annals of Otology, Rhinology and Laryngology*, 91, 20–24.

Gimsing, S., & Bergholtz, L. M. (1983). Otoscopy compared with tympanometry. *Journal of Laryngology, Otology, and Rhinology*, 97, 387–391.

Green, K. W., & Margolis, R. H. (1983). The ipsilateral acoustic reflex. In S. Silman (Ed.), *The acoustic reflex: Basic principles and clinical applications* (pp. 275–299). New York: Academic Press.

Gladstone, V. S., Less, S., & Wenger, A. P. (1980). Homograft tympanoplasty: Graft material effects on otoadmittance and audiometric measurements. *Ear and Hearing, 1,* 102–105.

Grimaldi, P. M. (1976). The value of impedance testing in diagnosis of middle ear effusion. *Journal of Laryngology and Otology, 90,* 141–152.

Groothuis, J. R., Sell, S. H., Wright, P. F., Thompson, J. M., & Altemeier, W. A., III. (1979). Otitis media in infancy: Tympanometric findings. *Pediatrics, 63,* 435–442.

Hall, J. W., & Weaver, T. (1979). Impedance audiometry in a young population. The effect of age, sex, and tympanogram abnormalities. *Journal of Otolaryngology, 8,* 210–222.

Hall, M., & Hughes, R. (1975). Maximum compliance and the symptom of fullness in Meniere's disease. *Archives of Otolaryngology, 101,* 227–228.

Haughton, P. (1977). Validity of tympanometry for middle ear effusions. *Archives of Otolaryngology, 100,* 505–513.

Haughton, P. M., & Pardoe, K. (1982). A comparison of otoscopy and tympanometry in the diagnosis of middle ear effusion. *Clinical Physiology Measures, 3,* 213–220.

Holmberg, K., Axelsson, A., Hansson, P., & Renvall, U. (1986). Comparison of tympanometry and otomicroscopy during healing of otitis media. *Scandinavian Audiology, 15,* 3–8.

Holt, G. R., Watkins, T. M., & Yoder, M. G. (1982). Assessment of tympanometry abnormalities of the tympanic membrane. *American Journal of Otolaryngology, 3,* 112–116.

Holt, G. R., Watkins, T. M., Yoder, M. G., & Garcia, A. (1981). The effect of tonsillectomy on impedance audiometry. *Otolaryngology, Head and Neck Surgery, 89,* 20–26.

Hopkinson, N., Schramm, V., Bosse, B., & Leggett, S. (1978). A comparison of results: Acoustic susceptance and otolaryngology. *Journal of the American Auditory Society, 3,* 191–199.

Howie, V. M., Ploussard, J. H., & Sloyer, J. (1975). The "otitis-prone" condition. *American Journal of Disease in Children, 129,* 676–678.

Isenberg, S. F., & Tubergen, L. B. (1980). An unusual congenital middle ear ossicular anomaly. *Archives of Otolaryngology, 106,* 179–181.

Ivey, R. (1975). Tympanometric curves and otosclerosis. *Journal of Speech and Hearing Research, 18,* 554–558.

Jacobson, J. T., & Mahoney, T. M. (1977). Admittance tympanometry in otosclerotic ears. *Journal of the American Auditory Society, 3,* 91–98.

Jerger, J. (1970). Clinical experience with impedance audiometry. *Archives of Otolaryngology, 92,* 311–324.

Jerger, J. (1975). Diagnostic use of impedance measures. In J. Jerger (Ed.), *Handbook of clinical impedance audiometry* (pp. 149–174). Dobbs Ferry, NY: American Electromedics.

Jerger, J., Anthony, L., Jerger, S., & Mauldin, L. (1974). Studies in impedance audiometry: Middle ear disorders. *Archives of Otolaryngology, 99,* 165–171.

Jerger, J., Jerger, S. J., & Mauldin, L. (1972). Studies in impedance audiometry: I. Normal and sensorineural ears. *Archives of Otolaryngology, 96,* 513–523.

Jerger, J., Mauldin, L., & Igarashi, M. (1978). Impedance audiometry in the squirrel monkey. Effect of middle ear surgery. *Archives of Otolaryngology, 104,* 214–224.

Jerger, S., Jerger, J., Mauldin, L., & Segal, P. (1974). Studies in impedance audiometry: II. Children less than six-years old. *Archives of Otolaryngology, 99,* 1–9.

Kobayashi, T., & Okitsu, T. (1986). Tympanograms in ears with small perforations of the tympanic membranes. *Archives of Otolaryngology, 112,* 642–645.

Lampe, R. M., & Weir, M. R. (1981). Tympanometry and otitis media [Letter]. *American Journal of Disabled Children, 135,* 864.

Lampe, R. M., Weir, M. R., McLeod, H., Aspinall, K., & Artalejo, L. (1981). Tympanometry in acute otitis media: Prognostic implications. *American Journal of Disabled Children, 135,* 233–235.

Leveque, H., Bialostozky, F., Blanchard, C. L., & Suter, C. M. (1979). Tympanometry in the evaluation of vascular lesions of the middle ear and tinnitus of vascular origin. *Laryngoscope, 89,* 1197–1218.

Liden, G. (1969). Test for stapes fixation. *Archives of Otolaryngology, 89,* 215–219.

Liden, G., Harford, E. R., & Hallen, O. (1974). Tympanometry for the diagnosis of ossicular disruption. *Archives of Otolaryngology, 99,* 23–29.

Liden, G., Peterson, J. L., & Bjorkman, G. (1969). Tympanometry. A method for analysis of middle-ear function. *Acta Otolaryngologica* (Stockholm), (Suppl. 263), 218–224.

Liden, G., Peterson, J. L., & Bjorkman, G. (1970). Tympanometry. *Archives of Otolaryngology, 92,* 248–257.

Lildholdt, T., Courtois, J., Kortholm, B., Schou, J. W., & Warrer, H. (1980). The diagnosis of negative middle ear pressure in children. The accuracy of symptoms and signs assessed by tympanometry. *Acta Otolaryngologica* (Stockholm), *89,* 459–464.

Lindeman, P., & Holmquist, J. (1982). Volume measurement of middle ear and mastoid air cell system with impedance audiometry on patients with eardrum perforation. *American Journal of Otology, 4,* 46–51.

Macrae, J. H. (1972). A theoretical investigation of cochlear effects on the acoustic impedance of the ear. *Journal of Auditory Research, 12,* 265–270.

Margolis, R. H. (1979). Tympanometry for prediction of middle ear effusion. [Letter]. *Archives of Otolaryngology, 105,* 225.

Margolis, R. H., Osguthorpe, J. D., & Popelka, G. R. (1978). The effects of experimentally-produced middle ear lesions on tympanometry in cats. *Acta Otolaryngologica* (Stockholm), *86,* 428–436.

Margolis, R. H., & Popelka, G. R. (1977). Interactions among tympanometric variables. *Journal of Speech and Hearing Research, 20,* 447–462.

McDermott, J. C., Giebink, S., Le, C. T., Harford, E. R., & Paparella, M. M. (1983). Children with persistent otitis media, audiometric and tympanometric findings. *Archives of Otolaryngology, 109,* 360–363.

Meistrup-Larsen, K. I., Andersen, M. S., Helweg, J., Deigaard, J., & Peitersen, E. (1981). Variations in tympanograms in children attending group-care during a one-year period. O. R. L. *Journal of Otorhinolaryngology and Related Specialties, 43*, 153–163.

Moffat, D. A., Ramsden, R. T., Rosenberg, J. N., Booth, J. B., & Gibson, W. P. (1977). Otoadmittance measurements in patients with rheumatoid arthritis. *Journal of Laryngology and Otology, 91*, 917–927.

Moller, P. (1981). Hearing, middle ear pressure and otopathology in a cleft palate population. *Acta Otolaryngologica, 92*, 521–529.

Moon, C. N., Jr., & Hahn, M. (1978). Pneumatic otoscopy and impedance studies in middle ear diagnosis. *Laryngoscope, 88*, 1439–1448.

Morioka, W. T., Neff, P. A., Boisseranc, T. E., Hartman, P. W., & Cantrell, R. W. (1976). Audiotympanometric findings on myasthenia gravis. *Archives of Otolaryngology, 102*, 211–213.

Neff, P. A., & Cantrell, R. W. (1977). Assessment of audiotympanometric testing: Three case reports. *Laryngoscope, 87*, 1052–1065.

Orchik, D. J., Dunn, J. W., & McNutt, L. (1978). Tympanometry as a predictor of middle ear effusion. *Archives of Otolaryngology, 104*, 4–6.

Orchik, D. J., Morff, R., & Dunn, J. W. (1978). Impedance audiometry in serous otitis media. *Archives of Otolaryngology, 104*, 409–412.

Orchik, D. J., Morff, R., & Dunn, J. W. (1980). Middle ear status at myringotomy and its relationship to middle ear immittance measurements. *Ear and Hearing, 1*, 324–328.

Osguthorpe, J. (1986). Effects of tympanic membrane scars on tympanometry: A study in cats. *Laryngoscope, 96*, 1366–1377.

Ostergard, C. A., & Carter, D. R. (1981). Positive middle ear pressure shown by tympanometry. *Archives of Otolaryngology, 107*, 353–356.

Paradise, J. L., Smith, C. G., & Bluestone, C. D. (1976). Tympanometric detection of middle ear effusion in infants and young children. *Pediatrics, 58*, 198–210.

Pollazzon, P., Narne, S., & Guariso, G. (1981). The importance of acoustic impedance measurements in middle ear pathology during acute viral respiratory illness in the first year of life. *International Journal of Pediatrics and Otorhinolaryngology, 3*, 319–325.

Renvall, U. (1975). Tympanometry in secretory otitis media. *Scandinavian Audiology, 4*, 83–88.

Renvall, U., & Holmquist, J. (1976). Tympanometry revealing middle ear pathology. *Annals of Otology, Rhinology and Laryngology, 85*(Suppl. 25), 209–215.

Renvall, U., Jarlstedt, J., & Holmquist, J. (1980). Identification of middle ear disease. *Acta Otolaryngologica, 90*, 283–289.

Renvall, U., Liden, G., Jungert, S., & Nilsson, E. (1975). Impedance audiometry in the detection of secretory otitis media. *Scandinavian Audiology, 4*, 119–124.

Reves, R., Budgett, R., Miller, D., Wadsworth, J., & Haines, A. (1985). Study of middle ear disease using tympanometry in general practice. *British Medical Journal, 290*(6486), 1953–1956.

Santos, B. B., & Rolisar, I. A. (1977). Brown's sign: A tympanographic documentation. *Ear, Nose and Throat Journal, 56,* 320–324.

Schwartz, D. M., & Schwartz, R. H. (1978). Acoustic impedance and otoscopic findings in young children with Down's syndrome. *Archives of Otolaryngology, 104,* 652–656.

Schwartz, D. M., & Schwartz, R. H. (1980). Acoustic immittance findings in acute otitis media. *Annals of Otology, Rhinology and Laryngology,* 89(Suppl. 68), 211–213.

Shurin, P. A., Pelton, S. I., & Klein, J. O. (1976). Otitis media in the newborn infant. *Annals of Otology, Rhinology and Laryngology,* (Suppl. 89), 211–213.

Smith, C. G., Paradise, J. L., & Young, T. I. (1982). Modified schema for classifying positive pressure tympanograms. *Pediatrics, 69,* 351–354.

Stool, E. S. (1984). Medical relevancy of immittance measures. *Ear and Hearing, 5,* 309–313.

Too-Chung, M. A. (1983). The assessment of middle ear function and hearing by tympanometry in children before and after early cleft palate repair. *British Journal of Plastic Surgery, 36,* 295–299.

Tos, M. (1980). Spontaneous improvement of secretory otitis and impedance screening. *Archives of Otolaryngology, 106,* 345–349.

Tos, M., & Poulsen, G. (1979). Tympanometry in 2-year-old children. Seasonal influence on frequency of secretory otitis and tubal function. *O. R. L. Journal for Oto-Rhino-Laryngology and Its Borderlands, 41,* 1–10.

Van Camp, K. J., Creten, W. L., Van de Heyning, P. H., & Vanpeperstrate, P. M. (1983). Optimizing tympanometric variables for detecting middle ear traumas. *Scandinavian Audiology,* (Suppl. 17), 7–10.

Van Camp, K. J., Creten, W. L., Vanpeperstraete, P. M., & Van de Heyning, P. H. (1979). Tympanometry: How not to overlook middle ear pathologies. In *The reflex.* Concord, MA: Grason-Stadler.

Van Camp, K. J., Creten, W. L., Vanpeperstraete, P. M., & Van de Heyning, P. H. (1980). Tympanometry—Detection of middle ear pathologies. *Acta Otorhinolaryngologica* (Belgium), *34,* 574–583.

Van Camp, K. J., Shanks, J. E., & Margolis, R. H. (1986). Simulation of pathological high impedance tympanograms. *Journal of Speech and Hearing Research, 29,* 505–514.

Van Camp, K. J., & Vogeleer, M. (1986). A tympanometric approach to otosclerosis. *Scandinavian Audiology, 15,* 109–114.

Van de Heyning, P. H., Van Camp, K. J., Creten, W. L., & Vanpeperstraete, P. M. (1982). Incudo-stapedial joint pathology: A tympanometric approach. *Journal of Speech and Hearing Research, 25,* 611–618.

Van Wagoner, R. S., & Campbell, J. D. (1976). The use of electro-acoustic impedance measurements in detecting early clinical otosclerosis. *Journal of Otolaryngology, 5,* 33–36.

Weir, M., & Lampe, R. (1984). Assessing middle ear disease: Beyond visual otoscopy. *American Family Physician, 30,* 201–210.

West, S. R., & Harris, B. J. (1983). Audiometry and tympanometry in children throughout one school year. *New Zealand Medical Journal,* 96(737), 603–605.

Wilber, L. (1972). Use of absolute and relative impedance in defining the nature of middle ear lesions in children. In D. Rose & L. Keating (Eds.), *Proceedings of the Mayo Impedance Symposium* (pp. 109–126). Rochester, MN: Mayo Foundation.

Williams, R. G., & Haughton, P. M. (1977). Tympanometric diagnosis of middle ear effusions. *Journal of Laryngology and Otology, 91*, 959–962.

5.4 Tympanogram Gradient/Width

Brooks, D. N. (1968). An objective method of detecting fluid in the middle ear. *Audiology, 7*, 280–286.

Brooks, D. N. (1969). The use of the electro-acoustic impedance bridge in the assessment of middle ear function. *Audiology, 8*, 563–569.

de Jonge, R. (1986). Normal tympanometric gradient: A comparison of three methods. *Audiology, 25*, 299–308.

Haughton, P. M. (1977). Validity of tympanometry for middle-ear effusions. *Archives of Otolaryngology, 103*, 505–513.

Koebsell, K. A., & Margolis, R. H. (1986). Tympanometric gradient measured from normal preschool children. *Audiology, 25*, 149–157.

Liden, G., Peterson, J., & Bjorkman, G. (1970). Tympanometry. *Archives of Otolaryngology, 92*, 248–257.

Margolis, R. H., & Heller, J. W. (1987). Screening tympanometry criteria for medical referral. *Audiology, 26*, 197–208.

Shanks, J. E., & Wilson, R. H. (1986). Effects of direction and rate of ear-canal pressure changes on tympanometric measures. *Journal of Speech and Hearing Research, 29*, 11–19.

6.0 EUSTACHIAN TUBE FUNCTION

Albin, N. (1984). The anatomy of the Eustachian tube. *Acta Otolaryngologica* (Stockholm), (Suppl. 414), 34–37.

Andreasson, L., & Ivarsson, A. (1976). On tubal function in the presence of central perforation of drum in chronic otitis media. *Archives of Otolaryngology, 82*, 1–10.

Beery, Q. C., Doyle, W. J., Bluestone, C. D., Cantekin, E. I., & Wiet, R. J. (1979). Eustachian tube function in an American Indian population. *Annals of Otology, Rhinology and Laryngology, 89*(Suppl. 68), 28–33.

Bluestone, C. D. (1971). Eustachian tube obstruction in the infant with cleft palate. *Annals of Otology, Rhinology and Laryngology, 80*(Suppl. 2), 1–30.

Bluestone, C. D. (1975). Assessment of Eustachian function. In J. F. Jerger (Ed.), *Handbook of clinical impedance audiometry* (pp. 127–148). Dobbs Ferry, NY: American Electromedics.

Bluestone, C. D. (1979). Eustachian tube dysfunction. In R. J. Wiet & S. W. Coulthard (Eds.), *Proceedings of Second National Conference on Otitis Media* (pp. 50–57). Columbus, OH: Ross Laboratories.

Bluestone, C. D. (1980). Assessment of Eustachian tube function. In J. Jerger & J. Northern (Eds.), *Handbook of clinical impedance audiometry* (2nd ed., pp. 83–108). Acton, MA: American Electromedics

Bluestone, C. D. (1983). Eustachian tube function: Physiology, pathophysiology and role of allergy in pathogenesis of otitis media. *Journal of Allergy and Clinical Immunology, 72*, 242–251.

Bluestone, C. D. (1985). Current concepts in Eustachian tube function as related to otitis media. *Auris Nasus Larynx, 12*(Suppl. 1), 81–84.

Bluestone, C. D., & Beery, Q. (1976). Concepts on the pathogenesis of middle ear effusions. *Annals of Otology, Rhinology and Laryngology, 85*(Suppl. 25), 182–186.

Bluestone, C. D., Beery, Q., & Andrus, W. (1974). Mechanics of the Eustachian tube as it influences susceptibility to and persistence of middle ear effusions in children. *Annals of Otolaryngology, 83*, 27–34.

Bluestone, C. D., Beery, Q., & Paradise, J. (1974). Audiometry and tympanometry in relation to middle ear effusions in children. *Laryngoscope, 83*, 594–604.

Bluestone, C. D., & Cantekin, E. (1981). Panel on experiences with testing Eustachian tube function tests. *Annals of Otolaryngology, 90*, 552–562.

Bluestone, C. D., Cantekin, E., & Beery, Q. (1977). Effect of inflammation on the ventilatory function of the Eustachian tube. *Laryngoscope, 82*, 1654–1670.

Bluestone, C. D., Cantekin, E., & Douglas, G. (1979). Eustachian tube function related to the results of tympanoplasty in children. *Laryngoscope, 89*, 450–458.

Bluestone, C. D., & Klein, J. D. (1983). Otitis media with effusion, atelectasis, and Eustachian tube dysfunction. In C. D. Bluestone & S.E. Stool (Eds.), *Pediatric otolaryngology* (Vol. 1, pp. 356–512). Philadelphia: Saunders.

Bluestone, C. D., Paradise, J. L., & Beery, Q. (1972). Physiology of the Eustachian tube in the pathogenesis and management of middle ear effusions. *Laryngoscope, 82*, 1654–1670.

Bluestone, C. D., Paradise, J., Beery, Q., & Wittel, R. (1972). Certain effects of cleft palate repair on Eustachian tube function. *Cleft Palate Journal, 9*, 183–193.

Bluestone, C. D., Wittel, R., & Paradise, J. (1972). Roentgenographic evaluation of Eustachian tube function in infants with cleft and normal palates. *Cleft Palate Journal, 9*, 93–100.

Bluestone, C. D., Wittel, R., Paradise, J., & Felder, H. (1972). Eustachian tube function as related to adenoidectomy for otitis media. *Transactions of the American Academy of Opthalmology and Otolaryngology, 76*, 1325–1339.

Buch, N., & Jorgensen, M. (1964). Eustachian tube and middle ear. *Archives of Otolaryngology, 79*, 472–480.

Buckingham, R., & Ferrer, J. (1973). Middle ear pressures in Eustachian tube malfunction: Manometric studies. *Laryngoscope, 83*, 1585–1593.

Bylander, A. (1980). Comparison of Eustachian function in children and adults with normal ears. *Annals of Otology, Rhinology and Laryngology, 89* (Suppl. 68), 20–24.

Bylander, A. (1984). Function and dysfunction of the Eustachian tube in children. *Acta Otorhinolaryngologica, 38*, 238–245.

Bylander, A. (1984). Upper respiratory tract infection and Eustachian tube function in children. *Acta Otolaryngologica, 97*, 343–349.

Bylander, A., Ivarsson, A., & Tjernstrom, O. (1981). Eustachian-tube function in normal children and adults. *Acta Otolaryngologica, 92*, 481–493.

Bylander, A., Tjernstrom, O., & Ivarsson, A. (1983). Pressure opening and closing functions of the Eustachian tube in children and adults with normal ears. *Acta Otolaryngologica, 95*, 55–62.

Bylander, A., & Tjernstrom, O. (1983). Changes in Eustachian tube function with age in children with normal ears. A longitudinal study. *Acta Otolaryngologica, 96*, 466–477.

Bylander, A., Tjernstrom, O., & Ivarsson, A. (1983). Pressure opening and closing function of the Eustachian tube by inflation and deflation by children and adults with normal ears. *Acta Otolaryngologica, 96*, 255–256.

Bylander, A., Tjernstrom, O., Ivarsson, A., & Andreasson, L. (1985). Eustachian tube function and its relation to middle ear pressure in children. *Auris Nasus Larynx, 12*(Suppl. 1), 843–845.

Cantekin, E. (1985). Eustachian tube function in children with tympanostomy tubes. *Auris Nasus Larynx, 12*(Suppl. 1), 846–848.

Cantekin, E., Bluestone, C. D., & Parker, L. (1976). Eustachian tube ventilatory function in children. *Annals of Otology, Rhinology and Laryngology, 85*(Suppl. 25), 171–177.

Cantekin, E., Bluestone, C. D., Saez, C., Doyle, W., & Phillips, D. (1977). Normal and abnormal middle ear ventilation. *Annals of Otolaryngology, 86*(Suppl. 41), 1–15.

Cantekin, E., Doyle, W., & Bluestone, C. D. (1983). Effect of levator veli palatini muscle excision on Eustachian tube function. *Archives of Otolaryngology, 109*, 281–284.

Cantekin, I., Doyle, W., Phillips, D., & Bluestone, C. (1980). Gas absorption in the middle ear. *Annals of Otolaryngology, 89*(Suppl. 68), 71–75.

Chan, K. G., Cantekin, E. I., Karnavas, W. J., & Bluestone, C. D. (1987). Auto-inflation of Eustachian tube in young children. *Laryngoscope, 97*, 668–674.

Chermack, G. D., & Moore, M. K. (1981). Eustachian tube function in the older adult. *Ear and Hearing, 2*, 143–147.

Cohn, A. (1977). Clinical assessment of Eustachian tube ventilatory function. *Laryngoscope, 87*, 1336–1358.

Cohn, A., Schwaber, M., Anthony, L., & Jerger, J. (1979). Eustachian tube function and tympanoplasty. *Annals of Otology, Rhinology and Laryngology, 88*, 339–347.

Diamant, M. (1977). New methods for the recording of the Eustachian tube function. *Acta Otolaryngologica, 348*, 7–34.

Diefendorf, A. O., Ferrell, C. J., & McCallen, P. (1986). Diagnostic implications of tympanometry in the presence of patent pressure-equalization tubes. *American Journal of Otology, 7*, 44–46.

Djeric, D., & Savic, D. (1985). Anatomical variations and relation of the bony portion of the Eustachian tube. *Acta Otolaryngologica, 99*, 543–550.

Donaldson, J. A. (1973). Physiology of the Eustachian tube. *Archives of Otolaryngology, 97*, 9–12.

Doyle, W. J. (1984). Functional Eustachian tube obstruction and otitis media in a primate model. *Acta Otolaryngologica* (Stockholm), (Suppl. 414), 52–57.

182 ACOUSTIC IMMITANCE MEASURES IN CLINICAL AUDIOLOGY

Doyle, W. J., Cantekin, E. I., & Bluestone, C. D. (1980). Eustachian tube function in cleft palate children. *Annals of Otology, Rhinology and Laryngology, 89*(Suppl. 68), 34–40.

Eden, A. R. (1981). Neural connections between the middle ear, Eustachian tube and brain. Implications for the reflex control of middle ear aeration. *Annals of Otology, Rhinology and Laryngology, 90,* 566–569.

Ekvall, L. (1970). Eustachian tube function in tympanoplasty. *Acta Otolaryngologica,* (Suppl. 263), 33–42.

Eliachar, I., Sando, I., & Northern, J. L. (1974). Measurement of middle ear pressure in guinea pigs. *Archives of Otolaryngology, 99,* 172–176.

Elner, A. (1976). Normal gas exchange in the human middle ear. *Annals of Otolaryngology, 85,* 161–164.

Elner, A., Ingelstedt, S., & Ivarsson, A. (1971). Indirect determination of the middle ear pressure. *Acta Otolaryngologica, 72,* 255–261.

Elner, A., Ingelstedt, S., & Ivarsson, A. (1971). The normal function of the Eustachian tube. *Acta Otolaryngologica, 72,* 320–328.

Falk, B. (1981). Negative middle ear pressure induced by sniffing: A tympanometric study in persons with healthy ears. *Journal of Otolaryngology, 10,* 299–305.

Falk, B. (1982). Sniff-induced negative middle ear pressure: Study of a consecutive series of children with otitis media with effusion. *American Journal of Otolaryngology, 3,* 155–162.

Falk, B. (1983). Variability of the tympanogram due to Eustachian tube closing failure. *Scandinavian Audiology,* (Suppl. 17), 11–15.

Falk, B. (1984). *Eustachian tube closing failure.* Study on sniff-induced negative middle-ear pressure. *Linkoping University (Sweden) Medical Dissertations, 174,* 1–107.

Falk, B., & Magnuson, B. (1984). Eustachian tube closing failure in children with persistent middle ear effusion. *International Journal of Pediatric Otorhinolaryngology, 7,* 97–106.

Falk, B., & Magnuson, B. (1984). Eustachian tube closing failure. Occurrence in patients with cleft palate and middle ear disease. *Archives of Otolaryngology, 240,* 10–14.

Falk, B., & Magnuson, B. (1984). Evacuation of the middle ear by sniffling: A cause of high negative pressure and development of middle ear disease. *Otolaryngology, Head and Neck Surgery, 92*(3), 312–318.

Falk, B., & Magnuson, B. (1984). Test-retest variability of Eustachian tube responses in children with persistent middle ear effusion. *Archives of Otolaryngology, 240,* 145–152.

Flisberg, K. (1964). Clinical assessment of tubal function. *Acta Otolaryngologica,* (Suppl. 188), 29–35.

Flisberg, K., & Ingelstedt, S. (1970). Middle-ear mechanics in patulous tube cases. *Acta Otolaryngologica, 263,* 18–22.

Flisberg, K., Ingelstedt, S., & Ortegren, U. (1963). On middle ear pressure. *Acta Otolaryngologica,* (Suppl. 182), 43–56.

Flisberg, K., Ingelstedt, S., & Ortegren, U. (1964). Controlled "ear aspiration" of air: A "physiological test of tubal function." *Acta Otolaryngologica,* (Suppl. 182), 35–38.

Flisberg, K., Jr. (1966). Ventilatory studies on the Eustachian tube. *Acta Otolaryngologica*, (Suppl. 219), 1–82.

Fowler, E. P. (1920). Drum tension and middle ear air pressures: Their determination significance and effect upon the hearing. *Annals of Otology, Rhinology and Laryngology*, 29, 688–694.

Gersdorff, M. C. (1977). An exploration method of the Eustachian tube for intact and perforated drums: Tubal-impedance-manometry. *Archives of Otorhinolaryngology*, 217, 391–407.

Givens, G., & Seidemann, M. (1984). Acoustic immittance testing of the Eustachian tube. *Ear and Hearing*, 5, 297–299.

Givens, G., & Seidemann, M. (1984). Bivariate tympanometric assessment of Eustachian tube patency. *Journal of Auditory Research*, 24, 320–328.

Gottshalk, H. G. (1962). Serous otitis: Treatment by controlled middle ear inflation. *Laryngoscope*, 72, 1379–1390.

Gottshalk, H. G. (1966). Further experience with controlled middle ear inflation in the treatment of serous otitis. *Eye, Ear, Nose & Throat Monthly*, 45, 49–51.

Gottshalk, H. G. (1980). Nonsurgical management of otitis media with effusion. *Annals of Otology, Rhinology and Laryngology*, 89(Suppl. 68), 301–302.

Gottshalk, H. G. (1984). The management of otitis media with effusion by controlled middle ear inflation. *American Journal of Otology*, 5, 248–252.

Graves, G., & Edwards, L. (1944). The Eustachian tube. *Archives of Otolaryngology*, 39, 359–397.

Groth, P., Ivarsson, A., & Tjernstrom, O. (1981). Comparison of Eustachian tube function measured by the microflow method and a new quantitative impedance method. *Aviation and Space Environmental Medicine*, 52, 540–544.

Groth, P., Ivarsson, A., & Tjernstrom, O. (1982). Reliability in tests of the Eustachian tube function. *Acta Otolaryngologica* (Stockholm), 93, 261–267.

Groth, P., Ivarsson, A., Tjernstrom, O., & White, P. (1985). The effect of pressure change rate on the Eustachian tube function in pressure chamber tests. *Acta Otolaryngologica* (Stockholm), 99, 67–73.

Gundersen, T., & Tonning, F-M. (1976). Ventilating tubes in the middle ear. Long term observations. *Archives of Otolaryngology*, 102, 198–199.

Gundersen, T., & Tonning, F-M. (1984). Ventilating tubes in the middle ear. *Archives of Otolaryngology*, 110, 783–784.

Hall, C. M., & Brackman, D. E. (1977). Eustachian tube blockage and Meniere's disease. *Archives of Otolaryngology*, 103, 355–357.

Harford, E. (1973). Tympanometry for Eustachian tube evaluation. *Archives of Otolaryngology*, 97, 17–20.

Haughton, P. M. (1977). Validity of tympanometry for middle ear effusions. *Archives of Otolaryngology*, 103, 505–513.

Hayashi, M., Takahashi, H., Sato, H., & Honjo, I. (1986). Clearance of the Eustachian tube under negative middle ear pressure. *American Journal of Otolaryngology*, 7, 399–401.

Holborow, C. (1970). Eustachian tube function. *Archives of Otolaryngology*, 92, 624–626.

Holmquist, J. (1968). The role of the Eustachian tube in myringoplasty. *Acta Otolaryngologica*, 66, 289–295.

Holmquist, J. (1969). Eustachian tube function assessed with tympanometry. *Acta Otolaryngologica*, 68, 501–508.

Holmquist, J. (1969). Eustachian tube function in patients with eardrum perforations following aspiration methods. *Acta Otolaryngologica*, 68, 391–401.

Holmquist, J. (1970). Middle ear ventilation in chronic otitis media. *Archives of Otolaryngology*, 92, 617–623.

Holmquist, J. (1972). Summary on Eustachian tube function. In D. E. Rose & L. Keating (Eds.), *Proceedings of the Mayo Impedance Symposium* (pp. 309–312). Rochester, MN: Mayo Foundation.

Holmquist, J. (1973). Eustachian tube function in patients with eardrum perforations following application. *Eye, Ear, Nose and Throat Monthly*, 52, 398–403.

Holmquist, J. (1976). Eustachian tube evaluation. In A. S. Feldman & L. A. Wilber (Eds.), *Acoustic impedance and admittance: The measurement of middle ear function* (pp. 156–174). Baltimore: Williams & Wilkins.

Holmquist, J. (1979). Tympanometric method for evaluation of Eustachian tube function [Letter]. *Annals of Otology, Rhinology and Laryngology*, 88, 297–298.

Holmquist, J. (1980). Middle ear ventilation. In B. Jazbi (Ed.), *Pediatric otorhinolaryngology: A review of ear, nose, and throat problems in children* (pp. 41–51). New York: Appleton-Century-Crofts.

Holmquist, J., & Larson, G. (1976). Eustachian tube dysfunction: A preliminary report of medical treatment. *Scandinavian Audiology*, 5, 107–111.

Holmquist, J., & Linderman, P. (1987). Eustachian tube function and healing after myringoplasty. *Otolaryngology, Head and Neck Surgery*, 96, 80–82.

Holmquist, J., & Miller, J. (1972). Eustachian tube evaluation using the impedance bridge. In D. E. Rose & L. Keating (Eds.), *Proceedings of the Mayo Impedance Symposium* (pp. 297–308). Rochester, MN: Mayo Foundation.

Holmquist, J., & Olen, L. (1980). Evaluation of Eustachian tube function. *Journal of Laryngology and Otology*, 94, 15–23.

Holmquist, J., & Strothers, G. (1972). The anatomy and physiology of the Eustachian tube: A review. In D. Rose & L. Keating (Eds.), *Proceedings of the Mayo Impedance Symposium* (pp. 287–296). Rochester, MN: Zenith Hearing Instrument.

Honjo, I. (1988). *Eustachian tube and middle ear diseases*. Tokyo: Springer-Verlag.

Honjo, I., Hayaski, M., Ito, S., & Takahashi, H. (1985). Pumping and clearance function of the Eustachian tube. *American Journal of Otolaryngology*, 6, 241–244.

Honjo, I., Kumazawa, T., & Honda, K. (1981). Simple impedance test for Eustachian tube function. *Archives of Otolaryngology, 107*, 221–223.

Honjo, I., Okazaki, N., & Kunazawa, T. (1979). Experimental study of the Eustachian tube function with regard to its related muscles. *Acta Otolaryngologica* (Stockholm), *87*, 84–89.

Honjo, I., Okazaki, N., & Kunazawa, T. (1980). Opening mechanism of the Eustachian tube: A clinical and experimental study. *Annals of Otology, Rhinology and Laryngology, 89*(Suppl. 68), 25–27.

Honjo, I., Okazaki, N., Nozoe, T., Ushiro, K., & Kumazawa, T. (1981). Experimental study of the pumping function of the Eustachian tube. *Archives of Otolaryngology, 91*, 85–89.

Honjo, I., Ushiro, K., Haji, T., Nozoe, T., & Matsui, H. (1983) Role of the tensor tympani muscle in Eustachian tube functioning. *Acta Otolaryngologica* (Stockholm), *95*, 329–332.

Honjo, I., Ushiro, K., Nozoe, T., & Okazaki, N. (1983). Cineroentgenographic and electromyographic studies of Eustachian tube function. *Archives of Otolaryngology, 238*, 62–67.

Ingelstedt, S., & Johnson, B. (1967). Mechanisms of the gas exchange in the normal human middle ear. *Acta Otolaryngologica*, (Suppl. 224), 452–461.

Ingelstedt, S., & Ortegren, U. (1963). Qualitative testing of the Eustachian tube function. *Acta Otolaryngologica* (Stockholm), (Suppl. 182), 7–23.

Ivarsson, A. (1980). A new impedance method for measuring middle ear mechanics and Eustachian tube function. *Annals of Otology, Rhinology and Laryngology, 89*(Suppl. 68), 207–210.

Jackler, R. K. (1985). Experimental evidence against middle ear oxygen absorption. *Laryngoscope, 90*, 1281–1282.

Jaumann, M. P., Steiner, W., & Berg, M. (1980). Endoscopy of the pharyngeal Eustachian tube. *Annals of Otology, Rhinology and Laryngology, 89*(Suppl. 68), 55.

Jonas, I., Mann, W., & Munker, G. (1970). Relationship between tubal function, craniofacial morphology and disorder of deglutition. *Archives of Otolaryngology, 92*, 311–324.

Jonathan, D., Chalmers, P., & Wong, K. (1986). Comparison of sonotubometry with tympanometry to assess Eustachian tube function in adults. *British Journal of Audiology, 20*, 231–235.

Kirchner, F. R., Robinson, R., & Smith, R. F. (1976). Study of the ventilation of middle ear using radioactive xenon. *Annals of Otology, Rhinology and Laryngology, 85*, 165–168.

Liden, G., Harford, E., & Hallen, O. (1974). Automatic tympanometry in clinical practice. *Audiology, 13*, 126–139.

Liden, G., Peterson, J., & Bjorkman, G. (1970). Tympanometry. *Archives of Otolaryngology, 92*, 248–257.

Lildholdt, T. (1980). Negative middle ear pressure. Variations by season and sex. *Annals of Otology, Rhinology and Laryngology, 89*(Suppl. 68), 67–70.

Lildholdt, T., Brask, T., & Hridegaard, T. (1984). Interpretation of sono-tubometry. A critical view of the acoustical measurement of the opening of the Eustachian tube. *Acta Otolaryngologica* (Stockholm), *98*, 250–254.

Lildholdt, T., Courtois, J., Kortholm, B., Schou, J. W., & Warrer, H. (1980). The diagnosis of negative middle ear pressure in children. The accuracy of symptoms and signs assessed by tympanometry. *Acta Otolaryngologica* (Stockholm), *89*, 459–464.

Lim, D. J. (1984). Functional morphology of the tubotympanum. *Acta Otolaryngologica* (Stockholm), (Suppl. 414), 13–18.

Lindeman, P., Holmquist, J., & Aberg, B. (1984). Ear drum mobility and middle ear volume measured with tympanometry. *Scandinavian Audiology*, *13*, 147–150.

MacBeth, R. (1960). Some thoughts of the Eustachian tube. *Proceedings of the Royal Society of Medicine*, *53*, 151–161.

Magnuson, B. (1981). On the origin of the high negative pressure in the middle ear space. *American Journal of Otolaryngology*, *2*, 1–12.

Magnuson, B. (1983). Eustachian tube malfunction and middle ear disease in new perspective. *Journal of Otolaryngology*, *12*, 187–193.

Magnuson, B., & Falk, B. (1984). Diagnosis and management of Eustachian tube malfunction. *Otolaryngologic Clinics of North America*, *17*, 659–671.

Malm, L. (1987). The influence of pregnancy on the Eustachian tube function in rats. *Acta Otolaryngologica*, *104*, 251–254.

McBride, T. P., Doyle, W. J., Hayden, F. H., & Gwaltney, J. M. (1989). Alterations of the Eustachian tube, middle ear, and nose in rhinovirus infection. *Archives of Otolaryngology*, *115*, 1054–1059.

McCurdy, J. (1980). Manometric measurements of Eustachian tube ventilatory function. *Laryngoscope*, *90*, 251–257.

McNicoll, W. (1983). Tympanic membrane mobility on otoscopy as an indicator of Eustachian tube function. *Laryngoscope*, *93*, 630–634.

Metz, O. (1953). Influence of the patulous Eustachian tube on the acoustic impedance of the ear. *Acta Otolaryngologica*, (Suppl. 109), 105–112.

Miller, G., Jr. (1965). Eustachian tubal function in normal and pathological ears. *Archives of Otolaryngology*, *81*, 41–48.

Miller, J. M., & Holmquist, J. (1974). An animal model for study of Eustachian tube and middle ear function. *Scandinavian Audiology*, *3*, 63–72.

Misurya, V. (1975). Physiologic Eustachian tube inflation. *Archives of Otolaryngology*, *101*, 730–732.

Moon, J., & Swanson, S. (1983). Passive Eustachian tube opening pressure. Its measurement, normal values, and clinical implications. *Archives of Otolaryngology*, *109*, 364–368.

Morimitsu, T., Enatsu, K., Matsumoto, I., & Ushisako, Y. (1981). A new test of Eustachian tube function with otoadmittance meter: Tubotympanometry. *Acta Otolaryngologica* (Stockholm), *91*, 207–214.

Murphy, D. (1979). Negative pressure in the middle ear by ciliary propulsion of mucus through the Eustachian tube. *Laryngoscope*, *89*, 954–961.

Murti, K. G., Cantekin, E. I., Stern, R. M., & Bluestone, C. D. (1980). Sonometric evaluation of Eustachian tube function using broadband stimuli. *Annals of Otology, Rhinology and Laryngology*, *89*(Suppl. 68), 178–184.

Newman, C., & Spitzer, J. (1981). Eustachian tube efficiency in geriatric subjects. *Ear and Hearing, 2,* 103–107.

Palva, T. (1980). Chronic tubal dysfunction (pathology and immunology in relation to the Eustachian tube and middle ear). *Journal of Laryngology and Otology, 94,* 9–13.

Parisier, S. C. (1973). A systematic approach for clinically evaluating Eustachian tube function: A preliminary report. *Transactions of the American Academy of Opthalmology and Otolaryngology, 77,* 117–123.

Perlman, H. (1939). The Eustachian tube. *Archives of Otolaryngology, 30,* 212–238.

Perlman, H. (1951). Observations on the Eustachian tube. *Archives of Otolaryngology, 55,* 370–385.

Proctor, B. (1967). Embryology and anatomy of the Eustachian tube. *Archives of Otolaryngology, 86,* 503–514.

Proctor, B. (1973). Anatomy of the Eustachian tube. *Archives of Otolaryngology, 97,* 2–8.

Rapport, P., Lim, D., & Weiss, H. (1975). Surface-active agent in Eustachian tube function. *Archives of Otolaryngology, 101,* 305–311.

Renvall, U., & Holmquist, J. (1974). Eustachian tube function in secretory otitis media. *Scandinavian Audiology, 3,* 87–91.

Renvall, U., Liden, G., Jungert, S., & Nilsson, E. (1975). Impedance audiometry in the detection of secretory otitis media. *Scandinavian Audiology, 4,* 119–124.

Rich, A. (1920). Physiological study of Eustachian tube and its related muscles. *Bulletin of Johns Hopkins Hospital, 31,* 206–214.

Riedel, C., Wiley, T., & Block, M. (1987). Tympanometric measures of Eustachian-tube function. *Journal of Speech and Hearing Research, 39,* 207–214.

Rood, S. (1986). Anatomy and physiology of the Eustachian tube. In C. Cummings, J. Fredrickson, L. Harken, C. Krause, & D. Schuller (Eds.), *Otolaryngology—Head and Neck Surgery* (pp. 2723–2732). St. Louis, MO: C. V. Mosby.

Rundcrantz, D. (1970). Posture and Eustachian tube function. *Acta Otolaryngologica, 263,* 15–17.

Sadé, J. (1984). Eustachian tube function. *Acta Otolaryngologica* (Stockholm), (Suppl. 414), 83–84.

Sadé, J., Wolfson, S., Sachs, Z., & Abraham, S. (1985). Caliber of the lumen of the Eustachian tube pre-isthmus in infants and children. *Archives of Oto-Rhino-Laryngology, 242,* 247–255.

Sadé, J., Wolfson, S., Sachs, Z., Levit, I., & Abraham, S. (1985). The human Eustachian tube lumen in children. *Acta Otolaryngologica, 99,* 305–309.

Schuchman, G., & Joachims, H. (1985). Tympanometric assessment of Eustachian tube function of divers. *Ear and Hearing, 6,* 325–328.

Schuknecht, H. F., & Kerr, A. G. (1967). Pathology of the Eustachian tube. *Archives of Otolaryngology, 86,* 497–502.

Schwartz, D., Schwartz, R., & Redfield, N. (1978). Treatment of negative middle ear pressure and serous otitis media with Politzer's technique. *Archives of Otolaryngology, 104,* 487–490.

Seidemann, M. F., & Givens, G. D. (1977). Tympanometric assessment of Eustachian tube patency in children. *Journal of Speech and Hearing Disorders, 42,* 487–497.

Seifert, M. W., Seidemann, M. F., & Givens, G. D. (1979). An examination of variables involved in tympanometric assessment of Eustachian tube function in adults. *Journal of Speech and Hearing Disorders, 44,* 388–396.

Shanks, J. E., & Wilson, R. H. (1986). Effects of direction and rate of ear-canal pressure changes on tympanometric measures. *Journal of Speech and Hearing Research, 29,* 11–19.

Shea, J. (1972). Autoinflation treatment of serous otitis media in children. *Journal of the Tennessee Medical Association, 64,* 104–108.

Sheehy, J. (1981). Testing Eustachian tube function. *Annals of Otolaryngology, 90,* 562–564.

Siedentop, K. H. (1977). Eustachian tube function. In B. Jaffe (Ed.), *Hearing loss in children* (pp. 381–395). Baltimore: University Park Press.

Siedentop, K. H., Lowey, A., Corrigan, R. A., & Osenar, S. B. (1978). Eustachian tube function assessed with tympanometry. *Annals of Otology, Rhinology and Laryngology, 87,* 163–169.

Siedentop, K. H., Tardy, E., & Hamilton, L. (1968). Eustachian tube function. *Archives of Otolaryngology, 88,* 386–395.

Spitzer, J. B., & Newman, C. W. (1984). Reliability of a measure of Eustachian tube function in normal subjects. *Annals of Otology, Rhinology and Laryngology, 93,* 48–51.

Square, R., Cooper, J. C., & Hearne, E. M. (1982). Eustachian-tube function. *Archives of Otolaryngology, 108,* 567–569.

Takahashi, H., Hayashi, M., Sato, H., & Honjo, I. (1989). Primary deficits in Eustachian tube function in patients with otitis media with effusion. *Archives of Otolaryngology, Head and Neck Surgery, 115,* 581–584.

Thomsen, K. A. (1955). Eustachian tube function tested by employment of impedance measuring. *Acta Otolaryngologica, 45,* 252–267.

Thomsen, K. A. (1957). Studies on the function of the Eustachian tube in a series of normal individuals. *Acta Otolaryngologica, 48,* 516–529.

Thomsen, K. A. (1958). Investigations of the tubal function and measurement of the middle ear pressure in pressure chamber. *Acta Otolaryngologica,* (Suppl. 140), 269–278.

Thomsen, K. A. (1960). Objective determination of middle ear pressure. *Acta Otolaryngologica,* (Suppl. 158), 212–216.

Tos, M., & Poulsen, G. (1979). Tympanometry in 2-year-old children. Seasonal influence on frequency of secretory otitis and tubal function. *O. R. L. Journal for Oto-Rhino-Laryngology and Its Borderlands, 41,* 1–10.

Toynbee, J. (1852). On the functions of the tympanic membrane, the ossicles, and the muscles of the tympanum and of the Eustachian tube in the human ear with an account of the muscles of the Eustachian tube and their action in different classes of animals. *Proceedings of the Royal Society of London, 6,* 217–221.

Virtanen, H. (1978). Sonotubometry: An acoustic method for objective measurement of auditory tubal opening. *Acta Otolaryngologica, 86,* 93–103.

Virtanen, H., & Marttila, T. (1982). Middle-ear pressure and Eustachian-tube dysfunction. *Archives of Otolaryngology, 108,* 766–769.
Virtanen, H., & Palva, T. (1982). The patulous Eustachian tube and chronic middle ear disease. *Acta Otolaryngologica, 93,* 49–53.
Virtanen, H., Palva, T., & Jauhiainen, T. (1980). Comparative preoperative evaluation of Eustachian function in pathological ears. *Annals of Otology, Rhinology and Laryngology, 89,* 360–369.
Westergaard, O. (1970). Tubal function in patients with chronic secretory otitis media. *Acta Otolaryngologica, 263,* 23–24.
Williams, P. S. (1975). Tympanometric pressure swallow test for the assessment of Eustachian tube function. *Annals of Otology, Rhinology and Laryngology, 84,* 339–343.
Wofford, M. (1981). Audiological evaluation and management of hearing disorders. In F. N. Martin (Ed.), *Medical audiology: Disorders of hearing* (pp. 145–173). Englewood Cliffs, NJ: Prentice-Hall

7.0 ACOUSTIC-REFLEX MEASURES

Alberti, P. W. (1978). The diagnostic role of stapedius reflex estimations. *Otolaryngologic Clinics of North America, 11,* 251–261.
Alford, B., Jerger, J. F., Coats, A., Peterson, S., & Weber, S. (1973). Neurophysiology of facial nerve testing. *Archives of Otolaryngology, 97,* 214.
Bates, M. A., Loeb, M., Smith, R., & Fletcher, J. L. (1970). Attempts to condition the acoustic reflex. *Journal of Auditory Research, 10,* 132–135.
Bauch, C. D., Olsen, W. O., & Harner, S. G. (1983). Auditory brainstem response and acoustic reflex tests. *Archives of Otolaryngology, 109,* 522–525.
Bench, J. (1971). Anticipatory elicitation of the middle-ear muscle reflex. *Journal of Laryngology and Otology, 85,* 1161–1165.
Blood, I. (1976). Dimensions of activating signals on the acoustic reflex. *Journal of Auditory Research, 16,* 83–88.
Borg, E. (1968). A quantitative study of the effect of the acoustic stapedius reflex on sound transmission through the middle ear of man. *Acta Otolaryngologica, 66,* 461–472.
Borg, E. (1971). On the non-linear dynamic properties of the acoustic middle ear reflex of unanesthetized animals. *Brain Research, 31,* 211–215.
Borg, E. (1972). Acoustic middle ear reflexes. *Acta Otolaryngologica* (Stockholm), *74*(Suppl. 304).
Borg, E. (1972). The dynamic properties of the acoustic middle ear reflex in non-anesthetized rabbits. Quantitative aspects of a polysynaptic reflex system. *Acta Physiologica* (Scandinavia), *86,* 366–387.
Borg, E. (1972). Excitability of the acoustic m. stapedius and m. tensor tympani reflexes in the nonanesthetized rabbit. *Acta Physiologica* (Scandinavia), *85,* 374–389.
Borg, E. (1972). On the change in the acoustic impedance of the ear as a measure of middle ear muscle reflex activity. *Acta Otolaryngologica* (Stockholm), *74,* 163–171.

Borg, E. (1976). Dynamic characteristics of the intra-aural muscle reflex. In A. Feldman & L. Wilber (Eds.), *Acoustic impedance and admittance: The measurement of middle ear function* (pp. 236–299). Baltimore: Williams & Wilkins.

Borg, E., & Moller, A. R. (1968). The acoustic middle ear reflex in unanesthetized rabbits. *Acta Otolaryngologica* (Stockholm), *65*, 575–585.

Brainerd, S. H., & Beasley, D. S. (1971). Respondent conditioning of the middle ear reflex. *Journal of Auditory Research*, *11*, 234–238.

Candiollo, L. (1967). The control mechanism of the middle ear transmission system: The middle ear muscles—In the morphology and function of auditory input control. *Translations of the Beltone Institute for Hearing Research*, *20*, 13–41.

Carmel, P. W., & Starr, A. (1963). Acoustic and nonacoustic factors modifying middle ear muscle activity in waking cats. *Journal of Neurophysiology*, *26*, 589–618.

Chiveralls, K., Fitzsimons, R., Beck, G. B., & Kernohan, H. (1976). The diagnostic significance of the stapedius reflex. *British Journal of Audiology*, *10*, 122–128.

Chobot, J. L., & Wilson, W. R. (1977). The effect of sensitization on the acoustic reflex as a function of frequency. *Journal of Auditory Research*, *17*, 99–104.

Clemis, J. D. (1984). Acoustic reflex testing in otoneurology. *Otolaryngology, Head and Neck Surgery*, *92*, 141–144.

Colletti, V. (1974). Biometric aspects of the stapedius reflex. *Acta Otorhinolaryngologica* (Belgium), *28*, 545–552.

Corcoran, A. L., Cleaver, V. C., & Stephens, S. D. (1980). Attention, eye closure and the acoustic reflex. *Audiology*, *19*, 233–244.

Counter, S. A., & Borg, E. (1982). The avian stapedius muscle. *Acta Otolaryngologica*, *94*, 267–274.

Cox, H. A. (1976). Acoustic reflex measurement [Letter]. *Archives of Otolaryngology*, *102*, 644.

Dallos, P. J. (1964). Dynamics of the acoustic reflex: Phenomenological aspects. *Journal of the Acoustical Society of America*, *36*, 2175–2183.

Downs, D. W., & Crum, M. A. (1980). The hyperactive acoustic reflex. Four case studies. *Archives of Otolaryngology*, *106*, 401–404.

Feldman, A. S., & Zwislocki, J. (1965). Effect of the acoustic reflex on the impedance at the eardrum. *Journal of Speech and Hearing Research*, *8*, 213–222.

Fisch, U., & van Schulthess, G. (1963). Electromyographic studies on the human stapedius muscle. *Acta Otolaryngologica*, *56*, 287–297.

Green, K. W., & Margolis, R. H. (1983). The ipsilateral acoustic reflex. In S. Silman (Ed.), *The acoustic reflex: Basic principles and clinical applications* (pp. 275–299). New York: Academic Press.

Greisen, O., & Neergaard, E. B. (1975). Middle ear reflex activity in the startle reaction. *Archives of Otolaryngology*, *101*, 348–353.

Hayes, D., & Jerger, J. (1982). Signal averaging of the acoustic reflex: Diagnostic applications of amplitude characteristics. *Scandinavian Audiology*, *17*, 31–36.

Hecker, M. H., & Kryter, K. D. (1965). A study of the acoustic reflex in infantrymen. *Acta Otolaryngologica* (Stockholm), (Suppl. 207), 1–16.

Hugelin, A., Dumont, S., & Paillas, N. (1960). Tympanic muscles and control of auditory input during arousal. *Science, 131,* 1371–1372.

Ison, J. R., & Krauter, E. E. (1975). Acoustic startle reflexes in the rat during consummatory behavior. *Journal of Comparative Physiology and Psychology, 89,* 39–49.

Jepsen, O. (1963). Middle ear muscle reflexes in man. In J. F. Jerger (Ed.), *Modern developments in audiology* (pp. 193–239). New York: Academic Press.

Kamerer, D. B. (1978). Electromyographic correlation of tensor tympani and tensor veli palatini muscles in man. *Laryngoscope, 88,* 651–662.

Kaplan, H., Babecki, S., & Thomas, C. (1980). The acoustic reflex in children without an hermetic seal. *Ear and Hearing, l,* 83–86.

Laws, D. W., & Moon, C. E. (1986). Effects of the menstrual cycle on the human acoustic reflex threshold. *Journal of Auditory Research, 26,* 197–206.

Lorente de No., R. (1933). The reflex contractions of the muscles of the middle ear as a hearing test in experimental animals. *Transactions of the American Laryngology, Rhinology, and Otology Society, 39,* 26–42.

Mangham, C., Burnett, P., & Lindeman, R. (1983). Evaluation of tensor tympani muscle dominance in the biphasic acoustic reflex. *Audiology, 22,* 105–119.

Mangham, C. A., & Miller, J. M. (1979). A case for further quantification of the stapedius reflex. *Archives of Otolaryngology, 105,* 593–596.

Marshall, L., Brandt, J. F., & Marston, L. E. (1975). Anticipatory middle-ear reflex activity from noisy toys. *Journal of Speech and Hearing Disorders, 40,* 320–326.

Martin, F. N., & Coombes, S. (1974). Effects of external ear canal pressure on the middle-ear muscle reflex threshold. *Journal of Speech and Hearing Research, 17,* 526–530.

McRobert, H. (1972). Summary on reflex. In D. E. Rose & L. Keating (Eds.), *Proceedings of the Mayo Impedance Symposium* (pp. 283–296). Rochester, MN: Mayo Foundation.

McRobert, H., Bryan, M. E., & Tempest, W. (1968). The acoustic stimulation of the middle ear muscles. *Sound and Vibration, 7,* 129–142.

Moller, A. (1958). Intra-aural muscle contraction in man examined by measuring acoustic impedance of the ear. *Laryngoscope, 68,* 48–62.

Moller, A. (1961). Bilateral contractions of the tympanic muscles in man examined by measuring acoustic impedance of the ear. *Annals of Otology, Rhinology and Laryngology, 70,* 735–753.

Moller, A. R. (1962). Acoustic reflex in man. *Journal of the Acoustical Society of America, 34,* 1524–1534.

Moller, A. (1962). The sensitivity of contraction of the tympanic muscles in man. *Annals of Otology, Rhinology and Laryngology, 71,* 86–95.

Perlman, H. B. (1960). The place of the middle ear muscle reflex in auditory research. *Archives of Otolaryngology, 72,* 201–206.

Peterson, J. L., & Liden, G. (1972). Some characteristics of the stapedial muscle reflex. *Audiology, 11,* 97–114.

Robinette, M. S., & Snyder, K. S. (1982). Effect of eye closure, mental concentration, and nonauditory sensory stimulation on the threshold and magnitude of the acoustic reflex. *Ear and Hearing, 3,* 220–226.

Sapper, H. (1977). The stapedius reflex. *Journal of Audiologic Technology, 16,* 47–60.

Sesterhenn, G., & Breuninger, H. (1976). The acoustic reflex at low sensation levels. *Audiology, 15,* 523–533.

Shearer, W. M. (1966). Behavior of middle ear muscle during stuttering. *Science, 152,* 1280.

Shearer, W. M., & Simmons, F. B. (1965). Middle ear activity during speech in normal speakers and stutterers. *Journal of Speech and Hearing Research, 8,* 203–207.

Simmons, F. B. (1959). Middle ear muscle activity at moderate sound levels. *Annals of Otology, Rhinology and Laryngology, 68,* 1126–1143.

Simmons, F. B. (1960). Middle ear protection from the acoustic trauma of loud continuous sound. *Annals of Otology, Rhinology and Laryngology, 69,* 1–9.

Simmons, F. B. (1963). Simultaneous transtympanic and electrophysiological indices of the acoustic reflex activity in the cat. *Acta Otolaryngologica, 55,* 309–314.

Simmons, F. B. (1964). Variable nature of the middle ear muscle reflex. *International Audiology, 3,* 136–146.

Simmons, F. B. Galambos, R., & Rupert, A. (1959). Conditioned response of middle ear muscles. *American Journal of Physiology, 197,* 537–538.

Stach, B., & Jerger, J. F. (1984). Acoustic reflex averaging. *Ear and Hearing, 5,* 289–296.

Starr, A., & Salomon, G. (1965). Electromyographic study of middle ear muscle activity during shock evoked motor activity in cats. *International Audiology, 4,* 28–30.

Stephens, S. D., Blegvad, B., & Krogh, H. J. (1977). Eye closure and the acoustic reflex threshold. *Journal of the American Auditory Society, 3,* 88–90.

Surr, R. K., & Schuchman, G. I. (1976). Measurement of the acoustic reflex without a pressure seal. *Archives of Otolaryngology, 102,* 160–161.

Terkildsen, K. (1975). Movements of the eardrum following interaural muscle reflexes. *Archives of Otolaryngology, 66,* 484–488.

Van Wagoner, R. S., & Goodwine, S. (1977). Clinical impressions of acoustic reflex measures in an adult population. *Archives of Otolaryngology, 103,* 322–325.

Wedeking, P., & Carlton, P. L. (1979). Habituation and sensitization in the modulation of reflex amplitude. *Physiology and Behavior, 22,* 57–62.

Woodford, C. M., Henderson, D., Hamernik, R. P., & Feldman, A. S. (1976). Acoustic reflex threshold of the chinchilla as a function of stimulus duration and frequency. *Journal of the Acoustical Society of America, 59,* 1204–1207.

Yonovitz, A. (1976). Classical conditioning of the stapedius muscle. *Acta Oto-laryngologica, 82,* 11–15.
Yonovitz, A., & Harris, J. D. (1976). Eardrum displacement following stapedius muscle contraction. *Acta Otolaryngologica* (Stockholm), *81,* 1–15.
Zakrisson, J. E., Borg, E., & Blom, S. (1974). The acoustic impedance change as a measure of stapedius muscle activity in man. *Acta Otolaryngologica, 78,* 357–364.
Zwillenberg, D., Kinkle, D. F., & Saunders, J. C. (1981). Measures of middle ear admittance during experimentally induced changes in middle ear volume in the hamster. *Otolaryngology, Head and Neck Surgery, 89,* 856–860.

7.1 Measurement Techniques

Advokat, C., & Carlton, P. L. (1978). Reflex modulation due to supplementary stimulation. *Behavioral Biology, 22,* 375–387.
Alberti, P. W., Fria, T. J., & Cummings, F. (1977). The clinical utility of ipsilateral stapedius reflex tests. *Journal of Otolaryngology, 6,* 466–472.
Bennett, M. J., & Weatherby, L. A. (1979). Multiple probe frequency acoustic reflex measurements. *Scandinavian Audiology, 8*(4), 233–239.
Blood, I. M., & Greenberg, H. J. (1981). Low-level acoustic reflex thresholds. *Audiology, 20,* 244–250.
Casselbrant, M., Ingelstedt, S., & Ivarsson, A. (1977). Volume displacement of the tympanic membrane as a function of middle ear muscle activity. A quantitative microflow method. *Acta Otolaryngologica* (Stockholm), *84,* 402–413.
Casselbrant, M., Ingelstedt, S., & Ivarsson, A. (1978). Volume displacement of the tympanic membrane at stapedius reflex activity in different postures. Studies on variations in perilymphatic pressure. *Acta Otolaryngologica* (Stockholm), *85,* 1–9.
Cohill, E. N., & Greenberg, H. J. (1979). Acoustic reflex thresholds using conventional and tracking methods. *Journal of the American Auditory Society, 5,* 149–150.
Counter, S. A., Borg, E., & Engstrom, B. (1989). Acoustic middle ear reflexes in laboratory animals using clinical equipment: Technical considerations. *Audiology, 28,* 135–143.
Cox, H. A. (1976). Acoustic reflex measurement [Letter]. *Archives of Otolaryngology, 2,* 644.
Danaher, E. M., & Pickett, J. M. (1974). Notes on an artifact in measurement of the acoustic reflex. *Journal of Speech and Hearing Research, 17,* 505–509.
Deutsch, L. J. (1972). The threshold of the stapedius reflex for pure tone and noise stimuli. *Acta Otolaryngologica* (Stockholm), *74,* 248–251.
Djupesland, G. (1964). Middle ear muscle reflexes elicited by acoustic and non-acoustic stimulation. *Acta Otolaryngologica,* (Suppl. 188), 287–292.
Djupesland, G., Flottorp, G., Sundby, A., & Szalay, M. (1973). A comparison between middle-ear muscle reflex thresholds for bone- and air-conducted pure tones. *Acta Otolaryngologica* (Stockholm), *75,* 178–183.

Ewertsen, H. W. (1973). Audiogram interpretation of symbols for stapedial reflexes. *Scandinavian Audiology, 1*, 61–63.

Feldman, A. S., & Williams, P. S. (1976). Tympanometric measurement of the transmission characteristics of the ear with and without the acoustic reflex. *Scandinavian Audiology, 5*, 43–47.

Gans, D. P., Sweetman, R. H., & Carlson, H. C. (1972). Use of high-speed photography in analysis of the acoustic reflex. *Journal of the Acoustical Society of America, 51*, 1826–1827.

Hayes, D., & Jerger, J. (1983). Signal averaging of the acoustic reflex: Diagnostic applications of amplitude characteristics. *Scandinavian Audiology*, (Suppl. 17), 31–36.

Ison, J. R., Reiter, L., & Warren, M. (1979). Modulation of the acoustic startle reflex in humans in the absence of anticipatory changes in the middle ear reflex. *Journal of Experimental Psychology, 5*, 639–642.

Kunov, H. (1977). The "eardrum artifact" in ipsilateral reflex measurements. *Scandinavian Audiology, 6*, 163–166.

Kunov, H. (1978). The ipsilateral acoustic impedance artifact and Rayleigh's radiation pressure. *Journal of Otolaryngology, 7*, 246–248.

Leis, B. R., & Lutman, M. E. (1979). Calibration of ipsilateral acoustic reflex stimuli. A comparison of loudness balance and equal reflex response methods. *Scandinavian Audiology, 8*, 93–99.

Lutman, M. E. (1980). Note on identification and rectification of the overshoot observed with the Grason-Stadler otoadmittance meter during acoustic reflex measurements. *Acta Otolaryngologica* (Stockholm), *89*, 63–65.

Lutman, M. E. (1980). Real-ear calibration of ipsilateral acoustic reflex stimuli from five types of impedance meters. *Scandinavian Audiology, 9*, 137–145.

Lutman, M. E., & Leis, B. R. (1980). Ipsilateral acoustic reflex artifacts measured in cadavers. *Scandinavian Audiology, 9*, 33–39.

Mahoney, T. (1981). Acoustic reflex crossover artifacts in infants and young children. *Archives of Otolaryngology, 107*, 363–366.

Mangham, C. A., & Miller, J. M. (1979). A case for further quantification of the stapedius reflex. *Archives of Otolaryngology, 105*, 593–596.

Margolis, R. H., Wilson, R. H., & Van Camp, K. J. (1982). A technique for detecting the ipsilateral acoustic reflex. *Journal of the Acoustical Society of America, 72*, 278–280.

Marsh, R. R., Hoffman, H. S., & Stitt, C. L. (1978). Reflex inhibition audiometry. A new objective technique. *Acta Otolaryngologica* (Stockholm), *85*, 336–341.

McPherson, D. L., & Thompson, D. (1978). Quantification of the threshold and latency parameters of the acoustic reflex in humans. *Acta Otolaryngologica* (Stockholm), *353*, 1–37.

Meeks, T., Owens, L., & Melnick, W. (1980). The effects of frequency modulation on middle ear reflex. *Otolaryngology, Head and Neck Surgery, 88*, 288–292.

Mendelson, E. S. (1957). A sensitive method for registration of human intratympanic muscle reflexes. *Journal of Applied Physiology, 11*, 499–502.

Mendelson, E. S. (1961). Improved method for studying tympanic reflexes in man. *Journal of the Acoustical Society of America, 33*, 146–152.

Metz, O. (1951). Studies on the contraction of the tympanic muscles as indicated by changes in the impedance of the ear. *Acta Otolaryngologica, 39,* 397–405.

Moller, A. (1958). Intra-aural muscle contraction in man, examined by measuring acoustic impedance of the ear. *Laryngoscope, 68,* 48–62.

Moller, A. R. (1978). A comment on H. Kunov: The "eardrum artifact" in ipsilateral reflex measurements. *Scandinavian Audiology, 7,* 61–64.

Newall, P., Royall, R. A., & Lightfoot, G. R. (1978). Some observations on the contralateral stapedial reflex artifact. *British Journal of Audiology, 12,* 78–82.

Niswander, P. S., & Ruth, R. A. (1976). An artifact in acoustic reflex measurement: Some further observations. *Journal of the American Auditory Society, 1,* 209–214.

Onchi, Y. (1963). Aural reflex indicator. *Transactions of the American Academy of Ophthalmology and Otolaryngology, 67,* 785–789.

Popelka, G. R. (1981). Instrumentation and procedures for measuring acoustic reflex thresholds. In S. R. Popelka (Ed.), *Hearing assessment with the acoustic reflex* (Chapter 4, pp. 47–58). New York: Grune & Stratton.

Popelka, G. R., & Dubno, J. R. (1978). Comments on the acoustic-reflex response for bone-conducted signals. *Acta Otolaryngologica, 86,* 64–70.

Reker, U. (1977). Normal values of the ipsilateral acoustic stapedius reflex threshold. *Archives of Otorhinolaryngology, 215,* 25–34.

Riedner, E., & Shimizu, H. (1976). Collapsing ears and acoustic reflex measurement with circumaural ear cushions. *Archives of Otolaryngology, 102,* 358–362.

Rizzo, S., Jr., & Greenberg, H. J. (1979). Influence of ear canal air pressure on acoustic reflex threshold. *Journal of the American Auditory Society, 5,* 21–24.

Ruth, R. A., Tucci, D. L., & Nilo, E. R. (1982). Effects of ear canal pressure on threshold and growth of the acoustic reflex. *Ear and Hearing, 3,* 39–41.

Salamon, D., & Starr, A. (1963). Electromyograph of middle ear muscles in man during motor activities. *Acta Neurologica* (Scandinavia), *39,* 161–168.

Sellari-Franceschini, S. (1986). Quantification of the parameters of the acoustic reflex in normal ears. *Audiology, 25*(3), 165–175.

Sohoel, T., & Arnesen, G. (1962). The choice of probe tube position and test frequency in determining the intra-aural reflexes. *Acta Otolaryngologica, 54,* 233–238.

Stach, B. A., & Jerger, J. (1984). Acoustic reflex averaging. *Ear and Hearing, 5,* 289–296.

Surr, R. K., & Schuchman, G. I. (1976). Measurement of the acoustic reflex without a pressure seal. *Archives of Otolaryngology, 102,* 160–161.

Terkildsen, K. (1957). Movements of the eardrum following inter-aural muscle reflexes. *Archives of Otolaryngology, 66,* 484–488.

Terkildsen, K. (1962). Intra-aural muscle reflex testing. *International Audiology, 1,* 228–230.

Zakrisson, J. E., Bork, E., & Blom, S. (1974). The acoustic impedance change as a measure of stapedius muscle activity in man. *Acta Otolaryngologica, 78,* 357–364.

Zito, R., & Roberto, M. (1980). The acoustic reflex pattern studied by the averaging technique. *Audiology*, *19*, 395–403.

7.2 Studies in Normal Subjects

Abahazi, D. A., & Greenberg, H. J. (1977). Clinical acoustic reflex threshold measurements in infants. *Journal of Speech and Hearing Disorders*, *42*, 514–519.

Barry, J., & Resnick, S. (1976). Comparison of acoustic reflex and behavioral thresholds as a function of stimulus frequency and duration. *Journal of the American Auditory Society*, *2*, 35–37.

Bennett, M. J. (1975). Acoustic impedance measurements with the neonate. *British Journal of Audiology*, *9*, 117–124.

Bennett, M. J., & Weatherby, L. A. (1982). Newborn acoustic reflexes to noise and pure tone signals. *Journal of Speech and Hearing Research*, *25*, 383–387.

Brask, T. (1978). Extratympanic manometry in man. Clinical and experimental investigations of the acoustic stapedius and tensor tympani contractions in normal subjects and in patients. *Scandinavian Audiology*, (Suppl. 7), 1–199.

Chiveralls, K., & Fitzimons, R. (1963). Stapedial reflex action in normal subjects. *British Journal of Audiology*, *7*, 105–110.

Cleaver, V. C. G., & Stephens, S. D. G. (1977). Observations on the clinical use of broad-band noise as an acoustic reflex stimulus. *British Journal of Audiology*, *11*, 22–24.

Colletti, V. (1974). Some stapedius reflex parameters in normal and pathological conditions. *Journal of Laryngology and Otology*, *88*, 127–137.

Creten, W. L., Vanpeperstraete, P. M., Van Camp, K. J., & Doclo, J. R. (1976). An experimental study on diphasic acoustic reflex patterns in normal ears. *Scandinavian Audiology*, *5*, 3–8.

Cunningham, D. (1976). Admittance values associated with the acoustic reflex and reflex decay. *Journal of the American Auditory Society*, *1*, 197–205.

Cunningham, D. R., & Porter, T. A. (1975). Susceptance and conductance changes in acoustic reflexometry. *Journal of the American Auditory Society*, *1*, 131–134.

Dallos, P. (1964). Dynamics of the acoustic reflex: Phenomenological aspects. *Journal of the Acoustical Society of America*, *36*, 2175–2183.

Deutsch, L. J. (1972). The threshold of the stapedius reflex for pure tone and noise stimuli. *Acta Otolaryngologica* (Stockholm), *74*, 248–251.

Djupesland, G. (1964). Middle ear muscle reflexes elicited by acoustic and non-acoustic stimulation. *Acta Otolaryngologica*, (Suppl. 188), 287–292.

Djupesland, G., Flottorp, G., & Winther, F. O. (1966). Size and duration of acoustically elicited impedance changes in man. *Acta Otolaryngologica* (Stockholm), (Suppl. 224), 220–228.

Djupesland, G., & Kvernvold, H. (1975). Acoustic impedance measured on ears with normal and diphasic impedance changes. *Scandinavian Audiology*, *4*, 39–43.

Feldman, A. S. (1967). Acoustic impedance studies of the normal ear. *Journal of Speech and Hearing Research*, *10*, 165–178.

Feldman, A. S. (1967). A report of further impedance studies of the acoustic reflex. *Journal of Speech and Hearing Research*, *10*, 616–622.

Feldman, A., & Williams, P. (1976). Tympanometric measurements of the transmission characteristics of the ear with and without the acoustic reflex. *Scandinavian Audiology*, *5*, 43–47.

Feldman, A. S., & Zwislocki, J. (1965). Effect of the acoustic reflex on the impedance at the eardrum. *Journal of Speech and Hearing Research*, *8*, 213–222.

Flottorp, G., Djupesland, G., & Winther, F. (1971). The acoustic stapedius reflex in relation to critical bandwidth. *Journal of the Acoustical Society of America*, *49*, 457–461.

Fria, T., LeBlanc, J., Kristensen, R., & Alberti, P. W. (1975). Ipsilateral acoustic reflex stimulation in normal and sensorineural impaired ears: A preliminary report. *Canadian Journal of Otolaryngology*, *4*, 695–703.

Gelfand, S. A. (1984). The contralateral acoustic-reflex threshold. In S. Silman (Ed.), *The acoustic reflex: Basic principles and clinical applications* (Chap. 5, pp. 137–186). New York: Academic Press.

Gelfand, S. A., & Piper, N. (1981). Acoustic reflex thresholds in young and elderly subjects with normal hearing. *Journal of the Acoustical Society of America*, *69*, 295–297.

Gelfand, S. A., & Piper, N. (1983). Acoustic reflex thresholds: Variability and distribution effects. *Ear and Hearing*, *5*, 228–234.

Gerber, S. E., Gong, E. L., & Mendel, M. I. (1984). Developmental norms for the acoustic reflex. *Audiology*, *23*, 1–8.

Gersdorff, M. C. (1977). Comparative study between the normally hearing child and the hard of hearing child, by acoustic impedance measurements of the ear. *Archives of Otorhinolaryngology* (New York), *217*, 13–31.

Green, G. G., & Kay, R. H. (1979). The dynamic characteristics of the stapedius reflex in humans [Proceedings]. *Journal of Physiology* (London), *296*, 15P–16P.

Green, K. W., & Margolis, R. H. (1983). The ipsilateral acoustic reflex. In S. Silman (Ed.), *The acoustic reflex: Basic principles and clinical applications* (pp. 275–299). New York: Academic Press.

Habener, S. A., & Snyder, J. M. (1974). Stapedius reflex amplitude and decay in normal hearing ears. *Archives of Otolaryngology*, *100*, 294–297.

Hung, I. J., & Dallos, P. J. (1972). Study of the acoustic reflex in human beings. I. Dynamic characteristics. *Journal of the Acoustical Society of America*, *52*, 1168–1180.

Iwamoto, V., & Pang-Ching, G. (1975). The acoustic reflex to air- and bone-conducted white noise. *Journal of Auditory Research*, *15*, 226–230.

Jepsen, O. (1951). The threshold of the reflexes of the intra-tympanic muscles in a normal material examined by means of the impedance method. *Acta Otolaryngologica, 39*, 406–408.

Jerger, J. (1979). Comments on "The effect of aging on the stapedius reflex thresholds." *Journal of the Acoustical Society of America, 66*, 908.

Jeter, I. K. (1975). Waveform patterns of reflex and voluntary contraction of the middle ear muscles. *Journal of Auditory Research, 16*, 183–192.

Johnsen, N. J., & Terkildsen, K. (1980). The normal middle ear reflex thresholds towards white noise and acoustic clicks in young adults. *Scandinavian Audiology, 9*, 131–135.

Johnson, D. W., & Sherman, R. E. (1979). Normal development and ear effect for contralateral acoustic reflex in children six to twelve years old. *Developmental Medicine and Child Neurology, 21*, 572–581.

Kankkunen, A., & Liden, G. (1984). Ipsilateral acoustic reflex thresholds in neonates and in normal-hearing and hearing impaired pre-school children. *Scandinavian Audiology, 13*, 139–144.

Keith, R. W., & Bench, R. J. (1978). Stapedial reflex in neonates. *Scandinavian Audiology, 7*, 187–191.

Keith, R. W., Murphy, K. P., & Martin, F. (1976). Acoustic impedance measurement in the otological assessment of multiply handicapped children. *Clinical Otolaryngology, 1*, 221–224.

Laukli, E., & Mair, I. W. (1980). Ipsilateral and contralateral acoustic reflex thresholds. *Audiology, 19*, 469–479.

Liden, G., Peterson, J. L., & Harford, E. R. (1969). Simultaneous recording of changes in relative impedance and air pressure during acoustic and non-acoustic elicitation of the middle-ear reflexes. *Acta Otolaryngologica* (Stockholm), (Suppl. 263), 208–217.

Lorente de No, R. (1933). The reflex contractions of the muscles of the middle ear as a hearing test in experimental animals. *Transactions of the American Laryngology, Rhinology, and Otology Society, 39*, 26–42.

Lorente de No, R., & Harris, A. S. (1933). Experimental studies in hearing. I. The threshold of the reflexes of the muscles of the middle ear. *Laryngoscope, 43*, 315–326.

Margolis, R. H., Dubno, J. R., & Wilson, R. H. (1980). Acoustic-reflex thresholds for noise stimuli. *Journal of the Acoustical Society of America, 68*, 892–895.

McMillan, P. M., Marchant, C. D., & Shurin, P. A. (1985). Ipsilateral acoustic reflexes in infants. *Annals of Otology, Rhinology and Laryngology, 94* (part 2), 145–148.

McPherson, D. L., & Thompson, D. (1977). Quantification of the threshold and latency parameters of the acoustic reflex in humans. *Acta Otolaryngologica*, (Suppl. 353), 1–37.

McRobert, H. (1968). The response of the tympanic muscles in human ears. *Sound, 2*, 71–76.

Metz, O. (1951). Studies on the contraction of the tympanic muscles as indicated by changes in the impedance of the ear. *Acta Otolaryngologica, 39*, 397–405.

Moller, A. (1961). *Bilateral contractions of the tympanic muscles in man,* (Rep. No. 18). Stockholm: Speech Transmission Laboratory of the Royal Institute of Technology.

Moller, A. (1962). The sensitivity of contraction of the tympanic muscles in man. *Annals of Otology, Rhinology and Laryngology, 71,* 86–95.

Morgan, D. E., Dirks, D. D., & Kamm, C. (1978). The influence of middle-ear muscle contraction on auditory threshold for selected pure tones. *Journal of the Acoustical Society of America, 63,* 1896–1903.

Osterhammel, D., & Osterhammel, P. (1979). Age and sex variations for the normal stapedial reflex thresholds and tympanometric compliance values. *Scandinavian Audiology, 8,* 153–158.

Peterson, J. L., & Liden, G. (1972). Some static characteristics of the stapedial muscle reflex. *Audiology, 11,* 97–114.

Popelka, G. R., Karlovich, S. R., & Wiley, T. L. (1974). Acoustic reflex and critical bandwidth. *Journal of the Acoustical Society of America, 55,* 883–885.

Reker, U. (1977). Methodological problems in the determination of homolateral stapedius reflex threshold. *Audiology, 16,* 487–498.

Richards, A. M., & Goodman, A. C. (1977). Threshold of the human acoustic stapedius reflex for short-duration bursts of noise. *Journal of Auditory Research, 17,* 183–189.

Robinson, D. O., & Allen, D. V. (1984). Racial differences in tympanometric results. *Journal of Speech and Hearing Disorders, 49,* 140–144.

Sato, R., & Ono, Y. (1968). The displacement of the stapes by the reflex of the human stapedius muscle. *Acta Otolaryngologica* (Stockholm), *68,* 509–513.

Schwartz, D. M., & Sanders, J. W. (1976). Critical bandwidth and sensitivity prediction in the acoustic stapedial reflex. *Journal of Speech and Hearing Disorders, 41,* 244–255.

Silman, S. (1979). The acoustic reflex, aging, and the distortion product: A reply to Jerger. *Journal of the Acoustical Society of America, 66,* 909–910.

Silman, S. (1979). The effects of aging on the stapedius reflex thresholds. *Journal of the Acoustical Society of America, 66,* 735–738.

Silverman, C. A., Silman, S., & Miller, M. H. (1983). The acoustic reflex threshold in aging ears. *Journal of the Acoustical Society of America, 73,* 248–255.

Sprague, B. H., Wiley, T. L., & Goldstein, R. G. (1985). Tympanometric and acoustic-reflex studies in neonates. *Journal of Speech and Hearing Research, 28,* 265–272.

Stream, R. W., Stream, K. S., Walker, J. R., & Breningstall, G. (1978). Emerging characteristics of the acoustic reflex in infants. *Otolaryngology, 86,* 628–636.

Terkildsen, K. (1960). Acoustic reflexes of the human musculus tensor tympani. *Acta Otolaryngologica,* (Suppl. 158), 230–238.

Terkildsen, K. (1960). The intra-aural muscle reflexes in normal persons and in workers exposed to intense noise. *Acta Otolaryngologica, 52,* 384–396.

Terkildsen, K. (1962). Intra-aural muscle reflex testing. *International Audiology, 1,* 228–230.

Updike, C. D., & Epstein, A. (1986). Characteristics of the acoustic reflex in response to narrow bands of noise. *Journal of Auditory Research, 26,* 147–156.

Van Wagoner, R. S., & Goodwine, S. (1977). Clinical impressions of acoustic reflex measures in an adult population. *Archives of Otolaryngology, 103,* 582–584.

Weatherby, L. A., & Bennett, M. J. (1980). The neonatal acoustic reflex. *Scandinavian Audiology, 9,* 103–110.

Weiss, H. S., Mundie, J. R., Cashin, J. L., & Shinabarger, E. W. (1962). The normal human intra-aural muscle reflex in response to sound. *Acta Otolaryngologica, 55,* 505–515.

Wersall, R. (1958). The tympanic muscles and their reflexes. *Acta Otolaryngologica,* (Suppl. 139), 1–112.

Wiley, T. L., & Block, M. G. (1984). Acoustic and nonacoustic reflex patterns in audiologic diagnosis. In S. Silman (Ed.), *The acoustic reflex: Basic principles and clinical applications* (pp. 387–411). New York: Academic Press.

Wiley, T. L., Oviatt, D. L., & Block, M. G. (1987). Acoustic-immitance measures in normal ears. *Journal of Speech and Hearing Research, 30,* 161–170.

Wilson, R. H. (1979). Factors influencing the acoustic-immitance characteristics of the acoustic reflex. *Journal of Speech and Hearing Research, 22,* 480–499.

Wilson, R. H., & McBride, L. M. (1978). Threshold and growth of the acoustic reflex. *Journal of the Acoustical Society of America, 63,* 147–154.

Wilson, R. H., Shanks, J. E., & Velde, T. (1981). Aural acoustic-immitance measurements: Inter-aural differences. *Journal of Speech and Hearing Research, 46,* 413–421.

Zakrisson, J. E., Borg, E., & Blom, S. (1974). The acoustic impedance change as a measure of stapedius muscle activity in man. *Acta Otolaryngologica, 78,* 357–364.

7.3 Studies in Pathologic Subjects

Ahuja, G. K., Verma, A., Ghosh, P., & Nagaraj, M. N. (1980). Stapedius reflexometry. A diagnostic test of myasthenia gravis. *Journal of Neurological Science, 46,* 311–314.

Bauch, C.D. (1983). Auditory brainstem responses and acoustic reflex tests. *Archives of Otolaryngology, 109,* 1–5.

Beagley, H. A. (1973). The role of electro-physiological tests in the diagnosis of non-organic hearing loss. *Audiology, 12,* 470–480.

Bel, J., Causse, J., Michaux, P., Cezard, R., Canut, Y. & Tapon, J. (1976). Mechanical explanation of the on-off effect (diphasic impedance change) in otospongiosis. *Audiology, 15,* 128–140.

Bergenius, J., Borg, E., & Hirch, A. (1983). Stapedius reflex test, brainstem audiometry and optovestibular test index of acoustic neuromas. *Scandinavian Audiology, 12,* 3–9.

Berlin, C. I. (1976). New developments in evaluating central auditory mechanisms. *Annals of Otology, Rhinology and Laryngology, 85,* 833–841.

Block, L. (1976). A comparison of the SISI and the stapedius reflex test in the differential diagnosis of cochlear pathology. *Journal of South African Speech and Hearing Association, 23,* 99–108.

Blom, S., & Zakrisson, J. E. (1974). The stapedius reflex in the diagnosis of myasthenia gravis. *Journal of Neurological Science, 21,* 71–76.

Borg, E. (1977). The intra-aural muscle reflex in retrocochlear pathology: A model study in the rabbit. *Audiology, 16,* 316–330.

Borg, E. (1982). Dynamic properties of the intra-aural reflex in lesions of the lower auditory pathway. An experimental study in rabbits. *Acta Otolaryngologica* (Stockholm), *93,* 19–29.

Borg, E., & Engstrom, B. (1982). Acoustic reflex after experimental lesions to inner and outer hair cells. *Hearing Research, 6,* 25–34.

Bosatra, A. (1976). Afflictions of the central nervous arc. In J. Jerger & J. Northern (Eds.), *Proceedings of the Third International Symposium of Impedance Audiometry* (pp. 51–58). Acton, MA: American Electromedics.

Bosatra, A. (1977). Pathology of the nervous arc of the acoustic reflexes. *Audiology, 16,* 307–317.

Bosatra, A., & Russolo, M. (1976). Oscilloscopic analysis of the stapedius muscle reflex in brain stem lesions. *Archives of Otolaryngology, 102,* 284–285.

Bosatra, A., Russolo, M., & Poli, P. (1980). Modifications of the stapedius muscle reflex under spontaneous and experimental brain-stem impairment. *Acta Otolaryngologica* (Stockholm), *80,* 61–66.

Brask, T. (1978). Extratympanic manometry in man. Clinical and experimental investigations of the acoustic stapedius and tensor tympani contractions in normal subjects and in patients. *Scandinavian Audiology,* (Suppl. 7), 1–199.

Bruschini, P., Sellari Franceschini, S., Bartalena, L., Aghini-Lombardi, F., Mazzco, S., & Martino, E. (1984). Acoustic reflex characteristics in hypo- and hyperthyroid patients. *Audiology, 23,* 38–45.

Bynke, O. (1980). Facial reflex examination. A clinical and neurophysiological study on acoustic tumours and brain displacement at the tentorial notch. *Acta Neurologica* (Scandinavia), (Suppl. 76), 1–127.

Chesnutt, B., Stream, R. W., Love, J. T., & McLarey, D. C. (1975). Otoadmittance measurements in cases of dual ossicular disorders. *Archives of Otolaryngology, 101,* 109–113.

Chiveralls, K. (1977). A further examination of the use of the stapedius reflex in the diagnosis of acoustic neuroma. *Audiology, 16,* 331–337.

Chiveralls, K., Fitzsimons, R., Beck, G. B., & Kernohan, H. (1976). The diagnostic significance of the stapedius reflex. *British Journal of Audiology, 10,* 122–128.

Clemis, J. D., & Mastricola, P. G. (1976). Special audiometric test battery in 121 proved acoustic tumors. *Archives of Otolaryngology, 102,* 654–656.

Cohen, M., & Prasher, D. (1988). The value of combining auditory brainstem responses and acoustic reflex threshold measurements in neuro-otological diagnosis. *Scandinavian Audiology, 17,* 153–162.

Collard, M. E., & Parker, W. (1984). Exaggerated acoustic reflex response in a patient with transient facial palsy and hyperacusis. *American Journal of Otology*, 5, 355–359.

Colletti, V. (1974). Some stapedius reflex parameters in normal and pathological conditions. *Journal of Laryngology and Otology*, 88, 127–137.

Colletti, V. (1975). Stapedius reflex abnormalities in multiple sclerosis. *Audiology*, 14, 63–71.

Coman, W. B., & Dale, B. A. (1968). Stapedectomy and the stapedius reflex. *Journal of Laryngology and Otology*, 82, 907–912.

Djupesland, G. (1964). Mechanical component to deafness in Meniere's disease. *Acta Otolaryngologica*, (Suppl. 188), 206–208.

Djupesland, G. (1976). Diagnostic implications of acoustic and nonacoustic reflex measurements. In J. Jerger & J. Northern (Eds.), *Proceedings of the Third International Symposium on Impedance Audiometry* (pp. 24–31). Acton, MA: American Electromedics.

Djupesland, G., & Kvernvold, H. (1973). A comparison between absolute and "relative" impedance measurement as a method of distinguishing between otosclerosis and ossicular chain discontinuity. *Scandinavian Audiology*, 2, 93–97

Djupesland, G., & Kvernvold, H. (1975). Acoustic impedance measured on ears with normal and diphasic impedance changes. *Scandinavian Audiology*, 4, 39–43.

Downs, D. W., & Crum, M. A. (1980). The hyperactive acoustic reflex. Four case studies. *Archives of Otolaryngology*, 106, 401–404.

Downs, D. W., Eskwitt, D. L., & Ferry, P. C. (1981). Acoustic reflex hyperactivity in an infant with meningitis. *Archives of Otolaryngology*, 107, 324–325.

Estrand, T., & Glitterstam, K. (1979). Bell's palsy—Prognostic value of the stapedius reflex with contralateral stimulation. *Journal of Laryngology and Otology*, 93, 271–275.

Feldman, A. S. (1977) Diagnostic application and interpretation of tympanometry and the acoustic reflex. *Audiology*, 16, 294–306.

Flottorp, G., & Djupesland, G. (1970). Diphasic impedance change and its applicability in clinical work. *Acta Otolaryngologica*, (Suppl. 263), 200–204.

Forquer, B. D., & Sheehy, J. L. (1981). Cochlear otosclerosis: Acoustic reflex findings. *American Journal of Otolaryngology*, 2, 297–300.

Forquer, B. D., & Sheehy, J. L. (1981). The negative on/off effect in cochlear and early stapedial otosclerosis. *Ear and Hearing*, 2, 256–259.

French-St. George, M., & Stephens, S. D. (1977). Acoustic reflex measures of cochlear damage—A normative study. *British Journal of Audiology*, 11, 11–119.

Freyss, G. E., Narcy, P. P., Manach, Y., & Toupet, M. G. (1980). Acoustic reflex as a predictor of middle ear effusion. *Annals of Otology, Rhinology and Laryngology*, 89(Suppl. 68), 196–199.

Fria, T., LeBlanc, J., Kristensen, R., & Alberti, P. W. (1975). Ipsilateral acoustic reflex stimulation in normal and sensorineural impaired ears: A preliminary report. *Canadian Journal of Otolaryngology*, 4, 695–703.

Gelfand, S. A. (1984). The contralateral acoustic-reflex threshold. In S. Silman (Ed.), *The acoustic reflex: Basic principles and clinical applications* (Chap. 5, pp. 137–186). New York: Academic Press.

Gelfand, S. A., & Silman, S. (1982). Acoustic reflex thresholds in brain damaged patients. *Ear and Hearing, 3,* 93–95.

Gersdorff, M. C. (1977). Comparative study between the normally hearing child and the hard of hearing child, by acoustic impedance measurements of the ear. *Archives of Otorhinolaryngology, 217,* 13–31.

Giacomelli, F., & Mozzo, W. (1965). An experimental and clinical study on the influence of the brainstem reticular formation on the stapedial reflex. *International Audiology, 9,* 42–44.

Gordon, A. G. (1981). Hyperactive acoustic reflexes and perilymphatic hypotension [Letter]. *Archives of Otolaryngology, 107,* 774.

Gordon, A. G. (1986). Abnormal middle ear muscle reflexes and audiosensitivity. *British Journal of Audiology, 20(2),* 95–99.

Gordon, A. S., & Friedberg, J. (1978). Current status of testing for seventh nerve lesions. *Otolaryngologic Clinics of North America, 11(2),* 25–261.

Gorga, M. P., & Stelmachowicz, P. G. (1983). Temporal aspects of the acoustic reflex in normal and hearing-impaired listeners. *Audiology, 22,* 120–127.

Greisen, O., & Rasmussen, P.E. (1970). Stapedius muscle reflexes and otoneurological examinations in brain-stem tumors. *Acta Otolaryngologica* (Stockholm), *70,* 366–370.

Grenman, R., Lang, H., Panelius, M., Salmivalli, A., Laine, H. & Rintamaki, J. (1984). Stapedius reflex and brainstem auditory evoked responses in multiple sclerosis patients. *Scandinavian Audiology, 13,* 109–113.

Gronas, H. E., Quist-Hanssen, S., & Bjelde, A. (1968). Delayed speech feedback in normal hearing and conductive hearing loss, with and without a functioning stapedius muscle. *Acta Otolaryngologica* (Stockholm), *66,* 241–247.

Hall, J. W. (1985). The acoustic reflex in central auditory dysfunction. In M. L. Pinheiro & F. E. Musiek (Eds.), *Assessment of central auditory dysfunction: Foundations and clinical correlations* (p. 103). Baltimore: Williams & Wilkins.

Hall, J. W., & Jerger, J. (1976). Acoustic reflex characteristics in spastic dysphonia. *Archives of Otolaryngology, 102,* 411–415.

Hammond, J. A., & Pang-Ching, G. K. (1979). Influence of acoustic reflex on pure-tone thresholds in sensorineural patients. *Journal of Auditory Research, 19,* 95–98.

Hannley, M., Jerger, J., & Rivera, V. (1983). Relationships among auditory brain stem responses, masking level differences and the acoustic reflex in multiple sclerosis. *Audiology, 22,* 20–33.

Harris, J. P., Davidson, T.M., May, M., & Fria, T. (1983). Evaluation and treatment of congenital facial paralysis. *Archives of Otolaryngology, 109,* 145–151.

Harrison, T., Silman, S., & Silvermann, C. A. (1989). Contralateral acoustic-reflex growth function in a patient with a cerebellar tumor: A case study. *Journal of Speech and Hearing Disorders, 54(4),* 505–509.

204 ACOUSTIC IMMITANCE MEASURES IN CLINICAL AUDIOLOGY

Hayes, D., & Jerger, J. (1981). Patterns of acoustic reflex and auditory brainstem response abnormality. *Acta Otolaryngologica* (Stockholm), *92*, 199–209.

Hecker, M. H. L., & Kryter, K. D. (1965). A study of the acoustic reflex in infantrymen. *Acta Otolaryngologica*, (Suppl. 207).

Hess, K. (1979). Stapedius reflex in multiple sclerosis. *Journal of Neurology, Neurosurgery, and Psychiatry*, *42*, 331–337.

Hirsch, A. (1983). Stapedius reflex tests in retrocochlear hearing disorders. *Audiology*, *22*, 463–470.

Hirsch, A., & Anderson, H. (1980). Audiologic test results in 96 patients with tumours affecting the eighth nerve. *Acta Otolaryngologica*, (Suppl. 369), 1–26.

Hirsch, A. & Anderson, H. (1980). Elevated stapedius reflex threshold and pathologic reflex decay. Clinical occurrence and significance. *Acta Otolaryngologica* (Stockholm), (Suppl. 368), 1–28.

Hirsch, A., & Lofqvist, L. (1986). The stapedius reflex test studied with laboratory and commercial equipment in acoustic neurinomas. *Scandinavian Audiology*, *15*(3), 147–150.

Horovitz, L. J., Johnson, S. B., Pearlman, R. C., Schaffer, E. J., & Hedin, A. K. (1978). Stapedial reflex and anxiety in fluent and disfluent speakers. *Journal of Speech and Hearing Research*, *21*, 762–767.

Igarashi, M., Mauldin, L., & Jerger, J. (1979). Impedance audiometry in the squirrel monkey. Effect of transection of crossed olivocochlear bundle. *Archives of Otolaryngology*, *105*, 258–259.

Jakimetz, J. J., Silman, S., Miller, M. H., & Silvermann, C. A. (1989). Some effects of signal bandwidth and spectral density on the acoustic-reflex threshold in the elderly. *Journal of the Acoustical Society of America*, *86*, 1783–1789.

Jastreboff, P. J. (1981). Cerebellar interaction with the acoustic reflex. *Acta Neurobiologica Experimenta* (Warsz), *41*, 279–298.

Jenkins, H. A., Morgan, D. E., & Miller, R. H. (1980). Intact acoustic reflexes in the presence of ossicular disruption. *Laryngoscope*, *90*, 267–273.

Jepsen, O. (1953). Intratympanic muscle reflexes in psychogenic deafness. *Acta Otolaryngologica*, (Suppl. 109), 61–69.

Jerger, J., Harford, E., Clemis, J., & Alford, B. (1974). The acoustic reflex in eighth nerve disorders. *Archives of Otolaryngology*, *99*, 409–413.

Jerger, J., & Hayes, D. (1983). Latency of the acoustic reflex in eighth nerve tumors. *Archives of Otolaryngology*, *109*, 1–6.

Jerger, J., Jenkins, H., Fifer, R., & Mecklenburg, D. (1986). Stapedius reflex to electrical stimulation in a patient with a cochlear implant. *Annals of Otology, Rhinology and Laryngology*, *95*, 151–157.

Jerger, J., Jerger, S. J., & Mauldin, L. (1972). Studies in impedance audiometry: I. Normal and sensorineural ears. *Archives of Otolaryngology*, *96*, 513–523.

Jerger, J., Mauldin, L., & Igarashi, M. (1978). Impedance audiometry in the squirrel monkey. Sensorineural losses. *Archives of Otolaryngology*, *104*, 559–563.

Jerger, J., Neely, G., & Jerger, S. (1980). Speech, impedance, and auditory brainstem response audiometry in brainstem tumors. *Archives of Oto-laryngology, 106*, 218–223.

Jerger, J., Oliver, T. A., & Jenkins, H. (1987). Suprathreshold abnormalities of the stapedius reflex in acoustic tumor: A series of case reports. *Ear and Hearing, 8*, 131–139.

Jerger, J., Oliver, T. A., Rivera, V., & Stach, B. A. (1986). Abnormalities of the acoustic reflex in multiple sclerosis. *American Journal of Otolaryngology, 7*, 163–176.

Jerger, S. (1980). Diagnostic application of impedance audiometry in central auditory disorders. In J. Jerger & J. L. Northern (Eds.), *Clinical impedance audiometry* (2nd ed., pp. 128–140). Acton, MA: American Electromedics.

Jerger, S., & Jerger, J. (1975). Extra- and intra-axial brain stem auditory disorders. *Audiology, 14*, 93–117.

Jerger, S., & Jerger, J. (1977). Diagnostic value of crossed vs uncrossed acoustic reflexes: Eighth nerve and brain stem disorders. *Archives of Otolaryngology, 103*, 445–453.

Jerger, S., Jerger, J., & Hall, J. (1979). A new acoustic reflex pattern. *Archives of Otolaryngology, 104*, 24–28.

Jerger, S., Neely, J. G., & Jerger, J. (1975). Recovery of crossed acoustic reflexes in brain stem auditory disorders. *Archives of Otolaryngology, 101*, 329–332.

Johns, M. E., Ruth, R. A., Jahrsdoerfer, R. A., & Cantrell, R. W. (1979). Stapedius muscle function tests in the diagnosis of neuromuscular disorders. *Otolaryngology, Head and Neck Surgery, 87*, 261–265.

Johnsen, N. J., Osterhammel, D., Terkildsen, K., Osterhammel, P., & Huis In't Veld, F. (1976). The white-noise middle ear muscle reflex threshold in patients with sensorineural hearing impairment. *Scandinavian Audiology, 5*, 131–135.

Kankkunen, A., & Liden, G. (1984). Ipsilateral acoustic reflex thresholds in neonates and in normal-hearing and hearing impaired pre-school children. *Scandinavian Audiology, 13*, 139–144.

Keating, L. W., Rose, D. E., Facer, D. W., Whicker, J. H., & Schreurs, K. (1972). Acoustic impedance measurements in the deaf. In D.E. Rose & L. Keating (Eds.), *Proceedings of the Mayo Impedance Symposium* (pp. 177–186). Rochester, MN: Mayo Foundation.

Keith, R. W. (1979). Loudness and the acoustic reflex: Cochlear-impaired listeners. *Journal of the American Auditory Society, 5*, 65–70.

Keith, R. W., Murphy, K. P., & Martin, F. (1976). Acoustic impedance measurement in the otological assessment of multiply handicapped children. *Clinical Otolaryngology, 1*, 221–224.

Keith, R. W., Murphy, K. P., & Martin, F. (1977). Acoustic reflex measurement in children with cerebral palsy. *Folia Phoniatrica* (Basel), *29*, 311–314.

Klockhoff, I. (1961). Middle ear reflexes in man: A clinical and experimental study with special reference to diagnostic problems in hearing impairment. *Acta Otolaryngologica*, (Suppl. 164), 1–91.

Kofler, B., Oberascher, B., & Pommer, B. (1984). Brain-stem involvement in multiple sclerosis: A comparison between brain-stem auditory evoked potentials and the acoustic stapedius reflex. *Journal of Neurology, 231,* 145–147.

Koike, M., Hojo, K., & Iwaski, E. (1977). Prognosis of facial palsy based on the stapedial reflex test. In U. Fisch (Ed.), *Facial nerve surgery.* Amstelveen: Kugler Medical Publishers.

Kramer, L. D., Ruth, R. A., Johns, M. E., & Sanders, D. B. (1981). A comparison of stapedial reflex fatigue with repetitive stimulation and single-fiber EMG in myasthenia gravis. *Annals of Neurology, 9,* 531–536.

Lamb, L., & Peterson, J. (1967). Middle ear reflex measurements in pseudohypacusis. *Journal of Speech and Hearing Disorders, 32,* 46–51.

Lamb, L., Peterson, J., & Hansen, S. (1968). Application of stapedius muscle reflex measures in the diagnosis of auditory problems. *International Audiology, 7,* 188–199.

Laukli, E., & Mair, I. W. (1980). Ipsilateral and contralateral acoustic reflex thresholds. *Audiology, 19,* 469–479.

Lehrer, J. F., & Poole, D. C. (1981). Abnormalities of the stapedius reflex in patients with vertigo. *American Journal of Otology, 3,* 96–103.

Liden, G. (1970). The stapedius muscle reflex used as an objective recruitment test: A clinical and experimental study. In G. E. W. Wolstenholme & J. Knight (Eds.), *Sensorineural hearing loss* (pp. 295–308). London: Churchill.

Liden, G. (1975). Application of tympanometry and acoustic reflex measurements. *Acta Otorhinolaryngologica* (Belgium), *29,* 802–813.

Liden, G., & Korsan-Bengtsen, M. (1973). Audiometric manifestations of retrocochlear lesions. *Scandinavian Audiology, 2,* 29–40.

Lindgren, F., Nilsson, R., & Axelsson, A. (1983). The acoustic reflex threshold in relation to noise-induced hearing loss. *Scandinavian Audiology, 12,* 49–56.

Lindstrom, D., & Liden, G. (1964). The tensor-tympani reflex in operative treatment of trigeminal neuralgia. *Acta Otolaryngologica,* (Suppl. 188), 271–274.

Lopes, Fo O., de Campos, C. A., de A. Quintanilha, R. F., & de Campos, C. C. (1978). Clinical investigation of the alteration in the middle ear impedance in patients with intracranial hypertension. *Journal of Otolaryngology, 7,* 439–443.

Love, J. T., Jr., & Stream, R. W. (1978). The biphasic acoustic reflex: A new perspective. *Laryngoscope, 88,* 298–313.

Lovrinic, J. H. (1977). Stapedial reflexes in normal versus recruiting ears. *Journal of Auditory Research, 17,* 251–261.

Macrae, J. H. (1972). Theoretical investigation of cochlear effects on the acoustic impedance of the ear. *Journal of Auditory Research, 12,* 265–270.

Macrae, J. H. (1973). Acoustic neuromas and acoustic impedance of the ear. *Journal of Speech and Hearing Disorders, 38,* 345–353.

Majkowski, J., Szwed, M., & Chadzypanagiotis, D. (1973). Effect of brainstem lesions on retention of a conditioned reflex in cats. *Physiological Behavior, 11,* 7–11.

Mangham, C. A. (1984). The effect of drugs and systematic disease on the acoustic reflex. In S. Silman (Ed.), *The acoustic reflex: Basic principles and clinical applications* (Chapter 13, pp. 441–468). New York: Academic Press.

Mangham, C. A., & Lindeman, R. C. (1980). The negative acoustic reflex in retrocochlear disorders. *Laryngoscope, 90,* 1753–1761.

Mangham, C., Lindeman, R., & Dawson, W. (1980). Stapedius reflex quantification in acoustic tumor patients. *Laryngoscope, 90,* 242–250.

Mangham, C. A., & Miller, J. M. (1977). Experimental acoustic neurinoma effects on the stapedius reflex in monkeys. *Transactions of the American Academy of Ophthalmology and Otolaryngology, 84,* 432–439.

May, M., Fria, T., Blumenthal, F., & Curtin, H. (1981). Facial paralysis in children: Differential diagnosis. *Otolaryngology, Head and Neck Surgery, 89,* 841–848.

May, M., & Hardin. (1978). Facial palsy interpretations of neurologic findings. *Laryngoscope, 88,* 1352–1362.

McCall, G. N. (1972). Acoustic impedance measurement in the study of phonatory disorders. In D. E. Rose & L. Keating (Eds.), *Proceedings of the Mayo Impedance Symposium* (pp. 225–230). Rochester, MN: Mayo Foundation.

McCall, G. N. (1973). Acoustic impedance measurement in the study of patients with spasmodic dysphonia. *Journal of Speech and Hearing Disorders, 38,* 250–255.

Mikaelian, D. O., Gamsey, H. B., Trocki, I., & Jassal, S. P. (1977). Acoustic reflex post-stapectomy: A preliminary report. *Transactions of the Pennsylvania Academy of Opthalmology and Otolaryngology, 30,* 161–166.

Morioka, W. T., Neff, P. A., Boisseranc, T. E., Hartman, P. W., & Cantrell, R. W. (1976). Audiotympanometric findings on myasthenia gravis. *Archives of Otolaryngology, 102,* 211–213.

Neff, P. A., Morioka, W. T., Sample, P. A., & Cantrell, R. W. (1980). Audiometric and tympanometric monitoring of a disease affecting nerve-muscle transmission. *Audiology, 19,* 293–309.

Noffsinger, D., Martinez, C. D., & Schaefer, A. B. (1982). Auditory brainstem responses and masking level differences from persons with brainstem lesion. *Scandinavian Audiology,* (Suppl. 15), 81–93.

Olsen, C. C., & Brandt, J. F. (1976). Middle ear muscle activity during speech in stapedectomized and laryngectomized subjects. *Journal of the American Auditory Society, 1,* 215–220.

Olsen, W. O., Bauch, C. D., & Harner, S. G. (1983). Application of Silman and Gelfand (1981) 90th percentile levels for acoustic reflex thresholds. *Journal of Speech and Hearing Disorders, 48,* 330–331.

Olsen, W. O., Noffsinger, D., & Kurdziel, S. (1975). Acoustic reflex and reflex decay. Occurrence in patients with cochlear and eighth nerve lesions. *Archives of Otolaryngology, 101,* 622–625.

Osterhammel, D., & Christau, B. (1980). High frequency audiometry and stapedius muscle reflex thresholds in juvenile diabetics. *Scandinavian Audiology, 9,* 13–18.

Palva, T., Jauhianinen, T. Sjoblom, C. J., & Ylikoski, J. (1978). Diagnosis and surgery of acoustic tumors. *Acta Otolaryngologica* (Stockholm), *86*, 233–240.

Parving, A., & Bak-Pedersen, K. (1978). Clinical findings and diagnostic problems in sensorineural low frequency hearing loss. *Acta Otolaryngologica* (Stockholm), *85*, 184–190.

Peterson, J. L., & Lamb, L. E. (1967). Middle ear reflex measurements in pseudohypacusis. *Journal of Speech and Hearing Disorders*, *32*, 46–51.

Peterson, M. K. (1978). Impedance audiometry and the brain-damaged child. *Developmental Medicine and Child Neurology*, *20*, 800–802.

Prasansuk, S., & Hinchcliffe, R. (1972). Acoustic stapedius reflex elicited after stapedectomy. *Journal of Laryngology and Otology*, *86*, 637–641.

Rane, R. L., Yut, J. P., & Berger, K. W. (1978). Negative needle deflection of the acoustic reflex in otosclerotics. *Journal of the American Auditory Society*, *3*, 241–244.

Rasmy, E. (1986). Stapedius reflex after stapedectomy with preservation of the stapedius tendon. *Journal of Laryngology and Otology*, *100*, 521–527.

Rose, D. E., Keating, L. W., Facer, G. W., & Wicker, J. H. (1972). Reflex measures in various types of ear pathology. In D. E. Rose & L. Keating (Eds.), *Proceedings of the Mayo Impedance Symposium* (pp. 261–268). Rochester, MN: Mayo Foundation.

Rosen, G., & Sellars, S. L. (1980). The stapedius reflex in idiopathic facial palsy. *Journal of Laryngology and Otology*, *94*, 1017–1020.

Rossi, D. F., & Sims, D. G. (1977). Acoustic reflex measurement in the severely and profoundly deaf. *Audiology and Hearing Education*, *3*, 6–9.

Ruth, R. A., Nilo, E. R., & Mravec, J. J. (1978). Consideration of acoustic reflex magnitude (ARM) in cases of idiopathic facial paralysis. *Otolaryngology*, *86*, 215–220.

Sanders, J., Josey, A., Glasscock, M., & Jackson, C. (1981). The acoustic reflex test in cochlear and eighth nerve pathology ear. *Laryngoscope*, *91*, 787–793.

Saunders, A. Z., & Jackson, R. T. (1981). CPA tumors with normal routine audiometry and positive reflex and BSER tests. *American Journal of Otology*, *2*, 318–323.

Schwartz, D. M., & Bess, F. H. (1975). Acoustic reflex measurements in sensorineural hearing loss. *Maico Audiological Library Series*, *14*, Report 5.

Shapiro, I. (1979). Evaluation of the relationship between hearing threshold and loudness discomfort level in sensorineural hearing loss. *Journal of Speech and Hearing Disorders*, *44*, 31–36.

Shapiro, I., Canalis, R. F., Firemark, R., & Bahna, M. (1981). Ossicular discontinuity with intact acoustic reflex. *Archives of Otolaryngology*, *107*, 576–578.

Shearer, W. M. (1966). Speech: Behavior of middle ear muscle during stuttering. *Science*, *152*, 1280.

Sheehy, J. L., & Inzer, B. E. (1976). Acoustic reflex test in neuro-otologic diagnosis. A review of 24 cases of acoustic tumors. *Archives of Otolaryngology*, *102*, 647–653.

Sieminski, L. R., Durrant, J. D., Rosenberg, P. E., & Lourinic, J. H. (1977). Stapedial reflexes in normal vs. recruiting ears. *Journal of Auditory Research*, *17*, 251–261.

Silman, S., & Gelfand, S. A. (1981). The relationship between magnitude of hearing loss and acoustic reflex thresholds. *Journal of Speech and Hearing Disorders, 46*, 312–316.

Silman, S., Gelfand, S. A., & Chun, T. (1978). Some observations in a case of acoustic neuroma. *Journal of Speech and Hearing Disorders, 43*, 459–466.

Silman, S., Popelka, G. R., & Gelfand, S. A. (1978). Effect of sensorineural hearing loss on acoustic stapedius reflex growth functions. *Journal of the Acoustical Society of America, 64*, 1406–1411.

Silman, S., Silverman, C. A., Gelfand, S. A., Lutolf, J., & Lynn, D. J. (1988). Ipsilateral acoustic-reflex adaptation testing for detection of facial-nerve pathology: Three case studies. *Journal of Speech and Hearing Disorders, 53*, 378–382.

Sleeckx, J. P., Shea, J. J., & Pitzer, F. J. (1967). Epitympanic ossicular fixation. *Archives of Otolaryngology, 85*, 619–631.

Spillman, T. (1964). The acoustic stapedial reflex threshold as an objective recruitment test in the differential diagnosis of sensorineural hearing loss. *Journal of Laryngology, Rhinology and Otology, 73*, 914–923.

Spitzer, J. B., & Ventry, I. M. (1980). Central auditory dysfunction among chronic alcoholics. *Archives of Otolaryngology, 106*, 224–229.

Stalberg, E. (1980). Clinical electrophysiology in myasthenia gravis. *Journal of Neurology, Neurosurgery, and Psychiatry, 43*, 622–633.

Suri'a, D., & Serra-Ravent'os, M. (1975). Acoustic impedance measurement and autistic children. *Folia Phoniatrica* (Basel), *27*, 387–388.

Terkildsen, K. (1960). The intra-aural muscle reflexes in normal persons and in workers exposed to intense noise. *Acta Otolaryngologica, 52*, 384–396.

Terkildsen, K., Osterhammel, P., & Bretlau, P. (1973). Acoustic middle ear muscle reflexes in patients with otosclerosis. *Archives of Otolaryngology, 89*, 152–155.

Thomas, W. G., McMurry, G., & Pillsbury, H. C. (1985). Acoustic reflex abnormalities in behaviorally disturbed and language delayed children. *Laryngoscope, 95*, 811–817.

Thomsen, J., & Terkildsen, K. (1975). Audiological findings in 125 cases of acoustic neuromas. *Acta Otolaryngologica* (Stockholm), *80*, 353–361.

Thomsen, K. A. (1955). Case of psychogenic deafness demonstrated by measuring of impedance. *Acta Otolaryngologica, 45*, 82–85.

Tonning, F. M. (1977). The reliability of level-diagnostic examinations in acute, peripheral facial palsy. *Acta Otolaryngologica* (Stockholm), *84*, 414–415.

Turner, J. S., & Saunders, A. Z. (1984). False positive stapedial reflexes and brainstem evoked response findings in patients with suspected retrocochlear lesions. *Laryngoscope, 94*, 910–913.

Turner, J. S., Jr., Saunders, A. Z., & Farrell, J. (1980). Audiometric and radiologic findings in acoustic tumor. *Southern Medical Journal, 73*, 3–5.

Uliel, S. (1980). Acoustic reflex measurements and the loudness function in sensorineural hearing loss. *South African Journal of Communicative Disorders, 27*, 58–77.

Van Camp, K. J., Van Peperstraete, P. M., Creten, W. L., & Vanhuyse, V. J. (1975). On irregular acoustic reflex patterns. *Scandinavian Audiology, 4*, 227–232.

Van Wagoner, R. S., & Goodwine, S. (1977). Clinical impressions of AR measures in an adult population. *Archives of Otolaryngology, 103,* 582–584.

Wiegand, D. A., & Poch, N. E. (1988). The acoustic reflex in patients with asymptomatic multiple sclerosis. *American Journal of Otolaryngology, 9,* 210–216.

Wiley, T. L., & Block, M. G. (1984). Acoustic and nonacoustic reflex patterns in audiologic diagnosis. In S. Silman (Ed.), *The acoustic reflex: Basic principles and clinical applications* (pp. 387–411). New York: Academic Press.

Yamane, M., & Nomura, Y. (1984). Analysis of stapedial reflex in neuromuscular diseases. *Otology, Rhinology, and Laryngology, 46,* 84–96.

Zakrisson, J. E., Borg, E., Diamant, H., & Miller, A. R. (1975). Auditory fatigue in patients with stapedius muscle paralysis. *Acta Otolaryngologica* (Stockholm), *79,* 228–232.

7.4 Acoustic Reflex Adaptation (Decay)

Alberti, P., & Kristensen, R. (1972). Stapedial reflex threshold and decay: Abnormal study in clinical practice. In D. Rose & L. Keating (Eds.), *Proceedings of the Mayo Impedance Symposium* (pp. 269–282). Rochester, MN: Mayo Foundation.

Anderson, H., Barr, B., & Wedenberg, E. (1969). Intra-aural reflexes in retrocochlear lesions. In C. A. Hamberger & J. Wersall (Eds.), *Nobel Symposium 10, Disorders of the Skull Base Region* (pp. 78–83). Stockholm: Almqvist & Wiksell.

Anderson, H., Barr, B., & Wedenberg, E. (1970). Early diagnosis of eighth nerve tumors by acoustic reflex tests. *Acta Otolaryngologica,* (Suppl. 263), 232–237.

Anderson, H., Barr, B., & Wedenberg, E. (1970). The early detection of acoustic tumors by stapedius reflex test. In G. E. W. Wolstenholme & J. Knight (Eds.), *Sensorineural hearing loss* (pp. 278–289). London: Churchill.

Borg, E., & Odman, B. (1979). Decay and recovery of the acoustic stapedius reflex in humans. *Acta Otolaryngologica* (Stockholm), *87,* 421–428.

Bosatra, A. (1983). Reflex delay in sensorineural hearing loss. *Scandinavian Audiology,* (Suppl. 17), 40–42.

Cunningham, D. R. (1976). Admittance values associated with the acoustic reflex and reflex decay. *Journal of the American Auditory Society, 1,* 197–205.

Dallos, P. J. (1974). Dynamics of the acoustic reflex: Phenomenological aspects. *Journal of the Acoustical Society of America, 36,* 2175–2183.

Djupesland, G., Flottorp, G., & Winther, F. O. (1967). Size and duration of acoustically elicited impedance changes in man. *Acta Otolaryngologica,* (Suppl. 224), 220–228.

Fowler, C., & Wilson, R. (1984). Adaptation of the acoustic reflex. *Ear and Hearing, 5,* 281–288.

Gerhardt, K. J., Melnick, W., & Ferraro, J. A. (1980). Acoustic reflex decay in chinchillas during a long-term exposure to noise. *Ear and Hearing, 1,* 33–37.

Givens, G. D., & Seidemann, M. F. (1979). A systematic investigation of measurement parameters of acoustic-reflex adaptation. *Journal of Speech and Hearing Disorders, 44,* 534–542.

Habener, S. A., & Snyder, J. M. (1974). Stapedius reflex amplitude and decay in normal hearing ears. *Archives of Otolaryngology, 100,* 294–297.

Hall, C. M. (1977). Stapedial reflex decay in retrocochlear and cochlear lesions. Review of procedures and methods for conducting SRD tests. *Annals of Otology, Rhinology and Laryngology, 86,* 219–222.

Hirsch, A. (1983). Stapedius reflex tests in retrocochlear hearing disorders. *Audiology, 22,* 463–470.

Hirsch, A., & Anderson, H. (1980). Audiologic test results in 96 patients with tumours affecting the eighth nerve. *Acta Otolaryngologica,* (Suppl. 369), 1–26.

Hirsch, A., & Anderson, H. (1980). Elevated stapedius reflex threshold and pathologic reflex decay. Clinical occurrence and significance. *Acta Otolaryngologica* (Stockholm), (Suppl. 368), 1–28.

Hirsch, A., & Lofqvist, L. (1986). The stapedius reflex test studied with laboratory and commercial equipment in acoustic neurinomas. *Scandinavian Audiology, 15,* 147–150.

Hung, I. J., & Dallos, P. (1972). Study of the acoustic reflex in human beings: I. Dynamic characteristics. *Journal of the Acoustical Society of America, 52,* 1168–1180.

Jerger, J., Harford, E., Clemis, J., & Alford, B. (1974). The acoustic reflex in eighth nerve disorders. *Archives of Otolaryngology, 99,* 409–413.

Jerger, J., & Jerger, S. (1983). Acoustic reflex decay: 10-second or 5-second criterion? *Ear and Hearing, 4,* 70–71.

Jerger, J., Oliver, T. A., & Jenkins, H. (1987). Suprathreshold abnormalities of the stapedius reflex in acoustic tumor: A series of case reports. *Ear and Hearing, 8,* 131–139.

Kaplan, H. J., Gilman, S., & Dirks, D. D. (1976). Dynamic properties of acoustic reflex adaptation. *Transactions of the American Academy of Ophthalmology and Otolaryngology, 82,* 368–374.

Kaplan, H., Gilman, S., & Dirks, D. D. (1977). Properties of acoustic reflex adaptation. *Annals of Otology, Rhinology and Laryngology, 86,* 348–356.

Klodd, D. A., & Nearhoff, D. J. (1977). Properties of acoustic reflex adaptation to pure tones and one-third octave bands of noise. *Journal of the American Auditory Society, 3,* 126–133.

Lutman, M. E., & Martin, A. M. (1978). Adaptation of the acoustic reflex to combinations of sustained steady state and repeated pulse stimuli. *Sound and Vibration, 56,* 137–150.

Olsen, W. O., Noffsinger, D., & Kurdziel, S. (1975). Acoustic reflex and reflex decay. Occurrence in patients with cochlear and eighth nerve lesions. *Archives of Otolaryngology, 101,* 622–625.

Olsen, W. O., Stach, B. A., & Kurdziel, S. A. (1981). Acoustic reflex decay in 10 seconds and in 5 seconds for Meniere's disease patients and for VIIIth nerve tumor patients. *Ear and Hearing, 2,* 180–181.

Olsen, W. O., Stach, B. A., & Kurdziel, S. A. (1983). Reply to Jerger and Jerger. *Ear and Hearing, 4,* 71.

Oviatt, D. L., & Kileny, P. (1984). Normative characteristics of ipsilateral acoustic reflex adaptation. *Ear and Hearing, 5,* 145–152.

Rodriguez, G. P., & Gerhardt, K. J. (1988). Adaptation properties of the acoustic reflex in response to continuous-, intermittent- and industrial-noise stimulation. *Audiology, 27,* 344–355.

Rosenhall, U., Liden, G., & Nilsson, E. (1979). Stapedius reflex decay in normal hearing subjects. *Journal of the American Audological Society, 4,* 157–162.

Segal, A. I. (1978). Definition of pathological reflex decay [Letter]. *Journal of the American Auditory Society, 3,* 227.

Sheehy, J., & Izner, B. (1976). Acoustic reflex test in neuro-otologic diagnosis. *Archives of Otolaryngology, 102,* 647–653.

Snashall, S. E. (1977). Bekesy audiometry and tone and reflex decay tests in diabetics. *Archives of Otolaryngology, 103,* 342–343.

Warren, W. R., Gutmann, L., Cody, R. C., Flowers, P., & Segal, A. T. (1977). Stapedius reflex decay in myasthenia gravis. *Archives of Neurology, 34,* 496–497.

Wiley, T. L., & Karlovich, R. S. (1975). Acoustic-reflex response to sustained signals. *Journal of Speech and Hearing Research, 18,* 148–157.

Wilson, R. H., McCullough, J., & Lilly, D. J. (1984). Acoustic-reflex adaptation: Morphology and half-life data for subjects with normal hearing. *Journal of Speech and Hearing Research, 27,* 586–595.

Wilson, R. H., Shanks, J. E., & Lilly, D. J. (1984). Acoustic-reflex adaptation. In S. Silman (Ed.), *The acoustic reflex: Basic principles and clinical applications* (pp. 329–386). New York: Academic Press.

Wilson, R. H., Steckler, J. F., Jones, H. C., & Margolis, R. H. (1978). Adaptation of the acoustic reflex. *Journal of the Acoustical Society of America, 64,* 782–791.

Zakrisson, J. E., & Borg, E. (1974). Stapedius reflex and auditory fatigue. *Audiology, 13,* 231–235.

7.5 Acoustic Reflex Growth

Block, M. G., & Wiley, T. L. (1979). Acoustic-reflex growth and loudness. *Journal of Speech and Hearing Research, 22,* 295–310.

Gelfand, S. A., Silman, S., & Silverman, C. A. (1981). Temporal summation in acoustic reflex growth functions. *Acta Otolaryngologica, 91,* 177–182.

Gersdorff, M. C. H. (1978). Impedancemetric study of the variations of the auditory reflex in man as a function of age. *Audiology, 17,* 260–270.

Gorga, M. P., Abbas, P. J., & Lilly, D. J. (1980). Magnitude of the acoustic reflex for either homophasic (0 degrees) or antiphasic (180 degrees) binaural activating signals presented in a background of noise. *Journal of the Acoustical Society of America, 67,* 589–593.

Habener, S. A., & Snyder, J. M. (1974). Stapedius reflex amplitude and decay in normal hearing ears. *Archives of Otolaryngology, 100,* 294–297.

Hall, J. W. (1982). Acoustic reflex amplitude. I. Effect of age and sex. *Audiology, 21,* 294–309.

Hall, J. W. (1982). Acoustic reflex amplitude. II. Effect of age-related auditory dysfunction. *Audiology, 21,* 386–399.

Hall, J. W., & Jerger, J. (1978). Central auditory function in stutterers. *Journal of Speech and Hearing Research, 21,* 324–337.

Harrison, T., Silman, S., & Silvermann, C. A. (1989). Contralateral acoustic-reflex growth function in a patient with a cerebellar tumor: A case study. *Journal of Speech and Hearing Disorders, 54,* 505–509.

Houghton, J. M., Greirlle, K. A., & Keith, W. J. (1988). Acoustic reflex amplitude and noise-induced hearing loss. *Audiology, 27,* 42–48.

Jerger, J., & Oliver, T. (1987). Interaction of age and intersignal interval on acoustic reflex amplitude. *Ear and Hearing, 8,* 322–325.

Jerger, J., Oliver, T. A., & Jenkins, H. (1987). Suprathreshold abnormalities of the stapedius reflex in acoustic tumor: A series of case reports. *Ear and Hearing, 8,* 131–139.

Robinette, M. S., & Brey, R. H. (1978). Effects of the visual modality on acoustic reflex magnitude. *Journal of the American Auditory Society, 4,* 6–10.

Robinette, M. S., & Snyder, K. S. (1982). Effect of eye closure, mental concentration, and nonauditory sensory stimulation on the threshold and magnitude of the acoustic reflex. *Ear and Hearing, 3,* 220–226.

Ruth, R. A., Nilo, E. R., & Mravec, J. J. (1978). Consideration of acoustic reflex magnitude (ARM) in cases of idiopathic facial paralysis. *Otolaryngology, 86,* 215–220.

Silman, S. (1984). Magnitude and growth of the acoustic reflex. In S. Silman (Ed.), *The acoustic reflex: Basic principles and clinical applications* (pp. 226–274). New York: Academic Press.

Silman, S., & Gelfand, S. A. (1981). Effect of sensorineural hearing loss on the stapedius reflex growth function in the elderly. *Journal of the Acoustical Society of America, 69,* 1099–1106.

Silman, S., Popelka, G. R., & Gelfand, S. A. (1978). Effect of sensorineural hearing loss on acoustic stapedius reflex growth functions. *Journal of the Acoustical Society of America, 64,* 1406–1411.

Sprague, B. H., Wiley, T. L., & Block, M. G. (1981). Dynamics of acoustic-reflex growth. *Audiology, 20,* 15–40.

Thompson, D. J., Sills, J. A., Recke, K. S., & Bui, D. M. (1980). Acoustic reflex growth in the aging adult. *Journal of Speech and Hearing Research, 23,* 405–418.

Wilson, R. H. (1981). The effects of aging on the magnitude of the acoustic reflex. *Journal of Speech and Hearing Research, 24,* 406–414.

Wilson, R. H., & McBride, L. M. (1978). Threshold and growth of the acoustic reflex. *Journal of the Acoustical Society of America, 63,* 147–154.

7.6 Temporal Characteristics

Borg, E. (1972). The dynamic properties of the acoustic middle ear reflex in non-anesthetized rabbits. Quantitative aspects of a polysynaptic reflex system. *Acta Physiologica* (Scandinavia), *86*, 366–387.

Borg, E. (1980). Recovery of the human intra-aural muscle reflex after "pauses" of various depth. *Acta Otolaryngologica* (Stockholm), *90*, 1–5.

Borg, E. (1982). Time course of acoustic intra-aural muscle reflex in non-anesthetized rabbits, normative data. *Acta Otolaryngologica* (Stockholm), *93*, 161–167.

Borg, E. (1982). Time course of the human acoustic stapedius reflex. *Scandinavian Audiology*, *11*, 237–245.

Bosatra, A., Russolo, M. & Silverman, C. A. Acoustic-reflex latency: State of the art. In S. Silman (Ed.), *The acoustic reflex: Basic principles and clinical applications* (pp. 302–328). New York: Academic Press.

Church, G. T., & Cudahy, E. A. (1984). The time course of the acoustic reflex. *Ear and Hearing*, *5*, 235–241.

Clemis, J. D., & Sarno, C. N. (1980a). The acoustic reflex latency test: Clinical application. *Laryngoscope*, *90*, 601–611.

Clemis, J. D., & Sarno, C. N. (1980b). Acoustic reflex latency test in the evaluation of nontumor patients with abnormal brainstem latencies. *Annals of Otology, Rhinology and Laryngology*, *89*, 296–302.

Gorga, M., & Stelmachowicz, P. (1983). Temporal characteristics of the acoustic reflex. *Audiology*, *22*, 120–127.

Jerger, J., & Hayes, D. (1983). Latency of the acoustic reflex in eighth-nerve tumors. *Archives of Otolaryngology*, *190*, 1–6.

Jerger, J., Oliver, T. & Stach, B. (1986). Problems in the clinical measurement of the acoustic reflex latency. *Scandinavian Audiology*, *15*, 31–40.

Letien, W. C., & Bess, F. H. (1975). Acoustic reflex relaxation in sensorineural hearing loss. *Archives of Otolaryngology*, *101*, 617–621.

Ljubin, C., Licul, F., & Ljubin, N. (1981). Dependence of latency upon acoustic stimuli in the audiomotor reflex (AMR). *Electromyography Clinical Neurophysiology*, *21*, 267–278.

Mangham, C. A., Jr., Burnett, P. A., & Lindeman, R. C. (1982). Standardization of acoustic reflex latency: A study in humans and nonhuman primates. *Annals of Otology, Rhinology and Laryngology*, *91*, 169–174.

Mangham, C., Lindeman, R., & Dawson, W. (1980). Stapedius reflex quantification in acoustic tumor patients. *Laryngoscope*, *90*, 242–250.

McPherson, D. L., & Thompson, D. (1977). Quantification of the threshold and latency parameters of the acoustic reflex in humans. *Acta Otolaryngologica*, (Stockholm), *353*, 1–37.

Neergaard, E. B., & Rasmussen, P. E. (1966). Latency of the stapedius muscle reflex in man. *Archives of Otolaryngology*, *84*, 173–180.

Nellis, R. A., & Wiley, T. L. (1979). Recovery characteristics of the acoustic reflex. *Journal of the American Auditory Society*, *4*, 184–189.

Norris, T. W., Stelmachowicz, P., Bowling, C., & Taylor, D. (1974). Latency measures of the acoustic reflex. Normal versus sensorineural. *Audiology*, *13*, 464–469.

Norris, T. W., Stelmachowicz, P. G., & Taylor, D. J. (1974). Acoustic reflex relaxation to identify sensorineural hearing impairment. *Archives of Otolaryngology*, *99*, 194–197.

Ruth, R. A., & Niswander, P. S. (1976). Acoustic reflex latency as a function of frequency and intensity of eliciting stimulus. *Journal of the American Auditory Society*, *2*, 54–60.

7.7 Assessment of Hearing Loss

Brooks, D. N., & Ghosh, S. (1982). Assessment of hearing level by means of the acoustic reflex. *Ear and Hearing*, *3*, 320–324.

Gelfand, S. A., Piper, N., & Silman, S. (1983). Effects of hearing levels at the activator and other frequencies on the expected levels of the acoustic reflex threshold. *Journal of Speech and Hearing Disorders*, *48*, 11–17.

Givens, G., & Bronerwine, L. (1983). Estimation of auditory sensitivity from the acoustic reflex with mentally deficient children. *Journal of Auditory Research*, *23*, 109–117.

Green, K. W., & Margolis, R. H. (1983). Detection of hearing loss with ipsilateral acoustic reflex thresholds. *Audiology*, *22*, 471–479.

Hall, J. W. (1978). Predicting hearing level from the acoustic reflex. A comparison of three methods. *Archives of Otolaryngology*, *104*, 601–605.

Hall, J. W. (1980). Predicting hearing loss from the acoustic reflex. In J. Jerger & J. L. Northern (Eds.), *Clinical impedance audiometry* (2nd ed., pp. 141–163). Acton, MA: American Electromedics.

Hall, J. W. (1981). Hearing loss prediction by the acoustic reflex in a young population: Comparison of seven methods. *International Journal of Pediatric Otorhinolaryngology*, *3*, 225–243.

Hall, J. W., Berry, G. A., & Olsen, K. (1982). Identification of serious hearing loss with acoustic reflex data. *Scandinavian Audiology*, *11*, 251–257.

Hall, J. W., & Bleakney, M. E. (1981). Hearing loss prediction by the acoustic reflex: Comparison of seven methods. *Ear and Hearing*, *2*, 156–164.

Hall, J. W., & Koval, C. B. (1982). Accuracy of hearing prediction by the acoustic reflex. *Laryngoscope*, *92*, 140–149.

Handler, S. D., & Margolis, R. H. (1977). Predicting hearing loss from stapedial reflex thresholds in patients with sensorineural impairment. *Transactions of the American Academy of Ophthalmology and Otology*, *84*, 425–431.

Hyde, M. L., Alberti, P. W., Morgan, P. P., Symons, F., & Cummings, F. (1980). Pure-tone threshold estimation from acoustic reflex thresholds—A myth? *Acta Otolaryngologica* (Stockholm), *89*, 345–357.

Jerger, J., Burney, P., Mauldin, L., & Crump, B. (1974). Predicting hearing loss from the acoustic reflex. *Journal of Speech and Hearing Disorders*, *39*, 11–22.

Jerger, J., Hayes, D., & Anthony, L. (1978). Effect of age on prediction of sensorineural hearing level from the acoustic reflex. *Archives of Otolaryngology*, *104*, 393–394.

Jerger, J., Hayes, D., Anthony, L., & Mauldin, L. (1978). Factors influencing prediction of hearing level from the acoustic reflex. *Monographs in Contemporary Audiology, 1.* Minneapolis, MN: Maico Hearing Instruments.

Keith, R. W. (1977). An evaluation of predicting hearing loss from the acoustic reflex. *Archives of Otolaryngology, 103,* 419–424.

Kobrak, H. G., Lindsay, J. R., & Perlman, H. B. (1935). Value of the reflex contraction of the muscles of the middle ear as an indicator of hearing. *Archives of Otolaryngology, 21,* 663–676.

Lindsay, J. R., Kobrak, H., & Perlman, H. B. (1936). Relation of the stapedius reflex to hearing sensation in man. *Arch Otolaryngologica, 23,* 671–678.

Margolis, R. H., & Fox, C. M. (1977). A comparison of three methods for predicting loss from acoustic reflex thresholds. *Journal of Speech and Hearing Research, 20,* 241–253.

Margolis, R. H., Fox, C., Lilly, D. J., Popelka, G. R., Silman, S., & Trumpf, A. (1981). The bivariate plotting procedure for hearing assessment with acoustic reflex threshold measures. In S. R. Popelka (Ed.), *Hearing assessment with the acoustic reflex* (pp. 59–84). New York: Grune & Stratton.

Miller, R., Davies, C. B., & Gibson, W. P. R. (1976). Using the acoustic reflex to predict the pure tone threshold. *British Journal of Audiology, 10,* 51–54.

Niemeyer, W. (1976). Predicting sensorineural hearing loss from acoustic reflex threshold. In J. Jerger & J. Northern (Eds.), *Proceedings of the Third International Symposium on Impedance Audiometry* (pp. 32–40). Acton, MA: American Electromedics.

Niemeyer, W., & Sesterhenn, G. (1974). Calculating the hearing threshold from the stapedius reflex threshold for different sound stimuli. *Audiology, 13,* 421–427.

Niswander, P. S., & Ruth, R. A. (1977). Prediction of hearing sensitivity from acoustic reflexes in mentally retarded persons. *American Journal of Mental Deficiencies, 81,* 474–481.

Poland, R. M., Wells, D. H., & Ferlauto, J. J. (1980). Methods for detecting hearing impairment in infancy. *Pediatric Annals, 9,* 31–32, 37–44.

Poole, P. B., Sheeley, E. C., & Hannah, J. E. (1982). Predicting hearing sensitivity and audiometric slope for mentally retarded persons. *Ear and Hearing, 3,* 77–82.

Popelka, G. R. (1981). *Hearing assessment with the acoustic reflex.* New York: Grune & Stratton.

Rizzo, S. R., Jr., & Greenberg, H. J. (1981). Predicting hearing loss from the acoustic reflex. *Journal of Auditory Research, 21,* 207–215.

Schwartz, D. M., & Sanders, J. W. (1976). Critical bandwidth and sensitivity prediction in the acoustic stapedial reflex. *Journal of Speech and Hearing Disorders, 41,* 244–255.

Sesterhenn, G., & Breuninger, H. (1977). Determination of hearing threshold for single frequencies from the acoustic reflex. *Audiology, 16,* 201–214.

Silman, S., & Gelfand, S. A. (1979). Prediction of hearing levels from acoustic reflex thresholds in persons with high-frequency hearing losses. *Journal of Speech and Hearing Research, 22,* 697–707.

Silman, S., & Gelfand, S. A. (1981). The relationship between magnitude of hearing loss and acoustic reflex threshold levels. *Journal of Speech and Hearing Disorders, 46,* 312–316.

Silman, S., Gelfand, S. A., Howard, J.C ., & Showers, T. J. (1982). Clinical application of the bivariate plotting procedure in the prediction of hearing loss. *Scandinavian Audiology*, *11*, 115–125.

Silman, S. S., Gelfand, S. A., Piper, N., Silverman, C. A., & Frank, L. V. (1984). Prediction of hearing loss from the acoustic reflex threshold. In S. Silman (Ed.), *The acoustic reflex: Basic principles and clinical applications* (pp. 188–225). New York: Academic Press.

Silman, S., Silverman, C. A., Showers, T., & Gelfand, S. A. (1984). Effect of age on prediction of hearing loss with the bivariate-plotting procedure. *Journal of Speech and Hearing Research*, *27*, 12–19.

Tsappis, A. (1977). Prediction of auditory sensitivity. Small sample confirmation using acoustic reflex thresholds. *Archives of Otolaryngology*, *103*, 322–325.

7.8 *Hearing Aid Selection*

Berger, K. (1976). The use of uncomfortable loudness level in hearing aid fitting. *Maico Audiological Library Series*, *15*. Minneapolis, MN: Maico Hearing Instruments.

Bragg, V. C. (1977). Toward a more objective hearing aid fitting procedure. *Hearing Instruments*, *28*(9), 6–9.

Cole, W. A. (1975). Hearing aid gain: A functional approach. *Hearing Instruments*, *26*, 22–24.

Greenfield, D. G., Wiley, T. L., & Block, M. G. (1985). Acoustic-reflex dynamics and the loudness-discomfort level. *Journal of Speech and Hearing Disorders*, *50*, 14–20.

Hall, J. W. III, & Ruth, R. A. (1985). Acoustic reflexes and auditory evoked responses in hearing aid evaluation. *Seminars in Hearing*, *6*, 251–273.

Horning, J. (1975). Tympanometry and hearing aid selection. *Hearing Aid Journal*, *28*, 8, 50.

Jerger, J., Oliver, T. A., & Chmiel, R. A. (1988). Prediction of dynamic range from stapedius reflex in cochlear implant patients. *Ear and Hearing*, *9*, 4–8.

Keith, R. W. (1979). An acoustic reflex technique of establishing hearing aid settings. *Journal of the American Auditory Society*, *5*, 71–75.

Keith, R. W., & Sininger, L. (1978). New ideas in hearing aid selection. *Hearing Instruments*, *29*, 6–8, 34.

Kiessling, J. (1980). Input-output function of the acoustic reflex and objective hearing aid evaluation. *Audiology*, *19*, 480–494.

Northern, J. L. (1978). Hearing aids and acoustic impedance measurements. *Monographs in Contemporary Audiology*, *1*.

Preves, D., & Orton, J. (1978). Use of acoustic impedance in hearing aid fitting. *Hearing Instruments*, *29*(6), 22–24.

Rainville, M. (1976). Hearing aid fitting using stapedial reflex measurements. In J. Jerger & J. Northern (Eds.), *Proceedings of the Third International Symposium on Impedance Audiometry* (pp. 49–50). Acton, MA: American Electromedics.

Rappaport, B. Z., & Tait, C. A. (1976). Acoustic reflex threshold measurement in hearing aid selection. *Archives of Otolaryngology*, *102*, 129–132.

Schwartz, D. M., & Larson, V. D. (1977). Hearing aid selection and evaluation procedures in children. In F. H. Bess (Ed.), *Childhood deafness: Causation, assessment and management* (pp. 217–233). New York: Grune & Stratton.

Snow, T., & McCandless, G. (1976). The use of impedance measures in hearing aid selection. *Hearing Aid Journal, 29*, 7–32.

Tato, J. M., & Rainville, M. J. (1975). Utilisation du reflexe stapedien pour l'adaption des prostheses [The use of the stapedius reflex in the fitting of hearing aids]. *Audiology, 15*, 428–432.

Tonisson, W. (1975). Measuring in-the-ear gain of hearing aids by the acoustic reflex method. *Journal of Speech and Hearing Research, 18*, 17–30.

7.9 Pharmacologic Aspects

Bauch C., & Robinette, M. (1978). Alcohol and the acoustic reflex: Effects of stimulus spectrum, subject variability and sex. *Journal of the American Auditory Society, 4*, 104–112.

Borg, E., & Moller, A. R. (1967). Effect of ethyl alcohol and pentobarbital sodium on the acoustic middle ear reflex in man. *Acta Otolaryngologica* (Stockholm), *64*, 415–426.

Borg, E., & Moller, A. R. (1975). Effect of central depressants on the acoustic middle ear reflex in rabbit. A method for quantitative measurements of drug effect on the CNS. *Acta Physiologica* (Scandinavia), *94*, 327–338.

Cohill, E. N., & Greenberg, H. J. (1977). Effects of ethyl alcohol on the acoustic reflex threshold. *Journal of the American Auditory Society, 2*, 121–123.

Cohill, E. N., & Greenberg, H. J. (1979). Effects of ethyl alcohol on the contralateral and ipsilateral acoustic reflex threshold. *Journal of Speech and Hearing Research, 22*, 289–294.

Davis, M., & Aghajanian, G. K. (1976). Effects of apomorphine and haloperidol on the acoustic startle response in rats. *Psychopharmacology, 47*, 217–223.

Davis, M., & Sheard, M. H. (1976). p-Chloramphetamine (PCA): Acute and chronic effects on habituation and sensitization of the acoustic startle response in rats. *European Journal of Pharmacology, 35*, 261–273.

Davis, M., & Walters, J. K. (1977). Psilocybin: Biphasic dose-response effects on the acoustic startle reflex in the rat. *Pharmacology, Biochemistry and Behavior, 6*, 427–431.

Frye, G. D., Breese, G. R., Mailman, R. B., Vogel, R. A., Ondrusek, M. G., & Mueller, R.A. (1980). An evaluation of the selectivity of fenmetozole (DH-524) reversal of ethanol-induced changes in central nervous system function. *Psychopharmacology* (Berlin), *69*, 149–155.

Liden, G., Nilsson, E., Laaskineu, O., Roos, B. E., & Miller, J. (1974). The stapedius reflex and motor reaction time: A parallel investigation of the effect of drugs. *Scandinavian Audiology, 3*, 73–80.

Light, M. H., II, Ferrell, C. J., & Sandberg, R. K. (1977). The effects of sedation on the impedance test battery. *Archives of Otolaryngology, 103*, 235–237.

Mangham, C. A. (1984). The effect of drugs and systematic disease on the acoustic reflex. In S. Silman (Ed.), *The acoustic reflex: Basic principles and clinical applications* (Chap. 13, pp. 441–468). New York: Academic Press.

Niswander, P. S., & Helfner-Mitchell, F. (1988). Observations on the acoustic reflex threshold in institutionalized retarded adults taking Mellaril and/or Thorazine. *Ear and Hearing, 9*, 9–14.

Richards, G. B., Mitchell, O. C., & Speights, J. L. (1975). Effects of phenobarbital on intra-aural muscle reflexes in retarded children. *Eye, Ear, Nose and Throat Journal, 54*, 73–75.

Robinette, M. S., Alper, R. R., & Brey, R. H. (1981). The effects of alcohol on the acoustic reflex relaxation index. *Journal of Auditory Research, 21*, 159–165.

Robinette, M. S., & Brey, R. H. (1978). Influence of alcohol on the acoustic reflex and temporary threshold shift. *Archives of Otolaryngology, 104*, 31–37.

Robinette, M. S., Rhoads, D. P., & Marion, M. W. (1974). Effects of secobarbital on impedance audiometry. *Archives of Otolaryngology, 100*, 351–354.

Ruth, R. A., Arora, N. S., & Gal, T. J. (1982). Stapedius reflex in curarized subjects: An index of neuromuscular weakness. *Journal of Applied Physiology, 52*, 416–420.

Ruth, R. A., Johns, M. E., & Gal, T. F. (1980). Acoustic reflex response during curare-induced weakness. *Annals of Otology, Rhinology and Laryngology, 89*, 188–193.

Saarnivaara, L. (1974). Comparison of althesin and thiopentone in anaesthesia for pediatric out-patient otology. *British Journal of Anaesthesia, 46*, 268–272.

7.10 Psychoacoustic Correlates

Alberti, P. W. (1972). Stapedial reflex estimation and the loudness recruitment phenomenon. In D.E. Rose & L. Keating (Eds.), *Proceedings of the Mayo Impedance Symposium* (pp. 231–252). Rochester, MN: Mayo Foundation.

Barry, S. J., & Resnick, S. B. (1976). Comparison of acoustic reflex and behavioral thresholds as a function of stimulus frequency and duration. *Journal of the American Auditory Society, 2*, 35–37.

Beedle, R. K., & Harford, E. R. (1973). A comparison of acoustic reflex and loudness growth in normal and pathological ears. *Journal of Speech and Hearing Research, 16*, 271–281.

Berger, K. W., Rane, R. L., & Hagberg, E. N. (1979). Comparisons of uncomfortable loudness levels and acoustic reflex thresholds. *Audiology and Hearing Education, 5*, 11–15.

Bernath, O. (1975). Experimental investigation on lateral inhibition by means of stapedius reflex threshold. *O.R.L. Journal of Oto-Rhino-Laryngology and Its Borderlands, 37*, 19–26.

Block, M., Greenfield, D., & Wiley, T. (1985). Acoustic-reflex dynamics and the loudness discomfort level. *Journal of Speech and Hearing Disorders, 50,* 14–20.

Block, M., & Wightman, F. (1977). A statistically based measure of the acoustic reflex and its relation to stimulus loudness. *Journal of the Acoustical Society of America, 61,* 120–125.

Block, M. G., & Wiley, T. L. (1979). Acoustic-reflex growth and loudness. *Journal of Speech and Hearing Research, 22,* 295–310.

Block, M. G., & Wiley, T. L. (1986). Acoustic-reflex growth for multitone complexes. *Journal of Speech and Hearing Research, 29,* 92–98.

Blood, I. M., & Greenberg, H. J. (1981). Low-level acoustic reflex thresholds. *Audiology, 20,* 244–250.

Borg, E. (1968). A quantitative study of the effect of the acoustic stapedius reflex on sound transmission through the middle ear of man. *Acta Otolaryngologica, 66,* 461–472.

Borg, E. (1972). Acoustic middle ear reflexes: A sensory control system. *Acta Otolaryngologica,* (Suppl. 304), 1–34.

Borg, E. (1972). On the use of acoustic middle ear muscle reflexes in studies of auditory function in nonanesthetized rabbits. *Acta Otolaryngologica, 74,* 240–247.

Borg, E. (1972). Regulation of middle ear sound transmission in the nonanesthetized rabbit. *Acta Physiologica* (Scandinavia), *86,* 175–190.

Borg, E. (1980). Processing of intensity-correlated information in an acoustic-autonomic reflex system. *Brain Research, 188,* 43–51.

Borg, E., Nilsson, R., & Liden, G. (1979). Fatigue and recovery of the human acoustic stapedius reflex in industrial noise. *Journal of the Acoustical Society of America, 65,* 846–848.

Borg, E., & Zakrisson, J.E. (1973). Stapedius reflex and speech features [Letter]. *Journal of the Acoustical Society of America, 54,* 525–527.

Borg, E., & Zakrisson, J.E. (1974). Stapedius reflex and monaural masking. *Acta Otolaryngologica* (Stockholm), *78,* 155–161.

Brasher, F., Coles, R. R. A., Elwood, M. A., & Ferres, H. M. (1969). Middle ear muscle activity and temporary threshold shift. *International Audiology, 8,* 579–584.

Brask, T. (1979). The noise protection effect of the stapedius reflex. *Acta Otolaryngologica* (Stockholm), (Suppl. 360), 116–117.

Chadwell, D. L., & Greenberg, H. J. (1979). Speech intelligibility in stapedectomized individuals. *American Journal of Otolaryngology, 1,* 103–108.

Charuhas, P. A., Chung, D. Y., & Barry, S. (1978). Relationship between uncomfortable loudness level and acoustic reflex threshold as a function of hearing loss. *Journal of Auditory Research, 18,* 237–242.

Chobot, J. L., & Wilson, W. R. (1977). The effect of sensitization on the acoustic reflex as a function of frequency. *Journal of Auditory Research, 17,* 99–104.

Citron, D., III, & Adour, K. K. (1978). Acoustic reflex and loudness discomfort in acute facial paralysis. *Archives of Otolaryngology, 104,* 303–306.

Coles, R. R. A. (1969). Middle ear muscle activity as a possible index of susceptibility to temporary threshold shift. *Sound, 3,* 72–74.

Counter, S. A., Borg, E., & Engstrom, B. (1989). Acoustic middle ear reflexes in laboratory animals using clinical equipment: Technical considerations. *Audiology, 28,* 135–143.

Cox, H. A., & Adelman, M. J. (1978). The differential loudness summation test. *Ear, Nose and Throat Journal, 57,* 35–42.

Cox, L. C., & Greenberg, H. J. (1977). Effects of human middle ear muscle contractions on speech intelligibility. *Journal of the American Auditory Society, 3,* 80–83.

Denenberg, L. J., & Altshuler, M. W. (1976). The clinical relationship between acoustic reflexes and loudness perception. *Journal of the American Auditory Society, 2,* 79–82.

Dix, M. R. (1968). Loudness recruitment and its measurement with special reference to the loudness discomfort level test and its value in diagnosis. *Annals of Otology, Rhinology and Laryngology, 77,* 1131–1151.

Djupesland, G., & Flottorp, G. (1970). Correlation between the Fowler Loudness Balance Test, the Metz Recruitment Test and the Flottorp-Opheim's Aural Harmonic Test in various types of hearing impairment. *International Audiology, 9,* 156–175.

Djupesland, G., Sundby, A., & Flottorp, G. (1973). Temporal summation in the acoustic stapedius reflex mechanism. *Acta Otolaryngologica* (Stockholm), *76,* 305–312.

Djupesland, G., Sundby, A., & Hogstad, K. E. (1975). A study of critical band-width in Meniere's syndrome using the acoustic stapedius reflex. *Scandinavian Audiology, 4,* 127–130.

Djupesland, G., & Zwislocki, J. (1971). Effect of temporal summation on the human stapedius reflex. *Acta Otolaryngologica, 71,* 262–265.

Djupesland, G., & Zwislocki, J. J. (1973). On the critical band in the acoustic stapedius reflex. *Journal of the Acoustical Society of America, 54,* 1157–1159.

Dorman, M., Cedar, I., Hannley, M., Leek, M., & Lindholm, J. M. (1986). Influence of the acoustic reflex on vowel recognition. *Journal of Speech and Hearing Research, 29,* 420–424.

Dudich, T. M., Keisler, M., & Keith, R. W. (1976). Some relationships between loudness and the acoustic reflex. *Impedance Newsletter, 4,* 12–15.

Durrant, J. D., & Shallop, J. K. (1969). Effects of differing states of attention on acoustic reflex activity and temporary threshold shift. *Journal of the Acoustical Society of America, 46,* 907–913.

Dykman, B. M., & Ison, J. R. (1979). Temporal integration of acoustic stimulation obtained in reflex inhibition in rats and humans. *Journal of Comparative Physiology and Psychology, 93,* 939–945.

Ewertsen, H. W., Filling, S., Terkildsen, K., & Tomsen, K. A. (1958). Comparative recruitment testing: An evaluation of some new and older methods. *Acta Otolaryngologica,* (Suppl. 140), 116–122.

Feldman, A. S., & Katz, D. (1978). Effects of stimulus duration and stimulus off time on the auditory and acoustic reflex thresholds. *Journal of Speech and Hearing Research, 21,* 74–78.

Ferraro, J. A., Melnick, W., & Gerhardt, K. R. (1981). Effects of prolonged noise exposure in chinchillas with severed middle ear muscles. *American Journal of Otolaryngology, 2,* 13–18.

Fitzzaland, R. E., & Borton, T. E. (1977). The acoustic reflex and loudness recruitment. *Journal of Otolaryngology, 6,* 460–465.

Fletcher, J. L., & Riopelle, A. J. (1960). Protective effect of the acoustic reflex for impulsive noises. *Journal of the Acoustical Society of America, 32,* 401–404.

Flottorp, G., Djupesland, G., & Winther, F. (1971). The acoustic stapedius reflex in relation to critical bandwidth. *Journal of the Acoustical Society of America, 49,* 457–461.

Forquer, B. D. (1979). The stability of and the relation between the acoustic reflex and uncomfortable loudness levels. *Journal of the American Auditory Society, 5,* 55–59.

Frank, T., & Karlovich, R. S. (1975). Effect of contralateral noise on speech detection and speech reception thresholds. *Audiology, 14,* 34–43.

Gelfand, S. A., Silman, S., & Silverman, C. A. (1981). Temporal summation in acoustic reflex growth functions. *Acta Otolaryngologica* (Stockholm), *91,* 177–182.

Gerhardt, K. D., & Hepler, E. L., Jr. (1983). Acoustic reflex activity and behavioral thresholds following exposure to noise. *Journal of the Acoustical Society of America, 74,* 109–114.

Gerhardt, K. J., Melnick, W., & Ferraro, J. A. (1979). Reflex threshold shift in chinchillas following a prolonged exposure to noise. *Journal of Speech and Hearing Research, 22,* 63–72.

Gerhardt, K. J., Melnick, W., & Ferraro, J. A. (1980). Acoustic reflex decay in chinchillas during a long-term exposure to noise. *Ear and Hearing, 1,* 33–37.

Gjaevenes, K., Gran, S., & Kollag, O. (1969). Contralateral remote masking and the aural reflex. *Journal of the Acoustical Society of America, 46,* 918–923.

Gjaevenes, K., & Sohoel, T. (1966). Reactivating the acoustic stapedius muscle reflex by adding a second tone. *Acta Otolaryngologica* (Stockholm), *62,* 213–216.

Gjaevenes, K., & Vigran, E. (1967). Contralateral masking: An attempt to determine the role of the aural reflex. *Journal of the Acoustical Society of America, 42,* 580–585.

Goodman, A. C., & Richards, A. M. (1977). Temporal summation of the human acoustic reflex: I. Variabilities. *Journal of Auditory Research, 17,* 193–203.

Gorga, M. P., Abbas, P. J., & Lilly, D. J. (1980). Magnitude of the acoustic reflex for either homophasic (0 degrees) or antiphasic (180 degrees) binaural activating signals presented in a background of noise. *Journal of the Acoustical Society of America, 67,* 589–593.

Gorga, M. P., Lilly, D. J., & Lenth, R. V. (1980). Effect of signal bandwidth upon threshold of the acoustic reflex and upon loudness. *Audiology, 19,* 277–292.

Greenfield, D., Wiley, T. L., & Block, M. (1985). Acoustic-reflex dynamics and the loudness-discomfort level. *Journal of Speech and Hearing Disorders, 50,* 14–20.

Gronas, H. E., Quist-Hanssen, S., & Bjelde, A. (1968). Delayed speech feedback in normal hearing and conductive hearing loss, with and without a functioning stapedius muscle. *Acta Otolaryngologica* (Stockholm), *66,* 241–247.

Gunn, W. J. (1973). Loudness changes resulting from an electrically induced middle-ear reflex. *Journal of the Acoustical Society of America, 54,* 380–385.

Gunn, W. J. (1973). Possible involvement of the acoustic reflex in loudness shifts resulting from a remote masker. *Journal of Auditory Research, 13,* 10–13.

Haberfellner, H., & Muller, G. (1976). Bobath-therapy, tonic reflex-activities and processing of acoustic stimuli. *Neuropaediatrie, 7,* 379–383.

Hannley, M., & Jerger, J. (1981). PB rollover and the acoustic reflex. *Audiology, 20,* 251–258.

Hellman, R., & Scharf, B. (1984). Acoustic reflex and loudness. In S. Silman (Ed.), *The acoustic reflex: Basic principles and clinical applications* (pp. 469–516). New York: Academic Press.

Hilding, D. A. (1961). The protective value of the stapedius reflex: An experimental study. *Transactions-American Academy of Ophthalmology and Otolaryngology, 65,* 297–307.

Holmes, D. W., & Woodford, C. M. (1977). Acoustic reflex threshold and loudness discomfort level: Relationships in children with profound hearing losses. *Journal of the American Auditory Society, 2,* 193–196.

Hood, J., & Poole, J. P. (1966). Tolerance limit of loudness: Its clinical and physiological significance. *Journal of the Acoustical Society of America, 40,* 47–53.

Humes, L. E. (1978). The effects of middle ear muscle contraction on auditory and overload thresholds. *Audiology, 17,* 360–367.

Irvine, D. R. (1976). Effects of reflex middle-ear muscle contractions on cochlear responses to bone-conducted sound. *Audiology, 15,* 433–444.

Iwamoto, V., & Pang-Ching, G. (1975). The acoustic reflex to air- and bone-conducted white noise. *Journal of Auditory Research, 15,* 226–230.

Jakimetz, J. J., Silman, S., Miller, M. H., & Silvermann, C. A. (1989). Some effects of signal bandwidth and spectral density on the acoustic-reflex threshold in the elderly. *Journal of the Acoustical Society of America, 86,* 1783–1789.

Jerger, J., Mauldin, L., & Lewis, N. (1977). Temporal summation of the acoustic reflex. *Audiology, 16,* 177–200.

Jerlvall, L. B., & Lindblad, A. C. (1978). The influence of attack time and relapse time on speech intelligibility. A study of the effects of AGC on normal hearing and hearing impaired subjects. *Scandinavian Audiology* (Suppl. 6), 341–353.

Johansson, B., Kylin, B., & Langfy, M. (1967). Acoustic reflex as a test of individual susceptibility to noise: A preliminary report. *Acta Otolaryngologica* (Stockholm), *64,* 256–262.

Kamm, C., Dirks, D. D., & Mickey, R. (1978). Effects of sensorineural loss on loudness discomfort level. *Journal of Speech and Hearing Research, 21,* 668–681.

Karlovich, R. S., Osier, H. A., Gutnick, H. N., Ivey, R. G., Wolf, K., Schwimmer, S., Strennen, M. L., & Gerber, J. (1977). The acoustic reflex and temporary threshold shift: Temporal characteristics. *Journal of Speech and Hearing Research, 20,* 565–573.

Karlovich, R. S., & Wiley, T. L. (1974). Spectral and temporal parameters of contralateral signals altering temporary threshold shift. *Journal of Speech and Hearing Research, 17,* 41–50.

Kawata, S. (1958). Judgement of recruitment by means of measuring the retraction grade of the tympanic membrane. *Acta Otolaryngologica, 49,* 517–526.

Keith, R. (1979). Loudness and the acoustic reflex: Cochlear-impaired listeners. *Journal of the American Auditory Society, 5,* 65–70.

Keith, R. (1979). Loudness and the acoustic reflex: Normal-hearing listeners. *Journal of the American Auditory Society, 4,* 152–156.

Korabic, E., & Cudahy, E. (1984). Acoustic reflex temporal summation measured at threshold. *Ear and Hearing, 5,* 331–339.

Lalande, N. M., & Hetu, R. (1978). Recovery of the acoustic reflex response as a function of noise exposure and quiet interval. *Canadian Acoustics, 10,* 19–28.

Lawrence, M. (1965). Middle ear muscle influence on binaural hearing. *Archives of Otolaryngology, 82,* 478–482.

Liden, G., Norlund, B., & Hawkins, J. D., Jr. (1963). Significance of the stapedius reflex for the understanding of speech. *Acta Otolaryngologica,* (Suppl. 188), 275–279.

Lilly, D. J. (1966). Measurement of the acoustic reflex as an audiometric technique. *Science, 154,* 1228.

Loeb, M., & Riopelle, J. (1960). Influence of loud contralateral stimulation in the threshold and perceived loudness of low frequency tones. *Journal of the Acoustical Society America, 32,* 602–610.

Lovrinic, J. H. (1977). Stapedial reflexes in normal versus recruiting ears. *Journal of Auditory Research, 17,* 251–261.

Mahoney, T., Vernon, J., & Meikle, M. (1979). Function of the acoustic reflex in discrimination of intense speech. *Archives of Otolaryngology, 105,* 119–123.

Margolis, R. H., & Popelka, G. R. (1975). Loudness and the acoustic reflex. *Journal of the Acoustical Society of America, 58,* 1330–1332.

Martin, F. N., & Brunette, G. W. (1980). Loudness and the acoustic reflex. *Ear and Hearing, 1,* 106–108.

McCandless, G., & Miller, D. (1972). Loudness discomfort and hearing aids. *Hearing Aid Journal, 25*, 7–32.

McCarty, T. A., & Hamlet, S. L. (1978). Elicitation of the acoustic reflex with synthetically produced consonant and vowel stimuli. *Journal of the American Auditory Society, 3*, 235–240.

McDonald, J. M., & Newby, H. A. (1980). Effect of the acoustic reflex on the spondee threshold. *Ear and Hearing, 1*, 215–218.

McLeod, H. L., & Greenberg, H. J. (1979). Relationship between loudness discomfort level and acoustic reflex threshold for normal and sensorineural hearing-impaired individuals. *Journal of Speech and Hearing Research, 22*, 873–883.

McRobert, H., Bryan, M. E., & Tempest, W. (1969). The effect of middle ear muscle contraction on sound transmission through the human ear. *International Audiology, 8*, 557–562.

Mendelson, E. S., Fletcher, J. L., & Loeb, M. (1963). Noise exposure and individual alterations in middle ear muscle reflex activity. *Aerospace Medicine, 34*, 507–513.

Metz, O. (1952). Threshold of reflex contractions of muscles of the middle ear and recruitment of loudness. *Archives of Otolaryngology, 55*, 536–543.

Mills, J. H., & Lilly, D. J. (1971). Temporary threshold shifts produced by pure tones and by noise in the absence of an acoustic reflex. *Journal of the Acoustical Society of America, 50*, 1556–1558.

Morgan, D. E., & Dirks, D. D. (1975). Influence of middle ear muscle contraction on pure-tone suprathreshold loudness judgements. *Journal of the Acoustical Society of America, 57*, 411–421.

Morgan, D., Dirks, D., Bower, D., & Kamm, C. (1979). Loudness discomfort level and acoustic reflex threshold for speech stimuli. *Journal of Speech and Hearing Research, 22*, 849-861.

Morgan, D. E., Gilman, S., & Dirks, D. D. (1977). Temporal integration at the 'threshold' of the acoustic reflex. *Journal of the Acoustical Society of America, 62*, 168–176.

Morgan, D. E., Wilson, R. H., & Dirks, D. (1974). Loudness discomfort level: Selected methods and stimuli. *Journal of the Acoustical Society of America, 56*, 577-581.

Niemeyer, W. (1971). Relations between discomfort level and the reflex threshold of the middle ear muscles. *Audiology, 10*, 172–176.

Nilsson, R., Borg, E., & Liden, G. (1980). Fatigability of the stapedius reflex in industrial noise. *Acta Otolaryngologica* (Stockholm), *89*, 433–439.

Olsen, C. C., & Brandt, J. F. (1976). Middle ear muscle activity during speech in stapedectomized and laryngectomized subjects. *Journal of the American Auditory Society, 1*, 215–220.

Olsen, C. C., & Brandt, J. F. (1977). Influence of acoustic reflex on acquisition of temporary threshold shift from short duration noise bursts. *Journal of the American Auditory Society, 3*, 151–158.

Olson, A. E., & Hipskind, N. M. (1973). The relation between levels of pure tones and speech which elicit the acoustic reflex and loudness discomfort level. *Journal of Auditory Research, 13*, 71–76.

Popelka, G. R., Karlovich, S. R., & Wiley, T. L. (1974). Acoustic reflex and critical bandwidth. *Journal of the Acoustical Society of America, 55,* 883–885.

Popelka, G. R., Margolis, R. H., & Wiley, T. L. (1976). Effect of activating signal bandwidth on acoustic-reflex thresholds. *Journal of the Acoustical Society of America, 59,* 153–159.

Prather, W. F. (1961). Shifts in loudness of pure tones associated with contralateral noise stimulation. *Journal of Speech and Hearing Research, 4,* 182–193.

Reger, S. N. (1960). Effect of middle ear muscle action on certain psychophysical measurements. *Annals of Otology, Rhinology and Laryngology, 69,* 1179–1198.

Reger, S. N., Menzel, O. J., Ickes, W. K., & Steiner, S. J. (1963). Changes in air conduction and bone conduction sensitivity associated with voluntary contraction of middle ear musculature. In J. L. Fletcher (Ed.), *Middle ear function seminar* (pp. 171–180), (U.S. Army Med. Res. Lab. Report No. 576). Fort Knox, KY: U.S. Army.

Reiter, L. A., & Ison, J. R. (1979). Reflex modulation and loudness recruitment. *Journal of Auditory Research, 19,* 201–207.

Richards, A. M. (1975). Threshold of the acoustic stapedius reflex for short-duration tone bursts. *Journal of Auditory Research, 15,* 87–94.

Richards, A. M., & Goodman. A. C. (1977). Threshold of the human acoustic stapedius reflex for short-duration bursts of noise. *Journal of Auditory Research, 17,* 183–189.

Ritter, R., Johnson, R. M., & Northern, J. L. (1979). The controversial relationship between loudness discomfort levels and acoustic reflex thresholds. *Journal of the American Auditory Society, 4,* 123–131.

Ross, S. (1968). Impedance at the eardrum, middle-ear transmission and equal loudness. *Journal of the Acoustical Society of America, 43,* 491-505.

Ross, S. (1968). On the relation between the acoustic reflex and loudness. *Journal of the Acoustical Society of America, 43,* 768–779.

Rossi, G., & Solero, P. (1983). Acoustic reflex patterns according to different intensity and different duration of white noise stimuli. *Acta Otolaryngologica, 95*(5–6), 606-614.

Rossi, G., & Solero, P. (1984). Dynamic parameters of the stapedius muscle reflex in response to stimuli of varying duration but with the same energy content. *Acta Otolaryngologica, 97,* 460–466.

Rossi, G., Solero, P., & Penna, M. (1976). Changes in stapedius reflex amplitude and latency following exposure to urban traffic noise. *Acta Otolaryngologica* (Stockholm), (Suppl. 339), 14–18.

Rossi, G., Solero, P., & Rolando, M. (1985) Relationships between acoustic reflex patterns elicited by unfiltered white noise and narrow band noise stimuli of different duration but of the same intensity. *Journal of Laryngology and Otology, 99,* 857–886.

Scharf, B. (1976). Acoustic reflex, loudness summation, and the critical band. *Journal of the Acoustical Society of America, 60,* 753–755.

Scharf, B. (1978). Comparison of normal and impaired hearing. I. Loudness, localization. *Scandinavian Audiology,* (Suppl. 6), 49–79.

Schoenfeld, L. S., Cooper, J. C., Jr., & Martin, F. N. (1973). Recruitment, loudness and the stapedial reflex threshold under hypnosis. *Perception and Motor Skills, 36,* 420–422.

Schwartz, D. M., & Sanders, J. W. (1976). Critical bandwidth and sensitivity prediction in the acoustic stapedial reflex. *Journal of Speech and Hearing Disorders, 41,* 244–255.

Schwetz, F., Hloch, T., & Schewozik, R. (1979). Experimental exposure to impulse noise in especially pathogenic impact frequency range. *Acta Otolaryngologica* (Stockholm), *87,* 264–266.

Sesterhenn, G., & Breuninger, H. (1978). On the influence of the middle ear muscles upon changes in sound transmission. *Archives of Otorhinolaryngology, 221,* 47-60.

Shallop, J. (1973). Some relationships among speech reception, the dynamic range of intelligible speech and the acoustic reflex. *Scandinavian Audiology, 2,* 119–122.

Shapiro, I. (1979). Evaluation of the relationship between hearing threshold and loudness discomfort level in sensorineural hearing loss. *Journal of Speech and Hearing Disorders, 14,* 31–36.

Shearer, W. M. (1966). Speech: Behavior of middle ear muscle during stuttering. *Science, 152,* 1280.

Shearer, W. M., & Simmons, F. B. (1965). Middle ear activity during speech in normal speakers and stutterers. *Journal of Speech and Hearing Research, 8,* 203–207.

Sieminski, L. R., Durrant, J. D., Rosenberg, P. E., & Lovrinic, J. H. (1977). Stapedial reflexes in normal vs. recruiting ears. *Journal of Auditory Research, 17,* 251–261.

Silverman, S. R. (1947). Tolerance for pure tones and speech in normal and defective hearing. *Annals of Otology, Rhinology and Laryngology, 56,* 658–677.

Simmons, F. B. (1965). Binaural summation of the acoustic reflex. *Journal of the Acoustical Society of America, 37,* 834–836.

Singh, D., & Greenberg, H. J. (1976). Temporal summation of the acoustic reflex in normal and sensorineural hearing-impaired ears. *Journal of the American Auditory Society, 2,* 8–14.

Spitzer, J. B., Ventry, I. M., & Nicholas, J. A. (1978). The contribution of the acoustic reflex to the ascending-descending most comfortable loudness gap. *Audiology, 17,* 271–280.

Stelmachowicz, P. G., & Lilly, D. J. (1979). An indirect estimate of auditory-frequency selectivity from acoustic-reflex measurements. *Journal of the Acoustical Society of America, 65,* 1501–1508.

Stelmachowicz, P. G., & Seewald, R. C. (1977). Threshold and suprathreshold temporal integration function in normal and cochlear-impaired subjects. *Audiology, 16,* 94–101.

Stephens, S. D., Blegvad, B., & Krogh, H. J. (1977). The value of some suprathreshold auditory measures. *Scandinavian Audiology, 6,* 213–221.

Terkildsen, K. (1960). An evaluation of perceptive hearing losses in children based on recruitment determinations. *Acta Otolaryngologica, 51,* 476–484.

Thomsen, K. A. (1955). The Metz Recruitment Test and a comparison with the Fowler Method. *Acta Otolaryngologica, 45,* 544–552.

Uliel, S. (1980). Acoustic reflex measurements and the loudness function in sensorineural hearing loss. *South African Journal of Communicative Disorders, 27,* 58–77.

Ward, W. D. (1961). Studies on the aural reflex: I. Contralateral remote masking as an indicator of reflex activity. *Journal of the Acoustical Society of America, 33,* 1034–1045.

Ward, W. D. (1962). Studies on the aural reflex: II. Reduction of temporary threshold shift from intermittent noise by reflex activity: Implications for damage risk criteria. *Journal of the Acoustical Society of America, 34,* 234–241.

Ward, W. D. (1965). Temporary threshold shifts following monaural and binaural exposure. *Journal of the Acoustical Society of America, 38,* 121–125.

Ward, W. D. (1972). Psychophysical correlates of middle ear muscle action. In D. E. Rose & L. Keating (Eds.), *Proceedings of the Mayo Impedance Symposium* (pp. 211–224). Rochester, MN: Mayo Foundation.

Wiley, T. L., & Karlovich, R. S. (1975). Acoustic reflex response to sustained signals. *Journal of Speech and Hearing Research, 18,* 148–157.

Wiley, T. L., & Karlovich, R. S. (1978). Acoustic-reflex dynamics for pulsed signals. *Journal of Speech and Hearing Research, 21,* 295–307.

Woodford, C., Henderson, D., Hamernik, R., & Feldman, A. (1975). Threshold-duration function of the acoustic reflex in man. *Audiology, 14,* 53–62.

Woodford, C. M., Henderson, D., Hamernik, R. P., & Feldman, A. S. (1976). Acoustic reflex threshold of the chinchilla as a function of stimulus duration and frequency. *Journal of the Acoustical Society of America, 59,* 1204–1207.

Woodford, C., & Holmes, D. (1977). Relationship between loudness discomfort level and acoustic reflex threshold in a clinical population. *Audiology and Hearing Education, 3,* 9–11.

Zakrisson, J. E. (1975). The role of the stapedius reflex in poststimulatory auditory fatigue. *Acta Otolaryngologica* (Stockholm), *79,* 1–10.

Zakrisson, J. E. (1979). The effect of the stapedius reflex on attenuation and post-stimulatory auditory fatigue at different frequencies. *Acta Otolaryngologica* (Stockholm), (Suppl. 360), 118–121.

Zakrisson, J. E., & Borg, E. (1974). Stapedius reflex and auditory fatigue. *Audiology, 13,* 231–235.

Zakrisson, J. E., Borg, E., Liden, G., & Nilsson, R. (1980). Stapedius reflex in industrial impact noise: Fatigability and role for temporary threshold shift (TTS). *Scandinavian Audiology,* (Suppl. 17), 326–334.

8.0 NONACOUSTIC REFLEXES

Bosatra, A., Russolo, M., & Semeraro, A. (1975). Tympanic muscle reflex elicited by electric stimulation of the tongue in normal and pathological subjects. *Acta Otolaryngologica* (Stockholm), *79*, 334–338.

Bosatra, A., Russolo, M., & Semeraro, A. (1977). Bipolar electric stimulation to elicit an isolated tensor tympani reflex. *Acta Otolaryngologica, 83*, 391–392.

Bynke, O. (1980). Facial reflex examination. A clinical and neurophysiological study on acoustic tumours and brain displacement at the tentorial notch. *Acta Neurologica* (Scandinavia), (Suppl. 76), 1–127.

Carmel, P. W., & Starr, A. (1963). Acoustic and nonacoustic factors modifying middle ear muscle activity in waking cats. *Journal of Neurophysiology, 26*, 589–618.

Djupesland, G. (1962). Preliminary report on the intra-aural muscular reflexes elicited by air current stimulation of the external ear. *Acta Otolaryngologica, 54*, 143–153.

Djupesland, G. (1964). Middle ear muscle reflexes elicited by acoustic and non-acoustic stimulation. *Acta Otolaryngologica,* (Suppl. 188), 287–292.

Djupesland, G. (1967). Contractions of the tympanic muscles in man. *Norwegian Monograph on Medical Science.* Oslo: Universitetsforlaget.

Djupesland, G. (1976). Diagnostic implications of acoustic and nonacoustic reflex measurements. In J. Jerger & J. Northern (Eds.) *Proceedings of the Third International Symposium on Impedance Audiometry* (pp. 24–31). Acton, MA: American Electromedics.

Djupesland, G. (1976). Nonacoustic reflex measurement-Procedures, interpretations and variables. In A. S. Feldman & L. A. Wilber (Eds.), *Acoustic impedance and admittance: The measurement of middle ear function* (pp. 217–235). Baltimore: Williams & Wilkins.

Djupesland, G., Flottorp, G., & Sundby, A. (1977). Impedance changes elicited by electrocutaneous stimulation. *Audiology, 16*, 355–364.

Djupesland, G., & Tvete, O. (1979). Impedance changes elicited by tactile and electrocutaneous stimulation. *Scandinavian Audiology, 8*, 243–245.

Fee, W. (1981). Clinical applications of nonacoustic middle ear muscle stimulation. *Archives of Otolaryngology, 107*, 224–227.

Fee, W. E., Jr., Dirks, D. D., & Morgan, D. E. (1975). Nonacoustic stimulation of the middle ear muscle reflex. *Annals of Otology, Rhinology and Laryngology, 84*, 80–87.

Gersdorff, M. C. (1980). Dynamic study of the acoustico-facial reflex by impedance measurement. *Archives of Otorhinolaryngology, 228*, 101–112.

Jerger, J., Jenkins, H., Chmiel, R., & Oliver, T. A. (1987). Electrically-elicited stapedius reflex and preferred listening level in a patient with cochlear implant. *Annals of Otology, Rhinology and Laryngology,* (Suppl. 128), 99-100.

Jerger, J., Oliver, T., & Chmiel, R. (1988). Prediction of dynamic range from stapedius reflex in cochlear implant patients. *Ear and Hearing, 9*, 4–8

Jeter, I. K. (1975). Waveform patterns of reflex and voluntary contraction of the middle ear muscles. *Journal of Auditory Research, 16,* 183–192.

Klockhoff, I., & Anderson, H. (1959). Recording of the stapedius reflex elicited by cutaneous stimulation. *Acta Otolaryngologica, 50,* 451–454.

Klockhoff, I., & Anderson, H. (1960). Reflex activity in the tensor tympanic muscle recorded in man: A preliminary report. *Acta Otolaryngologica, 51,* 184–189.

Liden, G., Peterson, J. L., & Harford, E. R. (1969). Stimultaneous recording of changes in relative impedance and air pressure during acoustic and non-acoustic elicitation of the middle-ear reflexes. *Acta Otolaryngologica,* (Suppl. 263), 208–217.

Macrae, J. H. (1970). A discussion of non-acoustic methods of eliciting the middle-ear muscle reflexes. *Journal of the Otolaryngological Society of Australia, 3,* 102–105.

Macrae, J. H. (1971). An investigation of the tympanic muscle reflexes elicited by acoustic and meatal tactile stimulation. *Journal of the Otolaryngological Society of Australia, 3,* 221–225.

McCall, G. N., & Rabuzzi, D. D. (1973). Reflex contraction of middle-ear muscles secondary to stimulation of laryngeal nerves. *Journal of Speech and Hearing Research, 16,* 56–61.

McDaniel-Bacon, L., Fulton, R. T., & Laskowski, R. P. (1980). Conditioning the middle ear reflex at sensation levels below reflex threshold: Air jet and electrical stimulation. *Ear and Hearing, 1,* 249–258.

Molina, P., Hardy, J., & Bertrand, R. A. (1978). Contribution of trigeminal and facial reflexes to the localization of Vth, VIIth and VIIIth cranial nerve dysfunction. *Applied Neurophysiology, 41,* 157–168.

Russolo, M., & Semeraro, A. (1977). Value of the isolated tensor tympani muscle reflex elicited by electrical lingual stimulation. *Audiology, 16,* 373–379.

Stephan, K., Welzl-Muller, K, & Stiglbrummer, H. (1988). Stapedius reflex threshold in cochlear implant patients. *Audiology, 27,* 227–233.

Tanabe, M., Kitajima, K., & Gould, W. J. (1975). Laryngeal phonatory reflex. The effect of anesthetization of the internal branch of the superior laryngeal nerve: Acoustic aspects. *Annals of Otology, Rhinology and Laryngology, 84,* 206–212.

Wiley, T. L., & Block, M. G. (1983). Acoustic and nonacoustic reflex patterns in audiologic diagnosis. In S. Silman (Ed.), *The acoustic reflex: Basic principles and clinical applications* (pp. 387–411). New York: Academic Press.

9.0 SCREENING

American Speech-Language-Hearing Association. (1979). Guidelines for acoustic immittance screening of middle-ear function. *Asha, 21,* 283–298.

American Speech-Language-Hearing Association. (1990). Guidelines for screening for hearing impairment and middle-ear disorders, *Asha, 32*(Suppl. 2), 17–24.

Aniansson, G. (1986). Screening diagnosis of secretory otitis media. *Scandinavian Audiology,* (Suppl. 26), 65–69.

Armstrong, B. W. (1962). Secretory otitis media: Problems and pitfalls. *Journal of the American Medical Association, 179,* 505–513.

Berry, Q., Andrus, W., & Bluestone, C. (1973). Tympanometry in relation to middle ear effusions in children. *Pediatric Clinics of North America, 21,* 398–390.

Brooks, D. N. (1971). A new approach to identification audiometry. *Audiology, 10,* 334–339.

Brooks, D. (1976). Mass screening with acoustic impedance. In J. Jerger & J. Northern (Eds.), *Proceedings of the Third International Symposium on Impedance Audiometry* (pp. 18–23). Acton, MA: American Electromedics.

Brooks, D. N. (1977). Middle-ear impedance measurements in screening. *Audiology, 16,* 228–293.

Cadman, D., Chambers, L., Feldman, W., & Sackett, D. (1984). Assessing the effectiveness of community screening programs. *Journal of the American Medical Association, 251,* 1580–1585.

Fitzzaland, R. E., & Zink, G. D. (1984). A comparative study of hearing screening procedures. *Ear and Hearing, 5,* 205–210.

Freyss, G., & Pialoux, P. (1977). Impedance measurement in the diagnosis of serous otitis. Description of a new test. Star. *Annales Otolaryngologie et Chirurgie Cervicofaciale, 94,* 259–269.

Gersdorff, M. C. (1977). Personal results, trial of classification and standardization in clinical impedancemetry. *Journal of Otolaryngology, 6* (Suppl. 5), 5–20.

Gimsing, S., & Bergholtz, L. M. (1983). Otoscopy compared with tympanometry. A study evaluating the accuracy of otoscopy in 1702 unselected ears. *Journal of Laryngology and Otology, 97,* 587–591.

Glebink, G. S., Heller, K. A., & Le, C. T. (1983). Prediction of serous versus purlent otitis media by otoscopy and tympanometry in an animal model. *Laryngoscope, 93,* 208–211.

Glorig, A., & House, H. P. (1947). A new concept in auditory screening. *Archives of Otolaryngology, 66,* 228–232.

Grimaldi, P. M. (1976). The value of impedance testing in the diagnosis of middle ear effusion. *Journal of Laryngology and Otology, 90,* 141–152.

Harker, L. A., & Van Wagoner, R. (1974). Application of impedance audiometry as a screening instrument. *Archives of Otolaryngology* (Stockholm), *77,* 198–220.

Haughton, P. M. (1977). Validity of tympanometry for middle ear effusion. *Archives of Otolaryngology, 101,* 469–473.

Holte, L., & Margolis, R. H. (1987). Screening tympanometry. *Seminars in Hearing, 8,* 329–337.

Kokko, E. (1974). Chronic secretory otitis media in children. A clinical study. *Acta Otolaryngologica* (Stockholm), (Suppl. 327), 1–44.

Lewis, N., Dugdale, A., Canty, A., & Jerger, J. (1975). Open-ended tympanometric screening: A new concept. *Archives of Otolaryngology, 101,* 722–725.

Lucker, J. (1980). Application of pass-fail criteria to middle ear screening results. *Asha, 22,* 839–840.

Margolis, R. H., & Heller, J. W. (1987). Screening tympanometry: Criteria for medical referral. *Audiology, 26,* 197–208.

McCandless, G. A., & Thomas, G. K. (1974). Impedance audiometry as a screening procedure for middle ear disease. *Transactions of the American Academy of Opthalmology and Otolaryngology, 78,* 98–102.

Painton, S. W. (1989). Automatic immittance audiometry on children with transtympanic ventilation tubes. *Ear and Hearing, 10,* 209–210.

Parving, A. (1985). Hearing disorders in childhood, some procedures for detection, identification and diagnostic evaluation. *International Journal of Pediatric Otorhinolaryngology, 9,* 31–57.

Renvall, U., & Holmquist, J. (1976). Tympanometry revealing middle ear pathology. *Annals of Otology, Rhinology and Laryngology, 85,* 209–215.

Renvall, U., & Liden, G. (1980). Screening procedure for detection of middle ear and cochlear disease. *Annals of Otology, Rhinology and Laryngology, 89*(Suppl. 68), 214–216.

Roberts, M. E. (1976). Comparative study of pure-tone, impedance, and otoscopic hearing screening methods. *Archives of Otolaryngology, 102,* 690–694.

Roeser, R. J., Soh, J., Dunckel, D. C., & Adams, R. (1977). Comparison of tympanometry and otoscopy in the establishment pass/fail referral criteria. *Journal of the American Auditory Society, 3,* 20–25.

Schwartz, D. M., & Redfield, N. P. (1976). Evaluation of automatic screening tympanometry in the identification of middle ear pathology. *Journal of the Auditory Society, l,* 276–279.

Shurin, P. A., Pelton, S. I., & Finkelstein, J. (1977). Tympanometry in the diagnosis of middle ear effusion. *New England Journal of Medicine, 296,* 412–417.

Wachtendorf, C. A., Lopez, L. L., Cooper, J. C., Hearn, E. M., & Gates, G. A. (1984). The efficacy of school screening for otitis media. In D. J. Lim, C. D. Bluestone, J. O. Klein, & J. D. Nelson (Eds.), *Recent advances in otitis media with effusion* (pp. 242–246). Philadelphia: B.C. Decker.

Zaller, M. K., Ruhe, D. J., & Dunster, J. R. (1985). Tympanometry screening in developmentally delayed individuals. *Journal of Auditory Research, 25,* 15–25.

9.1 Neonates/Infants

Crowell, D. H., Pang-Ching, G., Anderson, R. E., Kapuniai, L. E., Teruya, K., Doo, G., Wright, P., & Stephens, J. K. (1980). Auditory screening of high risk infants with brainstem evoked responses and impedance audiometry. *Hawaii Medical Journal, 39,* 277–282.

Dedmon, D., & Robinette, M. (1973). The acoustic reflex as a tool for neonatal screening. *Audecibel, 22,* 202–210.

Forman-Franco, B., & Abramson, A. L. (1979). Audiometric evaluation of infants 12-18 months of age. *International Journal of Pediatric Otorhinolaryngology, 1,* 61–69.

Hall, J. W., & Weaver, T. (1979). Impedance audiometry in a young population. *Journal of Otolaryngology, 8,* 210–222.

Keith, R. W. (1973). Impedance audiometry with neonates. *Archives of Otolaryngology, 97,* 465–467.

Marchant, C. D., McMillan, P. M., Shurin, P. A., Johnson, C. E., Turczyic, V. A., Feinstein, J. C., & Panek, P. M. (1986). Objective diagnosis of otitis media in early infancy by tympanometry and ipsilateral acoustic reflex thresholds. *Journal of Pediatrics, 109,* 590–595.

Paradise, J. L., Smith, C. G., & Bluestone, C. D. (1976). Tympanometric detection of middle ear effusion in infants and young children. *Pediatrics, 58,* 198–210.

Poulsen, G., & Tos, M. (1980). Repetitive tympanometric screenings of two-year-old children. *Scandinavian Audiology, 9,* 21–28.

Tos, M., & Poulsen, G. (1980). Screening tympanometry in infants and two-year-old children. *Annals of Otology, Rhinology and Laryngology,* (Suppl. 68), 217-222.

Tos, M., Poulsen, G., & Hancke, A. B. (1979). Screening tympanometry during the first year of life. *Acta Otolaryngologica* (Stockholm), *88,* 388-394.

9.2 Preschool and School Age Children

Al-Fadala, S., & Holmquist, J. (1984). Otoscopy and tympanometry in screening for middle ear disorders in children. *Scandinavian Audiology, 13,* 297–299.

Barrett, K. A. (1985). Hearing and immittance screening in school-aged children. In J. Katz (Ed.), *Handbook of clinical audiology* (3rd ed., pp. 621–641). Baltimore, MD: Williams & Wilkins.

Bennett, M., & Mowat, L. (1981). Validity of impedance measurements and referral criteria in school hearing screening programmes. *British Journal of Audiology, 15,* 147–150.

Bess, F. H. (1980). Impedance screening for children. A need for more research. *Annals of Otology, Rhinology and Laryngology, 85*(Suppl. 68), 228–232.

Birch, L., & Elbrond, O. (1985). Daily impedance audiometric screening of children in a day-care institution. Changes through one month. *Scandinavian Audiology, 14,* 5–8.

Bjuro-Moller, M. (1978). School audiometry—Methods and goals. *Scandinavian Audiology, 8,* 13–18.

Bluestone, C. D., Beery, Q. C., & Paradise, J. L. (1974). Audiometry and tympanometry in relation to middle ear effusions in children. *Laryngoscope, 83,* 594–603.

Bluestone, C. D., Fria, T. J., Arjona, S. K., Casselbrant, M. L., Schwartz, D. M., Ruben, R. J., Gates, G. A., Downs, M. P., Northern, J. L., Jerger, J. F., Paradise, J. L., Bess, F. H., Kenworthy, O. T., & Rogers, K. D. (1986). Controversies in screening for middle ear disease and hearing loss in children. *Pediatrics, 77,* 57–70.

Brooks, D. N. (1971). A new approach to identification audiometry. *Audiology, 10,* 334–339.

Brooks, D. N. (1973). Hearing screening: A comparative study of an impedance method and pure tone screening. *Scandinavian Audiology, 2,* 67–76.

Brooks, D. N. (1974). Impedance measurement in screening for auditory disorders in children. *Hearing Instruments, 36,* 20–21.

Brooks, D. N. (1974). The role of the acoustic impedance bridge in pediatric screening. *Scandinavian Audiology, 3,* 99–104.

Brooks, D. N. (1976). School screening for middle ear effusions. *Annals of Otology, Rhinology and Laryngology, 85,* 223–228.

Brooks, D. N. (1978). Acoustic impedance testing for screening auditory function in school children. Part 1. *Maico Audiological Library Series, 15,* Report 9.

Brooks, D. N. (1978). Acoustic impedance testing for screening auditory function in school children. Part 2. *Maico Audiological Library Series, 15,* Report 9.

Brooks, D. N. (1979). Otitis media and child development. *Annals of Otology, Rhinology and Laryngology, 88,* 29–47.

Brooks, D. N. (1981). Development of school screening audiometry. *British Journal of Audiology, 15,* 283–290.

Brooks, D. N. (1985). Acoustic impedance measurement as screening procedure in children: Discussion paper. *Journal of the Royal Society of Medicine, 78,* 119–121.

Cantekin, E. I., Stool, S. E., Bluestone, C. D., Beery, Q. C., Fria, T. J., & Sabo, D. L. (1980). Identification of otitis media with effusion in children. *Annals of Otology, Rhinology and Laryngology, 89*(Suppl. 68), 190–195.

Carmody, P., Curotta, J., & Mackie, K. (1983). Pass/fail criteria in screening for otitis media in children with learning disorders. *International Journal of Pediatric Otorhinolaryngology, 6,* 151–162.

Causse, J., & Causse, B. (1983). Early detection of otosclerosis by impedance audiometry screening. *Scandinavian Audiology,* (Suppl. 17), 45–52.

Cody, R. C. (1977). Hearing screening in the schools. *Hearing Instruments, 23,* 6–7.

Cooper, J. C., Jr., Gates, G. A., Owen, J. H., & Dickson, H. D. (1975). An abbreviated impedance bridge for school screening. *Journal of Speech and Hearing Disorders, 40,* 260–269.

Corth, S. B., & Harris, R. W. (1984). Incidence of middle ear disease in Indochinese refugee schoolchildren. *Audiology, 23,* 27–37.

Cross, A. W. (1985). Health screening in schools. Part I. *Journal of Pediatrics, 107,* 487–494.

Djupesland, G., Nicklasson, B., Helland, S., & Hemsen, E. (1983). Hearing threshold level and middle ear pressure in children with phonetic/phonemic disability. *Scandinavian Audiology,* (Suppl. 17), 71–77.

Downs, M. P. (1980). Identification of children at risk for middle effusion problems. *Annals of Otology, Rhinology and Laryngology, 89*(Suppl. 68), 168–171.

Eagles, E., Wishik, S., & Doerfler, L. (1967). Hearing sensitivity and ear disease in children: A prospective study. *Laryngoscope,* (Monograph Suppl.), 1–274.

Felding, J. U. (1983). The longitudinal Hjorring population-study. Results of six years of follow-up. *Scandinavian Audiology,* (Suppl. 17), 53–57.

Feldman, A. S., Northern, J. L., Rosenberg, J., Wilber, L., & Howie, V. M. (1978). Impedance screening for children [Letter]. *Annals of Otology, Rhinology and Laryngology, 87,* 738–739.

Ferrer, H. P. (1974). Use of impedance audiometry in school children. *Public Health, 88,* 153–163.

Fiellau-Nikolajsen, M. (1979). Tympanometry in three-year-old children: II. Seasonal influence on tympanometric. *Scandinavian Audiology, 8,* 181–185.

Fiellau-Nikolajsen, M. (1983). Tympanometric prediction of the magnitude of hearing loss in preschool children with secretary otitis media. *Scandinavian Audiology,* (Suppl. 17), 66–70.

Findlay, R. C., Stool, S. E., & Svitko, C. A. Tympanometric and otoscopic evaluation of a school age deaf population: A longitudinal study. *American Annals of the Deaf, 122,* 407–413.

Fitzzaland, R. E., & Zink, G. D. (1984). A comparative study of hearing screening procedures. *Ear and Hearing, 5,* 205–210.

Fountain, D. C., Armstrong-Bednall, G., Majumdar, B., Neil, J. F., Polnay, L., & Pullan, C. R. (1986). Conductive hearing losses in a day nursery population—natural history and the role of tympanometry as a screening test. *Public Health, 100,* 214–218.

Freyss, G. E., Manac'h, Y., Philippe, P. N., & Toupet, M. G. (1980). Acoustic reflex as a predictor of middle ear effusion. *Annals of Otology, Rhinology and Laryngology, 89*(Suppl. 68), 196–199.

Gimsing, S., & Bergholtz, L. (1983). Audiological screening of school children: Preliminary results. *Scandinavian Audiology,* (Suppl. 17), 63–65.

Gimsing, S., & Bergholtz, L. M. (1983). Audiologic screening of seven- and ten-year-old children. *Scandinavian Audiology, 12,* 171–177.

Gimsing, S., & Bergholtz, L. M. (1983). Otoscopy compared with tympanometry. A study evaluating the accuracy of otoscopy in 1702 unselected ears. *Journal of Laryngology and Otology, 97,* 587–591.

Grosso, P., & Rupp, R. R. (1978). Pure-tone and tympanometric screening: An ideal pair in identification audiometry. *Journal of the American Auditory Society, 4,* 11–15.

Haggard, M. P., Wood, E. J., & Carroll, S. (1984). Speech, admittance, and tone tests in school screening: Reconciling economics with pathology and disability perspectives. *British Journal of Audiology, 18,* 133–150.

Hall, J. W., & Weaver, T. (1979). Impedance audiometry in a young population: Effects of age, sex, and minor tympanogram abnormality. *Journal of Otolaryngology, 8,* 210–222.

Hallett, C. P. (1982). The screening and epidemiology of middle-ear disease in a population of primary school entrants. *Journal of Laryngology and Otology, 96,* 899–914.

Harford, E., Bess, F. H., Bluestone, D. D., & Klein, J. O. (1978). *Impedance screening for middle ear disease in children.* New York: Grune & Stratton.

Holmes, A. E., Muir, K. C., & Kemker, F. J. (1989). Acoustic reflectometry versus tympanometry in pediatric middle ear screenings. *Language, Speech and Hearing Services in Schools, 20,* 41–49.

Hoover, K. M., Chermak, G. D., & Doyle, C. S. (1982). A comparative study of immitance screening procedures with preschool aged children. *American Journal of Otology, 4,* 142–147.

Hopkinson, N. T., & Schramm, V. L. (1979). Preschool otologic and audiologic screening. *Otolaryngology and Head and Neck Surgery, 87,* 246–257.

Koebsell, K. A., & Margolis, R. H. (1986). Tympanometric gradient measured from normal preschool children. *Audiology, 25,* 149–157.

Lescouflair, G. (1975). Critical view on audiometric screening in school. *Archives of Otolaryngology, 101,* 469–473.

Liden, G., & Renvall, U. (1980). Impedance and tone screening of school children. *Scandinavian Audiology, 9,* 121–126.

Lous, J. (1982). Three impedance screening programs on a cohort of seven-year-old children. *Scandinavian Audiology,* (Suppl. 17), 60–64.

Margolis, R. H., & Heller, J. W. (1987). Screening tympanometry: Criteria for medical referral. *Audiology, 26,* 197–208.

McCandless, G. A., & Thomas, G. K. (1974). Impedance audiometry as a screening procedure for middle ear disease. *Transactions of the American Academy of Opthalmology and Otolaryngology, 78,* 98–102.

McKenzie, E., Magian, V., & Stokes, R. (1982). A study of the recommended pass/fail criteria for impedance audiometry in a school screening program. *Journal of Otolaryngology, 11,* 40–45.

Northern, J. L. (1980). Impedance screening. An integral part of hearing screening. *Annals of Otology, Rhinology and Laryngology, 85*(Suppl. 68), 233–235.

Orchik, D. J., & Herdman, S. (1974). Impedance audiometry as a screening device with school age children. *Journal of Auditory Research, 14,* 283–286.

Paradise, J. L., & Smith, C. G. (1979). Impedance screening for preschool children. State of the art. *Annals of Otology, Rhinology and Laryngology, 88,* 56–65.

Paradise, J. L., Smith, C. G., & Bluestone, C. D. (1976). Tympanometric detection of middle ear effusion in infants and young children. *Pediatrics, 58,* 198–210.

Paulman, P. M., & Halm, D. E. (1984). Screening for middle ear fluid in an urban pre-school population. *Nebraska Medical Journal, 69,* 307.

Portoian-Shuhaiber, S., & Cullinan, T. R. (1984). Middle ear disease assessed by impedance in primary school children in south London. *Lancet, 19,* 1111–1112.

Poulsen, G., & Tos, M. (1978). Screening tympanometry in newborn infants and during the first six months of life. *Scandinavian Audiology, 7,* 159–166.

Renvall, U, Jarlstedt, J., & Holmquist, J. (1980). Identification of middle ear disease. *Acta Otolaryngologica* (Stockholm), *90,* 283–289.

Renvall, U., & Liden, G. (1979). Impedance screening for middle ear disease. *Acta Otolaryngologica* (Stockholm), (Suppl. 360), 190–191.

Renvall, U., Liden, G., Jungert, S., & Nilsson, E. (1973). Impedance audiometry as a screening method in school children. *Scandinavian Audiology, 2,* 133–137.

Rosenberg, P., Northern, J., & Lovrinic, J. (1974). Proceedings of the symposium on new advances in screening for auditory disorders in children with emphasis on impedance audiometry. *Hearing Instruments, 25,* 20–21.

Roush, J. & Tait, C. A. (1985). Pure-tone and acoustic immittance screening of preschool-aged children: An examination of referral criteria. *Ear and Hearing, 6,* 245–250.

Schwartz, D. M., & Redfield, N. P. (1976). Evaluation of automatic screening tympanometry in the identification of middle ear pathology. *Journal of the American Auditory Society, 1,* 276–279.

Stool, S. E., Craig, H. B., & Laird, M. A. (1980). Screening for middle ear diseases in a school for the deaf. *Annals of Otology, Rhinology and Laryngology, 89*(Suppl. 69), 172–177.

Summary Reports on National-International Conferences. (1978). Use of acoustic impedance measurement in screening for middle ear disease in children. *Annals of Otology, Rhinology and Laryngology, 87,* 288–292.

Task Force of the Symposium on Impedance Screening for Children. (1978). Use of acoustic impedance measurement in screening for middle ear disease in children. *Pediatrics, 62,* 570–573.

Thomsen, J., Tos, M., Hanke, A. B., & Melchiors, H. (1982). Repetitive tympanometric screenings in children followed from birth to age four. *Acta Otolaryngologica,* (Suppl. 386), 155–157.

Tos, M. (1980). Spontaneous improvement of secretory otitis and impedance screening. *Archives of Otolaryngology, 106,* 345–349.

Tos, M., & Poulsen, G. (1980). Screening tympanometry in infants and two-year-old children. *Annals of Otology, Rhinology and Laryngology,* (Suppl. 89), 217–222.

Tos, M., Stangerup, S. E., Holm-Jensen, S., & Sorensen, C. H. (1984). Spontaneous course of secretory otitis and changes of the eardrum. *Archives of Otolaryngology, 110,* 281–289.

Van den Borg, R. E. (1942). An investigation about the pressure in the tympanic cavity in school children and the consequences of an abnormal pressure for hearing. *Acta Otolaryngologica, 36,* 500–511.

Vooyt, G. R., Halama, A. R., & van der Merwe, C.A. (1986). Immittance screening in black preschool children attending day-care centers. *Audiology, 25,* 158–164.

West, S. R., & Harris, B. J. (1983). Audiometry and tympanometry in children throughout one school year. *New Zealand Medical Journal, 96,* 603–605.

Wishik, S., Kramm, E., & Koch, E. (1958). Audiometric testing of school children. *Public Health Reports, 73,* 265–278.

10.0 MISCELLANEOUS TEXTS AND REFERENCES

Adour, K. K. (1982). Current concepts in neurology: Diagnosis and management of facial paralysis. *The New England Journal of Medicine, 307,* 348–351.

Alberti, P., & Kristensen, R. (1970). The clinical application of impedance audiometry. *Laryngoscope, 80,* 735–746.

Anderson, H., & Wedenberg, E. (1968). Audiometric identification of normal hearing carriers of genes deafness. *Acta Otolaryngologica, 65,* 535–554.

Balkany, T. J. (1975). Pulsatile impedance tympanometry. *Impedance Newsletter, 4.*

Ballenger, J. J. (1985). Otosclerosis. In J. J. Ballenger (Ed.), *Diseases of the nose, throat, ear, head, and neck* (p. 1197). Philadelphia: Lea and Febiger.

Barajas, J. J., Olaizola, F., Tapia, M. C., Alarcon, J. L., & Alaminos, D. (1981). Audiometric study of the neonate: Impedance audiometry. Behavioural responses and brain stem audiometry. *Audiology, 20,* 41–52.

Beranek, L. (1954). *Acoustics.* New York: McGraw-Hill.

Bess, F. H., Lewis, H., Donnell, P., & Cialiczka, D. J. (1975). Acoustic impedance measurements in cleft palate children. *Journal of Speech and Hearing Disorders, 40,* 13-25.

Blood, I. M., & Greenberg. H. J. (1977). Acoustic admittance of the ear in the geriatric person. *Journal of the American Auditory Society, 2,* 185–187.

Bluestone, C. D., & Beery, O. (1976). Concepts of the pathogenesis of middle ear effusion. *Annals of Otolaryngology, 85,* 182–186.

Bluestone, C. D., & Klein, J. (1983). Otitis media with effusion, atelectasis, and Eustachian tube dysfunction. In C. Bluestone & S. Stool (Eds.), *Pediatric otolaryngology.* Philadelphia: W.B. Saunders.

Bluestone, C. D., & Shurin, P. A. (1974). Middle ear disease in children. *Pediatric Clinics of North Amanca, 2,* 379–400.

Brooks, D. N. (1968). Clinical use of the acoustic impedance meter. *Sound, 2* 40–43.

Brooks, D. N. (1969). The use of the electro-acoustic impedance bridge in the assessment of middle ear function. *International Audiology, 8,* 563–569.

Brooks, D. N., Wooley, H., & Kanjilak, G. C. (1972). Hearing loss and middle ear disorders in patients with Down's syndrome (mongolism). *Journal of Mental Deficiency Research, 16,* 21–27.

Buckingham, R. A. (1972). Kodachrome study of otitis media. In A. Glorig & K. S. Gerwin (Eds.), *Otitis media: Proceedings of the National Conference* (pp. 92–102). Springfield, IL: Charles C. Thomas

Burke, K. S., Nilges,, T. C., & Henry, G. B. (1970). Middle ear impedance measurements. *Journal of Speech and Hearing Research, 13,* 317–325

Chalmers, P., & Knight, J. J. (1981). Diagnostic acoustic impedance measurements in the United Kingdom, 1960–1980. In R. Penha & P. Pizarro (Eds.), *Proceedings of the Fourth International Symposium on Acoustic*

Impedance Measurements. Lisbon, Portugal: Universidade Nova De Lisboa.

Dallos, P. (1973). *The auditory periphery.* New York: Academic Press.

Daspit, C. P., Churchill, D., & Linthicum, F. H., Jr. (1980). Diagnosis of perilymph fistula using ENG and impedance. *Laryngoscope, 90,* 217–223.

Densert,, O., Ivarsson, A., & Pedersen, K. (1977). The influence of perilymphatic pressure on the displacement of the tympanic membrane. A quantitative study on human temporal bones. *Acta Otolaryngologica* (Stockholm), *84,* 220–226.

Di Carlo, L. M., Kendall, D. C., & Goldstein, R. (1962). Diagnostic procedures for auditory disorders in children. *Folia Phoniatrica 14,* 206–264.

Djupesland G. (1964). Mechanical component to deafness in Meniere's disease. *Acta Otolaryngologica,* (Suppl. 188), 206–208.

Djupesland,, G. (1969). Use of impedance indicator in diagnosis of middle ear pathology. *International Audiology, 8,* 570–579.

Djupesland, G. (1981). Diagnostic application of impedance audiometry testing the middle ear function. In R. Penha & P. Pizarro (Eds.), *Proceedings of the Fourth International Symposium on Acoustic Impedance Measurements* (pp. 217–289). Lisbon, Portugal: Universidade Nova De Lisboa.

Djupesland, G., & Zwislocki, J. (1972). Sound pressure distribution in the outer ear. *Scandinavian Audiology, 1,* 197–203.

Egan, J. J. (1979). Audiology. Impedance: Its present and full potential. *Ear, Nose and Throat Journal, 58,* 409–410.

Elner, A., Inglelstedt, S., & Ivarsson, A. (1971). A method for studies of the middle ear mechanics. *Acta Otolaryngologica, 72,* 191–200.

Facer, G. (1981). Facial nerve paralysis: Is it always Bell's Palsy? *Postgraduate Medicine, 69,* 206–208.

Feldman, A. (1964). Acoustic impedance measurements as a clinical procedure. *International Audiology, 3,* 1–11.

Feldman, A. S. (1969). Acoustic impedance measurement of post-stapedectomized ears. *Laryngoscope, 79,* 1132–1155.

Feldman, A. S. (1974). Eardrum abnormality and the measurement of middle ear function. *Archives of Otolaryngology, 99,* 211–217.

Feldman, A., & Wilber, L. (1976). *Acoustic impedance and admittance: The measurement of middle ear function.* Baltimore: Williams & Wilkins.

Feldmann, H. (1970). A history of audiology. *Translation of the Beltone Institute for Hearing Research, 22,* Tonndorf (Ed.), Chicago, 4201 W. Victoria St., 60646.

Forfar, J. O. (1973). Demography, vital statistics and the pattern of disease in childhood. In J. O. Forfar (Ed.), *Textbook of pediatrics* (p. 23). Edinburgh: Churchill Livingstone.

Frenckner, P. (1939). Movements of the tympanic membrane and of the malleus in normal cases and in cases of otosclerosis. *Acta Otolaryngologica,* 587–607.

Gardner, M., & Hawley, M. (1973). Comparison of network and real-ear characteristics of the external ear. *Journal of the Auditory Engineering Society, 21,* 158–165.

Ginsberg, I. A., & White, T. P. (1984). Otologic considerations in audiology. In J. Katz (Ed.) *Handbook of clinical audiology* (pp. 15–38). Baltimore: Williams & Wilkens.

Glasscock, M. E., Harris, P. F., & Newsome, G. (1974). Glomus tumors: Diagnosis and treatment. *Larngoscope, 84,* 2006–2032.

Goodhill, V. (1979). *Ear diseases, deafness, and dizziness.* New York: Harper and Row.

Grason-Stadler. (1972). *Otoadmittance handbook.* Conoord, MA: Author.

Grason-Stadler. (1973). *Otoadmittance handbook-2,* Form 1720-H-2. Concord, MA: Author.

Grimaldi, P. M. (1976). The value of impedance testing in diagnosis of middle ear effusion. *Journal of Laryngology and Otology, 90,* 141–152.

Hall, M., & Hughes, R. (1975). Maximum compliance and the symptom of fullness in Meniere disease. *Archives of Otolaryngology, 101,* 227–228.

Harford, E., Bess, F. H., Bluestone, C. D., & Klein, J. O. (1978). *Impedance screening for midde ear disease in children.* New York: Grune and Stratton.

Harper, A. R. (1961). Acouatic impedance as an aid to diagnosis in otology. *Journal of Laryngology and Otology, 75,* 614–620.

Harris, J., Davidson, T., May, M., & Fria, T. (1983). Evaluation and treatment of congenital facial paralysis. *Archives of Otolaryngology, 109,* 145–151.

Hayes, D., & Jerger, J. (1978). Impedance audiometry in otologic diagnosis. *Otolaryngology Clinics of North America, 11,* 759–767.

Hayes, D., & Jerger, J. (1980). The effect of degree of hearing loss on diagnostic test strategy. *Archives of Otolaryngology, 106,* 266–268.

Himelfarb, M. Z., Popelka, G. R., Weiser, A., & Shanon, E. (1981). The significance of acoustic admittance procedures in the audiologic evaluation of multiply handicapped children. *British Journal of Audiology, 15,* 21–24.

Himelfarb, M. Z., & Shanon, E. (1977). Otoadmittance in normal subjects. *Laryngoscope, 87,* 1125–1129.

Hughes, G. (1982). Electroneurography: Objective prognostic assessment of facial paralysis. *Journal of Otology, 4,* 73–76.

Ison, J. R., Reiter, L., & Warren, M. (1979). Modulation of the acoustic startle reflex in humans in the absence of anticipatory changes in the middle ear reflex. *Journal of Experimental Psychology, 5,* 639–642.

Jackson, G. (1980). Facial paralysis of neoplastic origin: Diagnosis and management. *Laryngoscope, 90,* 1581–1595.

Jerger, J. (1974). Second international symposium on impedance measurement, Houston, Texas. *Audiology, 13,* 271–274.

Jerger, J. (1975). *Handbook of clinical impedance audiometry.* Acton, MA: American Electromedics.

Jerger, J. (1976). Clinical applications of the acoustic reflex. *Proceedings of the third international symposium on impedance audiometry* (pp. 12–17). Acton, MA: American Electromedics.

Jerger, J., Mauldin, L., & Igarashi, M. (1978). Impedance audiometry in the sguirrel monkey. Effect of middle ear surgery. *Archives of Otolaryngology, 104,* 214–224.

Jerger, J. F., & Northem, J. L. (Chairmen). (1976). *Proceedings of the Third International Symposium on Impedance Audiometry.* Acton, MA: American Electromedics.

Jerger, J., & Northem, J. L. (1980).*Clinical impedance audiometry* (2nd ed.). Acton, MA: American Electromedics.

Jerger, S., & Jerger, J. (t981). *Auditory disorders: A manual for clinical evaluation.* Boston: Little, Brown.

Jordan, R. E. (1963). Secretory otitis media in etiology of cholesteatoma. *Archives of Otolaryngology, 78,* 261.

Keith, R. W. (1974). Applications of impedance audiometry with children. *Hearing Instruments, 25,* 22–23.

Kennelly, A. E., & Kurokawa, K. (1921). Acoustic impedance and its measurement. *Proceedings of the American Academy of Arts and Sciences, 56,* 1–42.

Kiang, N., Moxon, E., & Levine, R. (1970). Auditory nerve activity in cats with normal and abnormal cochleas. In G. Wolstenholme and J. Knight (Eds.), *Sensorineural hearing loss* (pp. 241–268). London: Churchill.

Klockhoff, I., Anggard, G., & Anggard, L. (1965). The acoustic impedance of the ear and cranio-labyrinthive pressure transmission. *Audiology, 4,* 45–49.

Kobrak, H. G. (1959). *The middle ear.* Chicago: University of Chicago Press.

Lamb, L., & Norris, T. (1970). Relative acoustic impedance measurement with mentally retarded children. *American Journal of Mental Deficiences, 75,* 51–56.

Liden, G. (1969). The scope and application of current audiometric tests. *The Journal of Laryngology and Otology, 83,* 507–520.

Liden, G. (1969). Test for stapes fixation. *Archives of Otolaryngology, 89,* 215–219.

Liden, G. (1975). Application of tympanometry and acoustic reflex measurements. *Acta Otorhinolaryngologica* (Belgium), *29,* 802–813.

Liden, G. (1977). Introduction to the round table on advances in acoustic impedance measurements. *Audiology, 16,* 273–277.

Liden, G. (1980). Impedance audiometry. *Annals of Otology, Rhinology and Laryngology, 89*(Suppl. 68), 53–58.

Liden, G., Bjorkman, G., Nyman, H., & Kunov, H. (1977). Tympanometry and acoustic impedance. *Acta Otolaryngologica, 83,* 140–145.

Liden, G., Peterson, J. L., & Bjorkman, G. (1970). Tympanometry: A method for analysis of middle ear function. *Acta Otolaryngologica* (Suppl. 263), 216–224.

Lindstrom, D., & Liden, G. (1964). The tensor-tympani reflex in operative treatment of trigeminal neuralgia. *Acta Otolaryngologica,* (Suppl. 188), 271–274.

Lloyd, L. (1975). Impedance measurements in the diagnosis of Meniere's (sic) disease. *Journal of the South African Speech and Hearing Association, 22,* 49–62.

Lopes O. (1972). The early diagnosis of glomic tumor in the middle ear by means of acoustic impedance. *Impedance Newsletter, 1.*

Lutman, M. E., & Martin, A. M. (1979). Development of an electroacoustic analogue model of the middle ear and acoustic reflex. *Sound and Vibration, 64,* 133–157.

Macrae, J. H. (1973). Neuromas and the acoustic impedance of the ear. *Journal of Speech and Hearing Disorders, 38,* 345–353.

Marquet, J., Van Camp, K. J., Creten, W. L., Decraemer, W. F., Wolff, H. B., & Schepens, P. (1973). Topics in physics and middle ear surgery. *Acta Otorhinolaryngologica* (Belgium), 27, 139–319.

Matz, G. T., Rattenborg, C. G., & Holaday, D. A. (1967). Effects of nitrous oxide on middle ear pressure. *Anesthesiology, 28,* 948–950.

McPherson D. L. (1971). Impedance audiometry. *Archives of Otolaryngology 93,* 338–339.

Metz, O. (1946). The acoustic impedance measured on normal and pathological ears. *Acta Otolaryngologica,* (Suppl. 63), 1–254.

Moller , A. R. (1964). The acoustic impedance in experimental studies on the middle ear. *Journal of International Audiology, 2,* 123–135.

Moller , A. (1965). An experimental study of the acoustic impedance of the middle ear and its transmission properties. *Acta Otolaryngologica, 60,* 129–149.

Neff, P. A., Morioka, W. T., Sample, P. A., & Cantrell, R. W. (1980). Audiometric and tympanometric monitoring of a disease affecting nerve-muscle transmission. *Audiology, 19,* 293–309.

Northern, J. L. (1976). Impedance measurements in otitis media. *Hearing Instruments, 27,* 6–7, 31.

Northern, J. L. (1976). *Selected readings in impedance audiometry.* Dobbs Ferry, NY: American Electromedics.

Northern J. L. & Bergstrom, L. (1973). Impedance audiometry. *Eye, Ear, Nose and Throat Journal, 52,* 404–406.

Onchi, Y. A. (1949). A study of the mechanism of the middle ear. *Journal of the Acoustical Society of America, 21,* 400–410.

Onchi, Y. (1961). Mechanism of the middle ear. *Journal of the Acoustical Society of America, 33,* 794–805.

Pearlman, R. C. (1980). Consultation: Impedance audiometry. *Nursing 10,* 86–92.

Pohlman, A. G., & Kranz, F. W. (1923). The effect of pressure changes in the external auditory canal on acuity and hearing. *Annals of Otology Rhinology and Laryngology, 32,* 545–553.

Pollack, M. C. (1975). *Amplification for the hearing impaired.* New York: Grune & Stratton.

Popelka, G. R. (1981). *Hearing assessment with the acoustic reflex.* New York: Grune & Stratton.

Priede, V. M. (1970). Acoustic impedance in two cases of ossicular discontinuity. *International Audiology, 9,* 127–136.

Priede, V. M. & Coles, R. R. A. (1971). On the value of acoustic impedance tests in the clinic [Letter]. *Audiology, 10,* 185–187.

Rabinowitz, W. M. (1981). Measurement of the acoustic input immittance of the human ear. *Journal of the Acoustical Society of America, 70,* 1025–1035.

Relkin, E. M., Saunders, J. C., & Konkle, D. F. (1979). The development of middle-ear admittance in the hamster. *Journal of the Acoustical Society of America, 66,* 133–139.

Robertson, E. O., Peterson, J. L., & Lamb, L. E. (1968). Relative impedance measurements in young children. *Archives of Otolaryngology, 88,* 162–168.

Rock E. (1974). Otologic applications and considerations in impedance audiometry. *Impedance Newsletter,* (Suppl. 13), 1–16.

Rock, E. H. (1976). The otolaryngologic, pediatric, and neurologic correlates of impedance audiometry. *Hearing Instruments, 27,* 14–15, 26.

Rose, D., & Keating, L. (Eds.). (1972). *Proceedings of the Mayo impedance symposium.* Rochester, MN: Mayo Foundation.

Sanders, J. W. (1982). Diagnostic audiology. In N. Lass, L. McReynolds, J. Northern, & D. Yoder (Eds.), *Speech, language and hearing* (pp. 1123–1143). Philadelphia: W.B. Saunders.

Schuknecht, H. F. (1974). *Pathology of the ear.* Cambridge, MA: Harvard University Press.

Shapiro, J. R., Pikus, A., Weiss, G., & Rowe, D. W. (1982). Hearing and middle ear function in osteogenesis imperfecta. *Journal of the American Medical Association, 247,* 2120–2126.

Silman, S. (1984). *The acoustic reflex: Basic principles and clinical applications.* New York: Academic Press.

Spector, G. J., Ciralsky, R. H., & Ogura, J. H. (1975). Glomus tumors in the head and neck. 3. Analysis of clinical manifestations. *Annals of Otology, Rhinology and Laryngology, 84,* 73–79.

Starr A. & Schwartzkroin , P. (1972). Cochlear microphonic and middle-ear pressure changes during nitrous oxide anesthesia in cats. *Journal of the Acoustical Society of America, 51*(Part 2), 1367–1368.

Stinson, M. R. (1982). The spatial distribution of sound pressure within scaled replicas of the human ear canal. *Journal of the Acoustical Society of America, 78,* 1596–1602.

Stone, G., & Feldman, A. S. (1971). Impedance measurements in normal and pathological ears. *Surgical Forum, 22,* 459–461.

Tato, J. M., Jr. (1976). Otologic manifestations and impedance audiometry. In J. Jerger & J. Northern (Eds.), *Proceedings of the Third International Symposium on Impedance Audiometry* (pp. 41–48). Acton, MA: American Electromedics.

Teele, D. W., Klein, J. O., & Rosner, B. A. (1980). Epidemiology of otitis media in children. *Annals of Otology, Rhinology and Laryngology, 89*(Suppl.68), 5–6

Terkildsen , K. Osterhammel, P., & Wielsen, S. (1970). Impedance measurements, probe-tone intensity, and middle ear reflexes. *Acta Otolaryngologica,* (Suppl. 263), 205–207.

Thomsen, J., Bretlau, P., Jorgensen, B. M., & Kristensen, H. K. (1974). Bone resorption in chronic otitis media. A historical and ultrastructural study. I. Ossicular necrosis. *Journal of Laryngology and Otology, 88*, 975–981.

Thomsen, J., Bretlau, P., & Kristensen, H. K. (1975). Bone resorption in chronic otitis media. *Acta Otolaryngologica, 79*, 400–408.

Thomsen, K. A. (1955). Case of psychogenic deafness demonstrated by measuring of impedance. *Acta Otolaryngologica* (Stockholm), *45*, 82–85.

Thomsen K. A. (1955). Employment of impedance measurement in otologic and oto-neurologic disorders. *Acta Otolaryngologica, 45*, 159–167.

Thomsen, K. A., Terkildsen, K., & Arnfred, I. (1965). Middle ear pressure variations during anesthesia. *Archives of Otolaryngology, 92*, 609–611.

Tomoyuki H. & Paparella , M. (1971). Middle ear muscle anomalies. *Archives of Otolaryngology, 94*, 235–239.

Toynbee, J. (1865). *Diseases of the ear.* Philadelphia: Blanchard and Lea.

Van Wagoner, R. S., & Campbell, J. D. (1976). The use of electro-acoustic impedance measurements in detecting early clinical otosclerosis. *Journal of Otolaryngology, 5*, 33–36.

von Békésy, G. (1960). *Experiments in hearing.* New York: McGraw-Hill.

Wedenberg, E. (1963). Objective auditory tests on non-cooperative children. *Acta Otolaryngologica*, (Suppl. 175), 1–32.

Wever, E. G., Bray, C. W., & Lawrence, M. (1942). The effect of pressure in the middle ear. *Journal of Experimental Psychology, 30*, 40–52.

Wever, E. G., & Lawrence, M. (1954). *Physiological acoustics.* Princeton, NJ: Princeton University Press.

Wever, E. G., Lawrence, M., & Smith, K. R. (1948). The effect of negative air pressure in the middle ear. *Annals of Otology, Rhinology and Laryngology, 57*, 418–428.

Wheatstone, C. (1827). Experiments in audition. *Quarterly Journal of Science, 4*, 67–72.

Wilson, R. H., & Nadol, J. B. (1983). *Hearing loss. Quick reference to ear, nose, and throat disorders* (pp. 34–35). Philadelphia: J.B. Lippincott.

Wollaston W. H. (1820). On sounds inaudible by certain ears. *Philosophical Transactions of the Royal Society of London, 110*, 306–314.

Wooten, P. G., Sheeley, E. C., & Hannah, J. E. (1975). Impedance audiometry with retardates. *Journal of Auditory Research, 15*, 156–161.

Yanagisawa, E., & Lee, K. J. (1987). Noninfectious diseases of the ear. In K. J. Lee (Ed.), *Essential otolaryngology: Head and neck surgery* (pp. 177–187). New York: Medical Examination.

Zito, M. R. (1983). Acoustic admittance measurements in human temporal bones. *Audiology, 22*, 438–450.

Zwislocki, J. J. (1968). On acoustic research and its clinical application. *Acta Otolaryngologica, 65*, 86–96.

Zwisiocki, J. J. (1982). Normal function of the middle ear and its measurement. *Audiology, 21*, 4–14.

Index

About the Authors

Terry L. Wiley, Ph.D.

Dr. Wiley is Professor of Audiology in the Department of Communicative Disorders, University of Wisconsin–Madison, where he has served on the faculty since 1972. He is an Affiliate Professor, Division of Otolaryngology, Department of Surgery, University of Wisconsin Medical School and the Institute on Aging at the University of Wisconsin–Madison. Dr. Wiley received his bachelor's degree from the University of Northern Iowa, his master's degree from Colorado State University and his doctorate from the University of Iowa. He is a Fellow of the American Speech-Language-Hearing Association and the American Academy of Audiology. Dr. Wiley is a former editor of both the *Journal of Speech and Hearing Disorders* and the *Journal of Speech and Hearing Research,* and he served two terms as an associate editor of the *Journal of Speech and Hearing Research.* Dr. Wiley received a 1983 national teaching award in audiology and he was elected to the Teaching Academy of the University of Wisconsin–Madison in 1995. He was the first author on a paper dealing with diagnostic audiology practices that received the Editor's Award for the article of highest merit published in the *American Journal of Audiology* during the 1995 publication year. The Wisconsin Speech-Language-Hearing Association awarded him the Honors of the Association in 1996. Dr. Wiley has taught and conducted research in the area of diagnostic audiology for over 25 years. Most relevant to the present text is a graduate course dealing with acoustic immittance measures that he developed and has taught for the past 15 years.

Cynthia G. Fowler, Ph.D.

Dr. Fowler is an Associate Professor in the Department of Communicative Disorders, University of Wisconsin–Madison, where she has been on the faculty since 1995. She was previously at the Veterans Affairs Medical Center, Long Beach, and the University of California, Irvine. She received her bachelor's degree from Emory University; her master's degree from Louisiana State University, Baton Rouge; and her doctorate from Northwestern University. She is a fellow of the American Speech-Language-Hearing Association and the American Academy of Audiology. She served as Feature Editor for the *American Journal of Audiology* and is an Associate Editor for the *Journal of Speech and Hearing Research*. Dr. Fowler has been actively involved in clinic, teaching, and research in the area of diagnostic audiology for over 17 years. She has written and contributed to numerous teaching materials, including tutorials, book chapters, and a CD ROM on diagnostic audiology.